Eating Disorders and the Brain

Eating Disorders and the Brain

Edited by

Bryan Lask
Regional Eating Disorders Service, Oslo, Norway
Ellern Mede Service for Eating Disorders, London, UK
Great Ormond Street Hospital for Children, London, UK

Ian Frampton
University of Exeter, Exeter, UK
Regional Eating Disorders Service, Oslo, Norway

WILEY-BLACKWELL

A John Wiley & Sons, Ltd., Publication

Library of Congress Cataloging-in-Publication Data
Eating disorders and the brain / [edited by] Bryan Lask and Ian Frampton. – 1st ed.
    p. ; cm.
  Includes bibliographical references and index.
  ISBN 978-0-470-67003-3 (cloth : alk. paper) – ISBN 978-1-119-99843-3 (ePDF) – ISBN 978-1-119-97364-5 (ePub) – ISBN 978-1-119-99840-2 (Wiley online library) – ISBN 978-1-119-97365-2 (mobi)
  1. Eating disorders–Pathophysiology. 2. Brain–Pathophysiology. I. Lask, Bryan. II. Frampton, Ian.
  [DNLM: 1. Eating Disorders–physiopathology. 2. Eating Disorders–psychology. 3. Brain–physiopathology. 4. Neurosciences. WM 175]
  RC552.E18E28257 2011
  616.85′26–dc22
                                                                                          2011006757

A catalogue record for this book is available from the British Library.

This book is published in the following electronic formats: ePDF 9781119998433; ePub 9781119973645; Wiley Online Library 9781119998402; Mobi 9781119973652

Set in 10/12pt Times by Laserwords Private Limited, Chennai, India
Printed and bound in Malaysia by Vivar Printing Sdn Bhd

First 2011

Cover design based on an illustration ©Ana Ribeiro

Bryan dedicates this book to Ana.
Ian dedicates this book to Katie, Ellie and Merryn.

Contents

Preface

Bryan Lask and Ian Frampton

The human brain is often described as 'the most complex structure in the universe, too complex for the human brain to understand' – a most delightful paradox. Eating disorders too are extraordinarily complex, difficult to understand, demanding to treat, have a poor prognosis and are themselves full of paradox. Surely then a union between these two unlikely bedfellows, as attempted in this book, cannot be an easy task? And perhaps this is why there have been relatively few such attempts to date. Yet, despite decades of effort, enormous amounts of research money and well over 100 000 publications, we still do not have an adequate understanding of the pathogenesis of eating disorders! We are still unable to explain why any one individual develops an eating disorder, while the majority do not, and we still do not have effective treatments. Until relatively recently, sociocultural attempts to elucidate the development of eating disorders have been the most influential. However, while offering a part-explanation, they have proved insufficient in accounting for the very specific phenomena so characteristic of these conditions.

In recent years, to an extent perhaps inspired by the 'decade of the brain', there has been more of a focus on what neuroscience might contribute to our understanding. And the results have been enlightening. For example, neuropsychological studies have shown impairments in different cognitive functions, especially executive and visuospatial skills, which appear to be trait- rather than state-related; in other words, they seem to predate the onset and therefore may actually be risk factors for the development of an eating disorder. Structural (anatomical) neuroimaging studies show cortical atrophy and ventricular enlargement, which do indeed reverse with refeeding and are therefore likely to be secondary to inadequate nutrition. However, functional neuroimaging consistently reveals regional and asymmetrical reduction in blood flow, suggesting dysfunction in specific brain regions, which is unlikely to be due simply to starvation and suggests regional dysfunction. This too may be a predisposing factor or a reflection of one. Neurochemistry studies show dysregulation within neurotransmitter systems, with effects upon the modulation of feeding, mood, anxiety, neuroendocrine control, metabolic rate, sympathetic tone and temperature. These studies indicate that neural mechanisms have a fundamental role in the origin and maintenance of the disorders. Thus we now have far more detailed information on the effects on the brain of starvation, overeating, chaotic eating and dehydration. Even more importantly, we now understand far more about the underlying brain abnormalities and dysfunctions that may contribute to the development of these serious disorders.

In this book we explore in depth how neuroscience knowledge informs our understanding of eating disorders and how it may be applied in clinical practice. We may have erred by focusing rather more on anorexia nervosa (AN) than the other eating disorders, but hope to be forgiven, because there is more neuroscience-based information available on this condition. The first chapter, by clinician David Wood, offers an invitation to fellow clinicians to become acquainted with the seemingly scary, but actually fascinating, world of neuroscience, as applied to eating disorders. In Chapter 2, Beth Watkins provides a meticulous review of the eating disorders – most of the information anyone is likely to need is contained therein. The next three chapters review in detail contemporary knowledge of neuroimaging (Tone Fugslet and Ian Frampton), neuropsychology (Joanna Steinglass and Deborah Glasofer) and neurochemistry and genetics (Ken Nunn). In Chapter 6, Maria Øverås explores how neuroscience contributes to our understanding of one of the core features of eating disorders, body-image disturbance. Mark Rose and Ian Frampton, in Chapter 7, explore and comment upon a number of neuroscience-based conceptual models of eating disorders. Each advances our understanding to some extent but none offers a full explanation of the pathogenesis, phenomenology and maintenance of any of the eating disorders. In Chapter 8, Ken Nunn, Ian Frampton and Bryan Lask attempt the seemingly impossible and propose just such a model for AN. It is for the reader, and subsequent testing of the model, to decide whether or not they have succeeded. The next two chapters explore the clinical relevance of neuroscience knowledge: Ilina Singh and Alina Wengaard (Chapter 9) consider the consequences of the development of neurobiological models for the understanding of eating disorders by patients and their families and their receptivity to treatment. Camilla Lindvall and Bryan Lask (Chapter 10) explore how this empirical knowledge can be converted into practice, with emphasis on its application in both an educational and a clinical context. In relation to the latter they offer a specific focus on cognitive remediation therapy. In the final chapter, the editors offer a summary of the contents of the previous chapters and explore how these findings might be investigated in the future, considering in turn each of the US National Institute of Mental Health Research Domain Criteria (RDoC) Project classes: genes, molecules, cells, neural circuits, behaviours and self-reports.

We hope that this volume will take us a small step forward in our understanding of the neuroscience of eating disorders and will open up an exciting and relevant avenue for all of its readers, regardless of their previous knowledge in the field.

List of contributors

Ian Frampton
College of Life and Environmental
  Sciences
University of Exeter
Exeter, EX4 4QG, UK

Regional Eating Disorders Service
Oslo University Hospital
Oslo Universitetssykehus HF
Ullevål, Bygg 37
0407 Oslo, Norway

Tone Seim Fuglset
Regional Eating Disorders Service
Oslo University Hospital
Oslo Universitetssykehus HF
Ullevål, Bygg 37
0407 Oslo, Norway

Deborah R. Glasofer
Columbia Center for Eating Disorders
Columbia University Medical Center/
  New York State Psychiatric Institute
New York, NY 10023, USA

Bryan Lask
Regional Eating Disorders Service
Oslo University Hospital
Oslo Universitetssykehus HF
Ullevål, Bygg 37
0407 Oslo, Norway

Ellern Mede Service
  for Eating Disorders
31 Totteridge Common
London, N20 8LR, UK

Great Ormond Street Hospital
  for Children
London, WC1N 3JH, UK

Camilla Lindvall
Regional Eating Disorders Service
Oslo University Hospital
Oslo Universitetssykehus HF
Kirkeveien 166 (Ullevål)
0407 Oslo, Norway

Kenneth Nunn
Molecular Neuropsychiatry Service
Department of Psychological Medicine
The Children's Hospital
  at Westmead
Westmead, NSW, 2145, Australia

School of Psychiatry
University of New South Wales
Sydney, 2052, Australia

Maria Øverås
Regional Eating Disorders Service
Oslo University Hospital
Oslo Universitetssykehus HF
Ullevål, Bygg 37
0407 Oslo, Norway

Mark Rose
Huntercombe Group, UK

Great Ormond Street Hospital
  for Children
London, WC1N 3JH, UK

Ilina Singh
London School of Economics
  and Political Science
London, WC2A 2AE, UK

Joanna E. Steinglass
Columbia Center for Eating Disorders
Columbia University Medical Center/
  New York State Psychiatric Institute
New York, NY 10032, USA

Beth Watkins
St George's University of London
Cranmer Terrace
London, SW17 0RE, UK

Great Ormond Street Hospital
  for Children
London, WC1N 3JH, UK

Alina Wengaard
Regional Eating Disorders Service
Oslo University Hospital
Oslo Universitetssykehus HF
Ullevål, Bygg 37
0407 Oslo, Norway

David Wood
Ellern Mede Service
  for Eating Disorders
31 Totteridge Common
London, N20 8LR, UK

Acknowledgements

Bryan wishes to thank:

Harold Behr for 40 years of monthly meetings, full of warm friendship and debate;
Isky Gordon, who dragged me screaming into the realms of neuroscience and insisted that this is where we would find the answer;
Rachel Bryant-Waugh, who has been such an excellent friend and supportive and stimulating colleague;
And finally, Ian Frampton, my co-editor, who has been so tolerant of my ignorance and patiently taught me so much.

Ian wishes to thank:

Bernadette Wren, who sparked my interest in why we should think about the brains of children with eating disorders;
Phil Yates for showing me how clinical psychologists can be neuropsychologists too;
Robert Goodman, who taught me so much about children's brains during my post-doctoral fellowship at the Institute of Psychiatry;
And finally, Bryan Lask, my co-editor, for all his wisdom and support over the past 20 years.

We both wish to thank:

Our fellow contributors, who have laboured selflessly and adhered so faithfully to deadlines.
Our brilliant colleagues in London and Oslo, and especially the participants in the UK and Norwegian Eating Disorders Neuro-Networks, the Ravello Collaboration and Project Jigsaw.
Kate Tchanturia for leading us into the exciting world of cognitive remediation therapy.
Roy Anderson and Heidi Langbakk Skille at RASP, Oslo University Hospital for their invaluable support of neuroscience research.
Helse Sør Øst, Norway, and the Huntercombe Group, the Ellern Mede Eating Disorders Service and Rosetree's Trust, UK, for generous financial support.

This book would not have been possible without Tone Fugslet, our editorial assistant, who has done such a wonderful job, with diligence, patience and humour – thank you, Tone.

And finally, special thanks to Ken Nunn, who has been beyond inspiration!

Bryan Lask and Ian Frampton
January 2011

1 Why clinicians should love neuroscience: the clinical relevance of contemporary knowledge

David Wood

Ellern Mede Service for Eating Disorders, London, UK

1.1 Introduction

Clinicians at times appear to have an uneasy relationship with neuroscience. At a superficial level it may seem that there might be little need to question whether the relationship between neuroscience and clinical work is problematic. However, despite their now reasonably lengthy coexistence, there still exists a tension between these two fields of endeavour. This leads to misunderstanding, and even distrust, which inhibits the undoubted opportunities – if not necessity – for creative and fruitful interaction. Questions are still asked within the clinical domain about the relevance of neuroscientific study, and neuroscientists can become so absorbed and fascinated with their subject that they lose sight of the clinical relevance of what they are studying. It is the contention of this chapter that the relationship between neuroscience and clinical work should not be problematic, and that those on both sides of the divide can learn, not only to live together, but also to admire each other's concepts.

Why should we love neuroscience? Of course, telling someone what he or she should love is a supremely arrogant and rather fruitless enterprise, as anyone who has tried to get their child to love eating, say, oysters will know. But neuroscience is not just an acquired taste; it does not require great familiarity to appreciate its qualities. It is certainly possible to comprehend the wonder, awe and excitement that this field of endeavour can evoke without having to fully understand its every detail. And without some appreciation of the currently available knowledge about the brain, clinicians are in danger of setting off down many a blind alley in carrying out clinical practice.

In order to support this argument, it is first necessary to review some fundamental problems. This will be followed by a brief, and highly condensed, overview of some

Eating Disorders and the Brain. Edited by Bryan Lask and Ian Frampton.
© 2011 John Wiley & Sons, Ltd. Published 2011 by John Wiley & Sons, Ltd.

current neuroscience facts, which will then be reviewed within the context of current developments within the field of eating disorders.

1.2 The legacy of mind–body dualism

The tension between clinical work and neuroscience would seem to be supported by the continuing predominance of dualistic thinking, not only within scientific discourse, but in postmodern culture more generally. Given the lengthy history of dualism, from Plato, down through Descartes, to William James and beyond, it is not surprising that it does not easily throw in the towel. The fundamental problem with which Homo sapiens has wrestled for so long is how can we reconcile our sense of ourselves as free agents, capable of choosing our path through life, with a notion of our bodies (including our brains) being constructed of physical stuff that obeys the deterministic laws of nature.

Plato considered that humans had earthly bodies and ethereal souls, and put the mental properties of reason, desire and appetite firmly in the domain of the soul. Indeed, Aristotle thought that the brain was merely an organ for cooling the blood and that the heart was really where the passions lay. Continuing in the Platonic tradition, Descartes, in his pamphlet 'On the Passions of the Soul' [1], decided that bodies were made up of stuff such as blood, muscles, nerves and so on, and were controlled by 'bodily spirits', whereas our thoughts and our passions belonged to the soul, and our mental experiences were instances of awareness of the movements of the bodily spirits via contact between soul and body in the pineal gland. It is hard to know what Plato would have made of someone whom we might now diagnose as suffering from anorexia nervosa (AN). It is reasonable to surmise that he would probably not have considered them to be suffering from an illness. More likely he would have marvelled at the way in which they were able, with so much stoicism, to conquer their appetites and disentangle themselves from the world of the senses, thus liberating their ethereal soul from the constraints of the material body. For Plato and his successors, the passions were seen as something that needed to be subjugated, brought under control, an idea that presages the current interest in emotion regulation and AN.

Dualist accounts, particularly of emotion, have been hard to shake off, and continue beyond Descartes, through Locke and Hume, to William James, Popper and Eccles [2], and even perhaps to some elements of modern emotion theory such as the somatic marker hypothesis [3–6]. They remain alive and well in some clinicians' apparently unshakeable belief that AN is a 'brain' disease, just as in others' similarly unshakeable beliefs that it is a 'mental' illness without physical correlates. But to argue either way implies a distinction between brain and mind that really can no longer be justified.

In essence, all dualist accounts come up against the difficulty that there is no convincing explanation of how, if brain and mind are of different stuff, they can interact, and how mental events can have a causative role in behaviour. There would seem to be little doubt that despite Cartesian dualism's refusal to go quietly, the general direction of neuroscientific endeavour has been inexorably towards a monist[1] position. However, this has brought with it new difficulties.

---

[1] The term 'monist' here refers to the view that the mind and the body are of one substance, as opposed to the two of the dualist position.

1.3   Free will and determinism

Despite the issue of free will and determinism having an indisputable and central relevance to ethical and legal debates about whether the state and its representatives have the right to intervene when a patient with AN asserts her right to starve herself to death, there is virtually no discussion of it in the clinical literature. The assertion that human beings are free[2] to choose their own destiny can really only be upheld if one espouses a dualist position. To be free is only possible if the mind is free of the body. It seems reasonable to suppose that much of the objection to a monist position arises because of fear of confronting the logical, determinist consequence of that position: that is, we are actually *not* free to choose, in the sense that we cannot choose whatever we want.

This issue generates a number of complicated problems in relation to 'mental' illness. For instance, if we define a wish (to exercise the 'freedom') to hurt oneself, or to be reckless of danger (such as when one is refusing to eat), as a characteristic of a mental illness, then we are denying that it is an act of free will and claiming that it is not an infringement of the patient's right to self-determination if we intervene. However, this often makes us uncomfortable, and if as a consequence we allow the patient to choose such a course of action, we can hardly define it as a sign of a mental illness.

If we accept that mind and body are two sides of a materialist, and hence deterministic, coin, then there can be no truly 'free' will, as any future event is deterministically caused by the past, and we have no control over that. Free will is incompatible with a materialist, monist position. Some authors have gone to considerable lengths to find a way out of this impasse. For instance, Hameroff and Penrose [7] have proposed that indeterminacy which can account for free will is introduced into a material deterministic system such as the brain by 'quantum effects in cytoskeletal microtubules within neurones'. But we do not need to go as far as this to find a way out of the problem. Let us instead take a simpler, clinically-based perspective.

1.4   Clinical implications

Let us consider a common clinical scenario of a teenage girl who has 'never been a problem' to her parents (by which it might be meant that she has not before asserted herself or easily engaged in conflict), has worked hard at school and achieved well, and has been compliant at home. She is likely to have been described as 'sensitive' in that she takes things to heart and can be quite easily hurt or upset by comments from friends. Not infrequently, her family has accommodated to her sensitivity by adapting to a life in which conflict is avoided, or in which, in order to avoid upset, her parents have become overly solicitous and protective.

Often, because of this previous experience of an ideal child, parents are deeply shocked and bewildered by what seems to be a very rapid change into someone they feel they hardly know. Compliance has been replaced by opposition, which at times is violent and extreme, although this may only occur in situations in which food is involved. Their sense of themselves as competent parents is under threat and they feel a bewildering range of emotions, including resentment, anger and frustration, about which they usually then feel guilty. What is the clinician to make of this?

---

[2] In the sense of not being bound by a physical deterministic universe.

Specialists in the field are now clear that what is disordered in 'eating disorders' is far more than attitudes to eating, food, weight and shape. But given their prominence, let us begin by considering the issue of food intake and energy balance.

1.5 Restriction of energy intake and increase in energy output

From a clinical perspective, the restriction of energy intake manifests itself in a number of different ways. The patient is often preoccupied with 'healthy eating' (which in reality is very unhealthy, in that the amount of energy that her diet is providing is substantially less than that required to sustain normal life). She will often have a particular fear of, or revulsion towards, energy-dense foods, which in essence means foods that contain fat. Very often she will have a belief that any fat that is consumed immediately reappears as fat on her body. Even when all fat has been eliminated from her diet, she will continue to reduce the amount of food consumed until either she has reached zero intake or she has been admitted to hospital. To the clinician it is obvious that this fear of energy intake is very far removed from the popular idea of someone who is dieting or slimming in order to lose weight. It has all the features of a genuine phobia with the attendant intense and frequently overwhelming anxiety that makes it impossible for the patient to approach food voluntarily.

Along with the avoidance of energy intake, those suffering with AN are frequently dominated by an intense drive to expend energy. Again, the intensity of this drive is far removed from the activity of those who want to 'get fit' or to use exercise as a way of losing a little weight. The activity can take almost any form. If she has previously enjoyed sport, the patient will intensify the amount of time she spends in swimming, running, cycling or gymnastics. It is clear that the motivation is no longer that of enjoyment. The patient is driven by something that has long since ceased to be under her control, and which leaves her feeling unbearably guilty, bad and lazy. It is extremely difficult for her to sit down for anything other than the briefest periods; she will be found doing her homework standing up, eating standing up, listening to the radio or watching television standing up – in fact, doing anything standing up that can be done standing up. Even when she does sit down she will often hold her body in a tense position, or will jiggle her legs up and down ceaselessly.

Patients with AN behave as if their homeostatic systems, which normally should be seeking a balance between energy input and output, have become reset, so that any situation in which input equals or exceeds output provokes extreme anxiety. Normally, when output exceeds input, these homeostatic systems should trigger activation of responses that are accompanied by subjective experiences of hunger and the initiation of food-seeking and eating behaviour. In this situation the survival goal is restoration of energy balance, and any activity that moves the organism back towards that goal should produce a positive emotional state, whereas activity that results in moving further away from that goal should produce a negative emotional state.

For the patient with AN, something has happened that has reset the desired goal away from energy balance, so that her emotional state becomes more negative the nearer she moves towards energy balance. And once a severe negative energy balance occurs, neurotransmitter imbalance dramatically complicates the situation (see Chapter 5).

1.6   Non-eating-related concerns

One of the advantages of working in an inpatient unit is that one spends a considerable amount of time in daily contact with patients in a way that is denied to those engaged exclusively in outpatient practice. This allows one to see even more clearly that their concerns are not just centred on food, weight and shape. Although there is no doubt that abnormal attitudes to energy intake and output (i.e. restricted food intake and increased activity) are central, patients with eating disorders invariably have serious difficulties with, amongst other things, perfectionism, rigidity, obsessionality, submissiveness, low self-esteem, sexuality and quite generalised difficulties with putting feelings into words (alexithymia).

One soon notices that patients not only deny themselves the comfort of food, but also the comfort of warmth, or of sitting on soft chairs. They find it very difficult to make eye contact, or to say 'hello' when greeted. Some may 'fly off the handle' for apparently obscure reasons. It is difficult for those who have not worked with patients with AN to comprehend their extreme sensitivity to the ways they respond to stimuli from the external world. It is as if the 'gain' on the input controls is turned up to maximum. Small changes in the external environment are experienced as 'catastrophic' and lead to massive reactions. If someone is only a minute or two late to an appointment it will be experienced as a major disaster and interpreted as evidence that the patient is not worth anything or that they are hated. A voice raised in mild irritation is experienced as a shout and a mild, relatively polite, justifiable criticism will be experienced as 'character assassination'.

It is frequently noted that people with AN evidence a strong need to feel in control of their environment. They find it difficult to allow others to make decisions and can very easily become upset if someone disagrees with them. Parents may be accused of 'not listening' when actually what is meant is that the parents are not obeying their demands. They insist on life being arranged the way they want it and often find it extremely difficult to understand why this might present problems for other people. It is virtually impossible to escape the conclusion that they find it difficult to regulate emotion. Things are always too hot or too cold, too hard or too soft, but never just right. They do not eat because if they do, they are at risk of experiencing 'unbearable' feelings, often of a kind related to 'badness' or guilt. If they eat they feel guilty (for being greedy); if they sit down they feel guilty (for being lazy); if they keep themselves warm they feel guilty (for being hedonistic). So why do they feel guilty? When asked, the patients do not know. However, it often seems that one answer to the question is that there has developed an internal imperative that is connected with the notion that to give in to such impulses or longings will result in a catastrophic loss of control. Any such submission to impulses is therefore experienced as being very bad. In other words, the rigid overcontrol is a desperate attempt to avoid the terrifying feelings that result from loss of control – the fear that if the patient relaxes her iron grip for even a second, everything will 'fall apart'.

This, in turn, begs the question of why loss of control should be experienced as so disastrous. One possible answer is that normal complex regulatory mechanisms have not developed, so that any loss of control results in the experience of chaos, with its attendant fear that the self will fall apart or be destroyed. This rather extreme language is used deliberately, for it feels to the patient that it is, absolutely, a matter of survival. And ironically, from the physical perspective, this desperate attempt to avoid the perceived destruction does indeed threaten survival.

So how can neuroscience add to our understanding of these issues?

1.7   In-the-beginning questions:[3] the problem of aetiology in eating disorders

We still do not fully understand why a 14-year-old girl might become so terrified of eating that she appears to be willing to risk starving to death. There is no doubt that psychology has developed theoretical models of the functioning of the human mind that are profound, useful and far-reaching. In relation to AN there are theories that variously implicate social and cultural attitudes, genetic endowment (although only in as-yet-unknown ways), trauma, and family and social relationships (although these last are more concerned with factors that maintain the condition rather than causing it). However, there remain few convincing *aetiological* accounts. The fact that AN is deemed to be a 'complex, multifactorial disorder', although undoubtedly true, is insufficient.

The interaction of aetiological factors can be considered in two dimensions: a temporal, 'vertical' dimension and a spatial, 'horizontal' dimension. In fact, these dimensions are not really distinct and they continuously interact, but they are useful in considering the complexity of aetiology (see Figure 1.1).

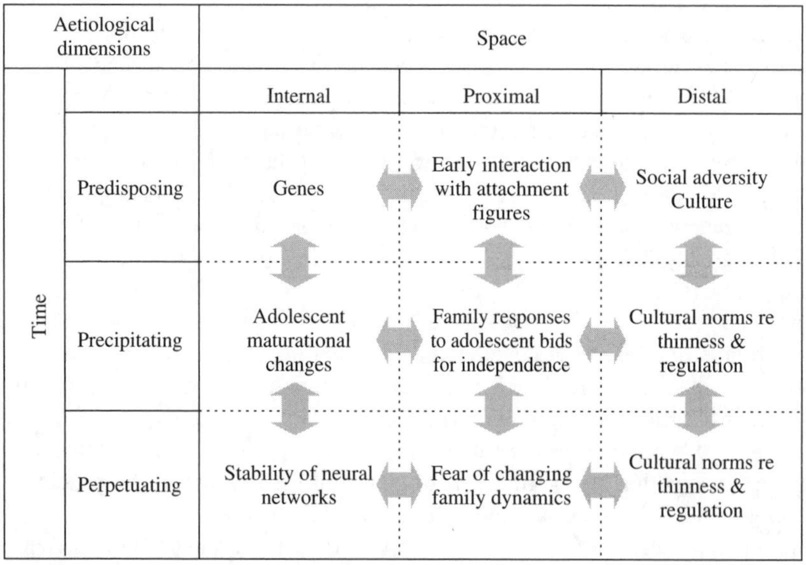

Aetiological dimensions		Space		
		Internal	Proximal	Distal
Time	Predisposing	Genes	Early interaction with attachment figures	Social adversity Culture
	Precipitating	Adolescent maturational changes	Family responses to adolescent bids for independence	Cultural norms re thinness & regulation
	Perpetuating	Stability of neural networks	Fear of changing family dynamics	Cultural norms re thinness & regulation

Figure 1.1   Interactions between aetiological dimensions.

---

[3] I am indebted to Earl Hopper for this phrase.

1.8   The temporal, 'vertical' aetiological dimension

One of the inherent problems in any temporal discussion of aetiology is that of *apperception*, the process by which new experience is *always* assimilated to, and transformed by, the residuum of past experience to form a new whole. Thus, to list these categories in reverse order, maintaining factors need to be seen in the light of the effect of precipitating factors and precipitating factors in the light of predisposing factors. In reality these categories cannot be separated out. But even today we still get stuck in discussions about 'Is there a gene for AN?', ignoring the fact that genes code for proteins and not for complex clusters of behavioural symptoms. Neurogenetics (that branch of genetics dealing with the action of genes in the nervous system) is rapidly developing accounts of how genes require very specific intracellular environments, which themselves contain information derived from the past (in the form of hormones, neurotransmitters and intracellular molecules produced as a result of the previous activity of perceptual systems), before they can be expressed in the production of specific proteins.

One that has received a great deal of attention is the serotonin transporter (5-HTT) gene, which determines the structure of an integral membrane protein that transports the neurotransmitter serotonin from synaptic spaces into presynaptic neurons, and thereby regulates the action of serotonin. Some people have a version of the gene (an allele) that produces a protein of shorter length, whereas others have a version that produces a longer protein, containing a greater number of repeating sequences of constituent amino acids.

Suomi's classic studies with rhesus monkeys (which have the same gene as humans) showed that those that carried the 'short' allele were significantly more affected by maternal deprivation than those that carried the 'long' form [8]. In humans a similar picture is found. In one study [9], people homozygous for the short allele of the 5-HTT gene had a 43% chance of becoming clinically depressed after four or more stressful events experienced between the ages of 21 and 26, whereas only 17% of those homozygous for the long allele became depressed. Those with the short allele were more likely to display abnormal levels of anxiety and to more readily acquire conditioned fear responses [10]. In this case, variation in only a single gene may explain why some people weather stressful events while others are plunged into depression. Kumsta *et al.* [11] have found a similar picture in Romanian orphans adopted into UK homes.

Importantly, however, the allele only reveals its influence when people experience adverse events, which include factors such as divorce, debt, unemployment or other occasions of 'threat, loss, humiliation or defeat' [12], over which they may have little or no control.

To put it more simply, genes need to interact with their environments in order to be expressed and gene–environment interactions are always recursive. Although it is obvious, it still needs to be stressed that the aetiology of any illness in which genes play an important role (and that is probably all illnesses) must be seen as the result of a complex recursive interaction between gene and environment. (For a more detailed discussion of these concepts, see Chapter 5.)

These understandings throw important light on more than a century of psychotherapeutic observation and theory building in relation to such concepts as transference,[4] unconscious fantasy and 'projective identification',[5] which are still widely misunderstood outside psychoanalytical discourse (and there continues to be debate about them even within psychoanalysis). However, psychoanalytical authors such as Quinidoz [13, 14] have argued that the above ideas provide a useful explanatory neuroscientific basis for the clinical observations.

Transference can now be understood as the inevitable outcome of the behaviour of a complex recurrent neural net.[6] That is, in any perception there is always an element of 'transference' in that when any 'input pattern of activation' arrives for processing, it activates those neural nets that most closely match (or will respond to) it, but their *subsequent* activity unfolds in a way that has more to do with the pattern of recurrent activity that has developed through training (learning) than with the stimulus itself [15].

Thus neuroanatomical evidence supports the psychoanalytical conclusion, initiated by Freud's observations, that there is *no such thing as an 'ahistorical' present* [12]: all one's current experience of the world is always and inevitably mediated through one's experience of the past. Likewise, *projection* and *projective identification* can be seen as phenomena arising from networks that behave in such a way that those encoding representations of the self are activated more easily than those encoding representations of the external world, leading to a perception of the outside world that is significantly distorted.

Neuroscientists would benefit from paying close attention to data derived from psychoanalytical observation, since the insights derived from the meticulous observation of transference phenomena made possible by skilled psychoanalytical technique give access to psychological processes that cannot be observed in any other way.

For example, Williams *et al.* [16, 17] explore some key themes observed in psychoanalytical work with patients with AN. These are:

1. difficulties in some aspects of early relationships, mostly connected to the idea of 'lack of fit',
2. fusion and projective identification (in which there is a lack of optimal differentiation between self and other),
3. attacks on paternal function (the function of the 'father' in helping the mother and infant differentiate) and
4. the presence of a destructive superego.

These elements, it is proposed, lead to the transformation of a healthy, nurturing, reciprocal relationship between self and other into a rather more 'receptacle/foreign body' type of relationship, and also to the lack of development of the space between two members of a dyad that allows them to become two identities instead of one single fused identity. In turn, these configurations predispose to subsequent difficulties,

---

[4] A term introduced by Freud to describe a situation that he observed in his clinical work with patients, in which the patient seemed to relate to him in ways that suggested that they were transferring attitudes, fantasies, thoughts and feelings connected to figures from the past on to their relationship with Freud in the present. Today the term is considered both in a restricted technical sense in relation to the phenomena occurring within the psychoanalytic treatment process and in a more general sense in relation to perception, and apperception, in general.

[5] A rather loosely and confusingly defined term referring to the attribution of disowned aspects of the self to the other in such a powerful way that the other unconsciously takes on those attributes.

[6] A neural net in which 'downstream' output neurons recurrently connect back on to input neurons.

particularly in relation to the negotiation of the boundary around the self, and the regulation of *what comes into or goes out* of the body/mind.

Although complex, to some clinicians these detailed psychoanalytical observations ring very true. Many, but not all, patients demonstrate some combination of these characteristics, but they are not specific to AN and are therefore not aetiologically satisfying. Minuchin famously described corresponding patterns of enmeshment in the families of AN patients, and distortions of healthy family structure [18], although whether these patterns are pathognomonic of AN was rightly challenged [19] and they were subsequently shown to be features of any family coping with a seriously ill child. Clinical accounts, however apt and illuminating, are not explanations, and although undeniably they have usefulness, they still lack the underlying coherence necessary to give a seriously satisfying aetiological framework. How might one relate these observations and formulations to underlying neurobiological processes?

The idea of 'lack of fit' suggests that there might be underlying neuropsychological problems that adversely affect the capacity to develop satisfactory attunement between mother and child. Subsequently, difficulties arise in developing optimal degrees of differentiation, as differentiation implies the development of sufficiently stable, coherent and robust self-representations that allow separation to occur without panic. The fact that this requires repeated consistent interaction implies that tuning of nascent neural networks is likely to be the underlying neurobiological process. It is likely that at least some of the genetic predispositions to the development of AN may act through their influence on, and possible disruption of, the formation of these early attuned networks, resulting in various compensatory strategies affecting subsequent personality formation.

Connan *et al.* [20] have proposed a complex neurodevelopmental model in which early stressful experience, such as suboptimal parenting, takes a central (but not sufficient) role in adjusting the 'sensitivity' of regulating systems. It is very important here to stress that 'suboptimal' in this sense does not mean 'bad' parenting. Many have correctly pointed out over the years that we must avoid blaming parents, not out of so-called political correctness, but because blame in this context is both unwarranted and unhelpful, and misses the point. However, at the same time we must not throw the baby out with the bath water. We must accept that trauma is ubiquitous in human experience. None of us have reached adulthood without experiencing it to some degree and in some form, and some of us may have needed to work very hard to overcome it. We must also remember that parents do not parent in isolation; they are part of a family and social context that may both help and hinder the extremely difficult task of parenting. A depressed mother may not have been able to provide her infant with optimal responsiveness, but she may be depressed for very good reasons and in circumstances over which she has little or no control.

Fonagy [21] has linked descriptions of analogous processes to neurobiological findings through Arnsten's [22] description of a 'biological switch'. Under conditions of stress, there is activation of limbic circuits and inhibition of prefrontal cortical circuits that contribute to a decrease in the capacity for 'mentalising' (a prefrontal cortical activity) and subsequent regression to two more primitive modes of functioning, termed either 'pretend' or 'psychic equivalence'. These two modes of functioning can be related to Hopper's [23] discussion of traumatic experience and to fears of annihilation resulting from experiences of extreme helplessness. These profound anxieties involve oscillating experiences of fears of falling apart, abandonment and so on (fission and fragmentation), and fears of suffocation, being trapped and so on (fusion and confusion).

Furthermore, they might be seen to link to properties of the two principle classes of anxious attachment strategies, avoidant (A) and ambivalent (C). Within that frame of reference, individuals who utilise type A strategies attempt to deactivate attachment behaviour in order to reduce exposure to the pain and distress caused by frustration of bids for proximity to attachment figures, perceived to be distant or rejecting. They tend to be self-reliant, excessively independent and avoidant of awareness of their own emotional reactions. Conversely, those utilising type C strategies attempt to keep attachment systems in a state of chronic hyperactivation, and tend to escalate emotion intensity in order to maintain proximity to attachment figures. When these strategies are utilised, negative experiences tend to be tightly bound together and, in terms of associative memory networks, 'one cognitive node with a negative emotional tag can automatically spread its activation to other negatively tinged cognitive nodes, causing all of them to become highly available to working memory' [24].

While Fonagy, Arnsten and Hopper describe these processes in relation to stress or traumatic experience, it needs to be remembered that any event can only be experienced through a 'filter' of tuned sensory neural networks. Some individuals may have more sensitively tuned networks than others, leading them to be more vulnerable to traumatic experience. In other words, some very highly sensitive individuals might have little option but to experience almost any interaction with the outside world as highly anxiety-provoking, in turn leading to consequent patterns of behaviour that have the characteristics described above.

Nelson *et al.* [25], in a review of social information processing in adolescence, identify three 'nodes': (i) a *detection* node, responsible for the detection of socially salient stimuli; (ii) an *affective* node, involved in the generation of emotional experience related to the stimulus; and (iii) a *cognitive* node, which is responsible for regulating the response to the stimulus. They make the point that the development of the affective node during adolescence is very much under the control of glucocorticoid hormones, whereas the cognitive regulatory node is learning-dependent and takes longer to mature. It therefore can be postulated that individuals with insufficiently developed cognitive regulatory capacities, who, until adolescence, have been very dependent on their parents to regulate their affect for them, can have this fragile equilibrium overturned by the hormonally dependent affective node developing more rapidly.

Thus when the hormonal changes of adolescence induce rapid development of the affective node, these early schematic appraisals of the self as being disgustingly greedy, enormous, too much for the carer to bear, and so on, surface through automatic or associative routes in the generation of the emotion of disgust directed towards the self later on in adolescence. Under these circumstances, starvation becomes not only the only option, but a very effective one. An early effect is that the ensuing loss of weight reverses the production of hormones and the brain regresses to its prepubescent state, minimising the dysregulation.

Neuroscience now offers a framework within which to more fully understand the aetiology of these complex behavioural phenotypes. At the same time, neurobiologists might study these detailed clinical observations and their associated theoretical elaborations as a means of generating further hypotheses about underlying neurobiological processes.

1.9   The spatial, 'horizontal' aetiological dimension

We now turn to the spatial dimension, composed of what are sometimes referred to as 'systemic' factors [26], which in turn can be divided into *internal factors* (within the individual), *proximal factors* (involving those close to the individual such as family and peers) and *distal* factors (which are more nebulous and involve culture and societal pressure).

A system can be defined as a set of components in mutual interaction [27]. A system exists if 'a set of elements within an environment relate to one another in such a way that changes in them can be predicted without reference to that environment'. However, 'the actual relationships between the elements of a system and between the system and its environment are always problematic' [12]. In other words, there is no such thing in reality as a fully closed system. Yet systems may be sufficiently closed for us to usefully consider them as systems, without having to always think of the whole universe when considering their behaviour. Because no system is ever truly closed, the relationship between a system and its environment, or between one system and another within an environment, allows us to consider systems as nested within other systems. We can then conceive of a hierarchy of systems at differing levels of complexity or abstraction. At each level, elements interact with one another in such a way that they become constituted as a new system. This new system in turn interacts with other systems at the same level to form the next level, and so on. One problem that arises is that when any system, or hierarchy of systems, exceeds a particular level of complexity, the consideration of it as a whole becomes exceedingly difficult or even impossible.

Until relatively recently we have not had sufficient understanding of how things work at the cellular or subcellular levels in brains to allow us to understand much about the relationship between brains, persons and societies. However, that has now changed. As an example, let us consider two levels of system which have not normally been seen as connected, and which have often been characterised as being in opposition: *cultural factors* and *neural circuitry* in AN. For many years the cultural factor that has been seen to be relevant to the genesis of AN has been the overvaluation within particular cultures of 'thinness'. Although this has been related to other causes, particularly the position of women in society and associated beliefs concerning a sense of agency, not much mention has been made of the issue of self-regulation. There would seem to be little doubt that over the last century there has been a crisis in industrialised societies in relation to the topic of regulation. Industrialisation has brought with it mass production, which in turn has brought the need to encourage consumers to consume, to consume more, and to consume still more. The idea that at some point one might feel satisfied with what one has got is not one that sits comfortably with the corporate need to achieve continuous and never-ending growth in profits.

There are also far fewer social constraints on all sorts of behaviour now than there were 50 years ago. For example, when the 'F word' was first used on British television in 1965, ripples of shock and horror spread throughout the country. Now it would be hard to get through an evening without hearing it several times. Parents do not have the support of social norms in the way that they did. In relation to the regulation of desire, they are actively undermined by a culture based on unbridled capitalism, which denies the possibility of having too many pairs of trainers, or that last month's computer already needs upgrading.

But how does this relate to neurones? In any complex nervous system, there will be circuits dedicated to control and regulation. In complex organisms such as humans, although many of these systems are innate, many need to be learned. This is almost certainly an evolutionary adaptation that allows flexibility and therefore increases survival value in environments where conditions vary. The principal source of learning, at least in the early years of life, is the family, but families are embedded in societies and recursively interact with them. For families embedded in modern post-industrial societies there is now a contradiction, in that parents want on the one hand to help their children learn to regulate themselves and their desires, and on the other to help their children fit in to a culture which demands they never feel satisfied. We need to be very concerned by the possibility that infants and toddlers may spend more time obtaining noncontingent feedback from a television than they do from their parents.

We now know that learning at the neural level involves physical changes in the structure of proteins involved in synapses that determine how easily or not an action potential will be created in the postsynaptic neurone (neuroplasticity). The more a particular neural net is activated, the more easily it becomes activated in future. This neural net may be involved in the recognition of one's mother's face, in the control of one's legs in learning to walk, in the learning of language or juggling or the ability to say 'no' to one's self, and all these actions involve changes in the ease with which a synapse transmits an impulse in any particular neural net. Thus, any particular cultural attribute, mediated by the transmission of culture through families and parents, becomes 'inscribed' physically in the neural circuitry of individuals. Living in a culture in which restraint and self-control are not encouraged surely must result in any individual within that culture having greater difficulty in developing functioning neural circuits that promote self-control than someone living in a highly regulated culture. It follows that control systems that are dependent on learning, such as those involving executive function, might be particularly affected. The point here is that 'cultural factors' need to be seen in a sophisticated way, not just as a somewhat ethereal background pressure, but as something real and tangible that becomes incorporated into the neural circuitry of our brains.

It is very easy to forget (or perhaps more accurately, it is easy to remain unaware, as we are rarely conscious of it in the first place) how much our culture becomes internalised. It is thus often easy to abdicate responsibility for it, to shrug our shoulders and say 'not my problem'. The point here is that we should not really be surprised that, if we allow commercial organisations in our society to spend millions of pounds on persuading children, through the medium of television advertising, that they need more, and that they should not be satisfied with what they have got, disorders of self-regulation became more common. We should not be surprised that if we contribute to, and support, an ethos that proclaims that social structures of authority are undesirable, and that we should be allowed to do more or less what we want, disorders of self-regulation became more common. We cannot and should not be seduced into absolving ourselves from responsibility by telling ourselves that culture and brains have no connection, and that because eating disorders have neurobiological substrates, culture does not really have a serious influence. Our brains physically develop within a culture that has real physical effects.

Thus, when considering 'cultural' factors in the genesis of eating disorders we should look beyond relatively simplistic notions of responses to depictions of thin models in the mass media. We should ask more complex questions such as why 'thinness' itself becomes so overvalued that it is a required attribute of those who are elevated to the status of cultural icons. It is at least worthy of serious consideration that thinness is overvalued as a sort of antidote to a constantly increasing underlying fear of dysregulation in postmodern societies. This fear is connected to, and exacerbated by, the fact that over the vast majority of the time in which our brains have been evolving, we have had to find ways of dealing with scarcity and lack in order to survive. Evolution through natural selection has endowed us with powerful behavioural systems whose goal is to maximise energy input. We are highly sensitive to lack, and behaviour that decreases the intensity of hunger is highly rewarding. Indeed, the need to have effective systems aimed at maximising energy input was so important that it is much easier to answer the question of which part of the brain is *not* concerned with eating and food (answer: almost none of it) than to decide which part *is* concerned, as these processes are widely distributed over the whole central nervous system [28].

On the other hand, overdoing it and taking in too much has not, from an evolutionary point of view, been much of a problem (although it may well have become one now), so systems for downregulating appetite are weaker than those involved in upregulating it. Thus the evolutionarily endowed, highly rewarding state of acquisitiveness is exploited by modern industrial societies for the purposes of economic growth. It is not that difficult to persuade people to want more: it is built into our behavioural systems. The price we pay for this is the troubling sense that we are not fully in control of ourselves. We do not like to feel that others are manipulating us and we want to maintain the fiction that we can resist if we want to. Thinness becomes a marker of those who are in control of themselves, those who are able to rise above the 'base' domination of appetitive desire, who can resist and stand firm against temptation. The ascetic ideal, persisting all the way down from Plato, in which emotions are seen as phenomena that need to be conquered, has been often admired. In the past this may have been a way of managing lack, and attempting to live with it, but now we are facing far greater difficulties from excess and having too much available, too much choice. Perhaps our evolutionarily adapted neurobiological systems are unable to deal with it.

1.10   The importance of a neuroscientific aetiological framework

All these ideas can be viewed as helpful elaborations of a more fundamental problem. This has to do with the disturbances in the formation of the self that result from very fundamental neurobiological abnormalities, related to the notion of *sensitivity*, that make the development of satisfactory self-regulatory systems very difficult. Self-regulation, or homeostasis, refers to the capacity of an organism to maintain its internal state within limits that are optimal for survival. In any complex organism it inevitably becomes an extremely complex process or set of processes, but one that is essential for survival and thus of central importance in the function of the organism.

The need for any organism to maintain its internal environment is obvious, and systems that have evolved in order to maintain this environment (homoeostatic systems) have been studied since physiology began. Just as there is a need to maintain the physical environment, there is also a need to maintain the psychological. Thus, in order to function well in our relationships and interactions, we need to be able to regulate our responses, to think before acting, to weigh up the costs and benefits of any particular course of action, to modulate what we say and how we say it, and so on. A particularly important regulatory mechanism involves knowing when we have had enough. Just as the initiation of behaviours is an important part of executive function, the decision as to when to stop and move on to something else is equally important.

Craig [29] has proposed that patterns of forebrain lateralisation originate from asymmetries in the peripheral autonomic nervous system. In his proposal, left-forebrain activity is particularly associated with parasympathetic activity and energy enrichment, and right-forebrain activity with sympathetic activity and energy expenditure. Of particular interest is the observation that this lateralisation seems to occur principally in the anterior insula, with the left anterior insula being activated predominantly by homeostatic afferents associated with parasympathetic functions (energy enrichment) and the right anterior insula being activated predominantly by homeostatic afferents associated with sympathetic functions (energy expenditure). Neuroimaging studies have commonly shown there to be significant asymmetries in insular activation in patients with AN [30–33] (see Chapter 3).

Emotions (consciously experienced as 'feelings') can now be considered a function of complex, high-level homeostatic systems, and many patients with AN have particular difficulty with emotion and emotion regulation. When considering the topic of emotion regulation, it is always important to remember that it is difficult to draw a distinction between the *generation* of emotion and the *regulation* of emotion [10]. 'Because emotions are multicomponent processes that unfold over time, emotion regulation involves changes in "emotion dynamics"' [34]. Emotion products (bodily sensations, facial expressions, actions, etc.) can also serve as stimuli for further emotion generation (such as becoming embarrassed about being frightened), which functions as part of the regulatory activity of the initial state.

The construction of a mental representation of one's own physical body is a complicated business and is vital to the development of a fully functioning self-representation. Longo *et al.* [35] have distinguished between the relatively well understood *somatosensation* (the initial sensory processing of somatic information in the primary somatosensory cortex) and two other, less well understood classes of higher-order processing: *somatoperception* (the process of perceiving the body itself and ensuring somatic perceptual constancy) and *somatorepresentation* (a combination of essentially cognitive, lexical-semantic knowledge about the body, emotions and attitudes about the body, and the link between the physical body and the psychological self). These correspond to the three levels of processing of any sensation: primary, reception; secondary, perception; and tertiary, interpretation and integration.

The relationship between emotion and the body is especially important and especially complex. Damasio's somatic marker hypothesis [3–6] is centrally concerned with the contribution to the *experience* of emotional states (feelings) by information about emotion-derived changes in the body conveyed back to the brain by somatic afferent pathways. It is likely that both somatoperception and somatorepresentation are significantly influenced by affects in a recursive fashion. If affect regulation is a serious difficulty, it makes sense to assume that the way the body is experienced is likely to be influenced. Clinical experience suggests that language is often used in a way that assigns physical properties to emotional states ('worrying about you is *too much* for me to bear', 'you are a *weight* on my mind', 'you occupy too much *space* in my head') [36–38]. This may reflect an underlying binding of insufficiently regulated (and hence very intense) emotion to lexical-semantic representations of the body as being 'too big', 'too heavy', 'too fat' and so on. It is as if the (somatoperceptive) physical self is not sufficiently distinguished from the (somatorepresentative) emotional self, and dysregulated 'big' or 'fat' emotions lead to the experience of 'big' or 'fat' bodies.

An association between alexithymia and AN (as well as many other conditions) has long been postulated [39–42]. Patients with AN appear to find it difficult to 'know' what they feel and to distinguish between one emotional state and another. Because of this, they cannot communicate in words about their current emotional state.

Alexithymia as a concept is poorly understood, and there is some question as to what it really means. That being said, there would seem to be reasonably good evidence to suggest that it reflects a valid concern about the way that patients with AN manage to communicate about feelings. In order to be able to put feelings into words (to ascribe lexical constructs to emotional experience) one first has to be able to consistently recognise and distinguish one emotional state from another. If there are serious difficulties in regulating emotions, it might therefore be difficult to find words for them. The attempt to regulate the emotional state itself may interfere with the ability to hold that state in awareness long enough to name it, given that naming it is almost certainly a high-level operation, requiring attention.

Perfectionism, an almost universal concomitant of AN, can be understood as an extreme way of avoiding unbearable feelings of failure and self-criticism, which again make sense if there is extreme sensitivity to negative emotion. Rather than accepting that one may be 'good enough', and thus not being too cast down by disappointment, any perceived negative judgement is appraised as catastrophic and therefore to be avoided at all costs.

Another common feature of AN, obsessionality, is still poorly understood, but it would seem to be clear that it is intimately connected with anxiety, and that obsessional mechanisms can function as ways of downregulating anxiety. 'Obsessional' mechanisms such as rituals are used under normal circumstances as ways of making the world seem well-ordered and predictable, and ritualised behaviour is a well-observed feature of normal development.

1.11   Conclusion

The key thesis of this chapter is that clinicians have nothing to fear from neuroscience; in fact, they have everything to gain. AN is an extremely complex disorder and to understand it we require complex and sophisticated models. Models developed before current neuroscience knowledge became available have provided useful insights into the phenomenology of AN but have had only very limited aetiological significance. There is no doubt that neuroscience is complex, but it need not be mysterious. It has provided, is providing and no doubt will continue to provide extraordinarily exciting and useful insights into why some people have the misfortune to develop such a devastating illness and others do not. Neuroscience allows us finally to dispense with the deeply unsatisfying dualism that has bedevilled psychiatry and related disciplines for decades. Mind and brain can now be integrated into a single, albeit complex, identity. Doing so helps us clarify the limits and constraints that apply to concepts such as freedom and self-determination, without which we struggle to know how to respond to the clinical dilemmas presented to us by our patients.

Clinical observation clearly demonstrates that AN is a disorder comprising far more than problems with eating, and that a range of experiential and behavioural symptoms are not easily integrated. It is through the insights that neuroscience is now providing that we are able to edge closer to a satisfactory underlying aetiological model that will inevitably allow us to build more effective treatments. Models are developing that elucidate the fundamental deficits and difficulties in the continuous and constant integration by our brains/minds of vast quantities of information, from both inside and outside our bodies. Such information helps explain how we can maintain our selves in an optimal relationship with our environment, and how we construct and maintain a coherent sense of self, both physical and psychological. While perhaps history teaches us to be wary of overoptimism, we have good reasons to feel that clinical work can now be more firmly grounded on a secure scientific basis.

References

1. Descartes, R. and Voss, S. (1989) *The Passions of the Soul*, Hackett Publishing Company, Indianapolis.
2. Popper, K.R. and Eccles, J.C. (1977) *The Self and Its Brain*, Springer International, New York.
3. Damasio, A.R. (1994) *Descartes' Error: Emotion, Reason, and the Human Brain*, Putnam, New York.
4. Damasio, A.R. (1999) *The Feeling of What Happens: Body and Emotion in the Making of Consciousness*, 1st edn, Harcourt Brace, New York.
5. Damasio, A.R. (2003) *Looking for Spinoza: Joy, Sorrow, and the Feeling Brain*, 1st edn, Harcourt, Orlando, FL.
6. Damasio, A.R. (2005) *Descartes' Error: Emotion, Reason, and the Human Brain*, Penguin, London.
7. Hameroff, S.R. and Penrose, R. (1996) Conscious events as orchestrated space-time selections. *Journal of Consciousness Studies*, **3**, 36–53.
8. Suomi, S.J. (2003) Gene-environment interactions and the neurobiology of social conflict. *Annals of the New York Academy of Sciences*, **1008**, 132–139.
9. Caspi, A., Sugden, K., Moffitt, T.E. *et al.* (2003) Influence of life stress on depression: moderation by a polymorphism in the 5-HTT gene. *Science*, **301** (5631), 386–389.
10. Gross, J.J. (2007) *Handbook of Emotion Regulation*, Guilford Press, New York.
11. Kumsta, R., Stevens, S., Brookes, K. *et al.* (2010) 5HTT genotype moderates the influence of early institutional deprivation on emotional problems in adolescence: evidence from the english and romanian adoptee (Era) study. *Journal of Child Psychology and Psychiatry*, **51** (7), 755–762.
12. Hopper, E. (2003) *The Social Unconscious: Selected Papers*, J. Kingsley Publishers, London, Philadelphia.

13. Quinodoz, J.M. (1997) Transitions in psychic structures in the light of deterministic chaos theory. *The International Journal of Psycho-Analysis*, **78** (Pt 4), 699–718.

14. Quinodoz, J.M. (2004) On chaotic possibilities: toward a new model of development. *The International Journal of Psycho-Analysis*, **85** (Pt 4), 1009–1010; author reply 10–12.

15. Churchland, P.M. (1995) *The Engine of Reason, the Seat of the Soul: A Philosophical Journey into the Brain*, MIT Press, Cambridge, MA.

16. Williams, G. *et al.* (eds) (2003) *Exploring Eating Disorders in Adolescents: The Generosity of Acceptance*, vol. **II**, Karnac Books, London.

17. Williams, G. *et al.* (eds) (2003) *Exploring Feeding Difficulties in Children: The Generosity of Acceptance*, vol. **I**, Karnac Books, London.

18. Minuchin, S., Rosman, B.L. and Baker, L. (1978) *Psychosomatic Families: Anorexia Nervosa in Context*, Harvard University Press, Cambridge, MA.

19. Dare, C., Le Grange, D., Eisler, I. and Rutherford, J. (1994) Redefining the psychosomatic family: family process of 26 eating disorder families. *The International Journal of Eating Disorders*, **16** (3), 211–226.

20. Connan, F., Campbell, I.C., Katzman, M. *et al.* (2003) A neurodevelopmental model for anorexia nervosa. *Physiology and Behavior*, **79** (1), 13–24.

21. Fonagy, P. (2005) Eating disorders and dysfunctional attachment: a focus on mentalization, *7th London International Conference on Eating Disorders, 2005*, Imperial College, London.

22. Arnsten, A. (1998) The biology of being frazzled. *Science*, **280**.

23. Hopper, E. (2003) *Traumatic Experience in the Unconscious Life of Groups: A Theoretical and Clinical Study of Traumatic Experience and False Reparation*, Jessica Kingsley Publishers, Philadelphia, PA.

24. Shaver, P.R. and Mikulincer, M. (2007) Adult attachment strategies and the regulation of emotion, in *Handbook of Emotion Regulation* (ed. J.J. Gross), The Guilford Press, New York.

25. Nelson, E., Leibenluft, E., McClure, E. and Pine, D. (2005) The social re-orientation of adolescence: a neuroscience perspective on the process and its relation to psychopathology. *Psychological Medicine*, **35**, 163–174.

26. Nicholls, D. (2007) Aetiology, in *Eating Disorders in Childhood and Adolescence* (eds B. Lask and R. Bryant-Waugh), Routledge, Hove.

27. von Bertalanffy, L. (1969) *General System Theory: Foundations, Development, Applications*, G. Braziller, New York.

28. Frampton, I. and Hutchinson, A. (2007) Eating disorders and the brain, in *Eating Disorders in Childhood and Adolescence* (eds B. Lask and R. Bryant-Waugh), Routledge, Hove.

29. Craig, A.D. (2005) Forebrain emotional asymmetry: a neuroanatomical basis? *Trends in Cognitive Sciences*, **9**, 566–571.

30. Chowdhury, U., Gordon, I., Lask, B. *et al.* (2003) Early-onset anorexia nervosa: is there evidence of limbic system imbalance? *The International Journal of Eating Disorders*, **33** (4), 388–396.

31. Lask, B., Gordon, I., Christie, D. *et al.* (2005) Functional neuroimaging in early-onset anorexia nervosa. *The International Journal of Eating Disorders*, **37** (S1), S49–S51.

32. Nunn, K., Frampton, I., Gordon, I. and Lask, B. (2008) The fault is not in her parents but in her insula: a neurobiological hypothesis of anorexia nervosa. *European Eating Disorders Review*, **16** (5), 355–360.

33. Gordon, I., Lask, B., Bryant-Waugh, R. and Christie, D. (1997) Childhood-onset anorexia nervosa: towards identifying a biological substrate. *International Journal of Eating Disorders*, **22** (2), 159–165.

34. Thompson, R.A. (1990) Emotion and self-regulation, in *Socioemotional Development Nebraska Symposium on Motivation* (ed. R.A. Thompson), University of Nebraska Press, Lincoln, pp. 367–467.

35. Longo, M.R., Azanon, E. and Haggard, P. (2009) More than skin deep: body representation beyond primary somatosensory cortex. *Neuropsychologia*, **48**, 655–668.
36. Skarderud, F. (2007) Eating one's words, part I: 'concretised metaphors' and reflective function in anorexia nervosa – an interview study. *European Eating Disorders Review*, **15** (3), 163–174.
37. Skarderud, F. (2007) Eating one's words, part II: the embodied mind and reflective function in anorexia nervosa – theory. *European Eating Disorders Review*, **15** (4), 243–252.
38. Skarderud, F. (2007) Eating one's words: part III: mentalisation-based psychotherapy for anorexia nervosa – an outline for a treatment and training manual. *European Eating Disorders Review*, **15** (5), 323–339.
39. Sifneos, P.E. (1973) The prevalence of 'alexithymic' characteristics in psychosomatic patients. *Psychotherapy and Psychosomatics*, **22** (2), 255–262.
40. Taylor, G.J. (1984) Alexithymia: concept, measurement, and implications for treatment. *The American Journal of Psychiatry*, **141** (6), 725–732.
41. Zonnevylle-Bender, M.J., van Goozen, S.H., Cohen-Kettenis, P.T. *et al.* (2004) Emotional functioning in anorexia nervosa patients: adolescents compared to adults. *Depression and Anxiety*, **19** (1), 35–42.
42. Zonnevylle-Bender, M.J., van Goozen, S.H., Cohen-Kettenis, P.T. *et al.* (2004) Emotional functioning in adolescent anorexia nervosa patients – a controlled study. *European Child and Adolescent Psychiatry*, **13** (1), 28–34.

2 Eating disorders: an overview

Beth Watkins

St George's University of London, London, UK

2.1 Introduction

This chapter provides an overview of the main eating disorders, including anorexia nervosa (AN), bulimia nervosa (BN) and eating disorder not otherwise specified (EDNOS), as well as atypical eating disorders that usually present in childhood, such as food-avoidance emotional disorder (FAED), selective eating and functional dypsphagia. The chapter will give clinical descriptions of each disorder and review their epidemiology, aetiology and risk factors, comorbidity, treatment, and course and outcome.

The eating disorders AN, BN and their variants are a major source of physical and psychological morbidity. Not only is there a central disturbance in eating habits and weight regulation, but a wide range of adverse physical, psychological and social consequences for sufferers of these disorders. Onset tends to be in adolescence and early adulthood, and as such, coincides with phases in life critical to personal development. Eating disorders, in particular AN and BN, principally affect adolescent girls and young-adult women. Indeed, women between the ages of around 15 and 35 represent the vast majority of those presenting with, and receiving treatment for, eating disorders [1].

Eating disorders have also been reported in men and boys [2–5], older women [6] and prepubertal children of both sexes [7–10]. The clinical picture in men and older women is very similar to that found in the adolescent and young-adult female population, and, indeed, it would appear that such cases fulfil existing accepted diagnostic criteria for AN or BN [11, 12]. The majority of studies employ the Diagnostic and Statistical Manual IV (DSM-IV) [11] criteria for these eating disorders and their variants, which are illustrated in Tables 2.1–2.3

Eating Disorders and the Brain. Edited by Bryan Lask and Ian Frampton.
© 2011 John Wiley & Sons, Ltd. Published 2011 by John Wiley & Sons, Ltd.

Table 2.1   DSM-IV diagnostic criteria for anorexia nervosa.

Refusal to maintain body weight at or above a minimally normal weight for age and height
(i.e. weight less than 85% of that expected).
Intense fear of gaining weight or becoming fat, even though underweight.
Disturbance in the way in which one's body weight or shape is experienced, undue influence
of body weight or shape on self-evaluation, or denial of the seriousness of the current low
body weight.
Amenorrhoea.

Table 2.2   DSM-IV diagnostic criteria for bulimia nervosa.

Recurrent episodes of binge eating.
Recurrent inappropriate compensatory behaviour in order to prevent weight gain.
The binge eating and inappropriate compensatory behaviours both occur, on average, at least
twice a week for three months.
Self-evaluation is unduly influenced by body shape and weight.
The disturbance does not occur exclusively during episodes of anorexia nervosa.

Table 2.3   DSM-IV examples of eating disorder not otherwise specified.

The EDNOS category is for disorders of eating that do not meet the criteria for any specific
eating disorder. For example:
For females, all of the criteria for AN are met except that the individual has regular
menses.
All of the criteria for AN are met except that, despite significant weight loss, the
individual's current weight is in the normal range.
All the criteria for BN are met except that the binge eating and inappropriate
compensatory behaviour mechanisms occur at a frequency less than twice a week or for
a duration of less than three months.
The regular use of inappropriate compensatory behaviours by an individual of normal body
weight after eating small amounts of food.
Repeatedly chewing and spitting out, but not swallowing, large amounts of food.
BED: recurrent episodes of binge eating in the absence of the regular use of inappropriate
compensatory behaviours characteristic of BN.

2.2   Clinical descriptions

Anorexia nervosa

AN is characterised by severe weight loss and a refusal to maintain body weight,
accompanied by abnormal cognitions leading to an overevaluation of the importance
of shape and weight. A combination of restriction of food intake, self-induced vomiting, laxative abuse and excessive exercise can contribute to weight loss and the
maintenance of a low weight, while preoccupation with shape and weight, dissatisfaction with shape and weight and an intense fear about gaining weight or get-
ting fat accompany the overvalued ideas about the importance of shape and weight.

Although amenorrhoea (the absence of at least three consecutive menstrual cycles) is a diagnostic criterion for AN, it is of questionable relevance and recent studies suggest that there are no meaningful differences between individuals with AN who do and do not menstruate [13, 14].

While AN in children has been shown to be strikingly similar to that in older adolescents and adults [15], it is important to note some fundamental developmental differences. For example, children with AN often fail to maintain hydration [16], and any weight loss, regardless of premorbid weight, during periods of expected growth should be treated with concern, even if the child remains within the healthy weight range [17].

There is little consistency in the literature to date with regard to terminology used to describe the onset of AN in children and adolescents under the age of 18 years. Some studies deem 'early onset' to simply mean an onset under the age of 18 years [18], while others describe those with an early onset to be aged 14 years or under [19]. Other studies attend to the pubertal status of the young person when applying the terms 'early onset' and 'late onset' [15]: Russell [20] noted that it is wise to consider the onset of AN as 'early' or 'late' in terms of pubertal development, as the age at onset of puberty varies from child to child, and it is a complex process which spans two to three years [21].

The question of whether the severity of earlier onset AN is similar to that seen in later onset has been raised, and findings are mixed. However, studies which used standardised assessment methods found similar severity levels in those with early and later onset [15, 22].

Bulimia nervosa

BN is an eating disorder characterised by recurrent episodes of overeating in which the person experiences a loss of control, coupled with accompanying compensatory behaviours to avoid weight gain, such as self-induced vomiting, laxative abuse, diuretic abuse and periods of fasting [23]. Weight and shape concern leading to an overevaluation of body shape and weight are core features, as in the case of AN, and those who suffer from BN usually experience high degrees of guilt and shame.

BN can be difficult to detect compared to AN, because those with BN tend to be of average or slightly above- or below-average weight.

Although rare, Bryant-Waugh and Lask [24] reported that 10% of their referrals to a specialist child and adolescent eating-disorder clinic comprised cases of BN with an onset below the age of 14 years. Cooper and colleagues [15] reported five cases of premenarcheal BN, in a consecutive series of 88 children diagnosed with an eating disorder, while Bryant-Waugh and Lask [25] reported a child aged seven who received a clinical diagnosis of BN.

Eating disorder not otherwise specified

The literature that describes the clinical features of EDNOS is consistent in suggesting that EDNOS closely resembles AN and BN [26–28]. Cases of EDNOS are often considered to be 'subthreshold' presentations of AN or BN, or present as a mix of the clinical features of both AN and BN [29]. Such presentations are often described as 'subclinical', 'partial' or 'atypical'. This falsely implies that they are less severe than the full syndromes of AN and BN [29].

Binge-eating disorder (BED) is characterised by recurrent binge eating in the absence of compensatory behaviours coupled with marked distressed about the eating behaviour. Binge-eating episodes are associated with eating until uncomfortably full, eating large amounts of food when not physically hungry, eating much more rapidly than normal, eating alone due to embarrassment about amounts eaten, and feeling disgusted or guilty after overeating. BED is included in the DSM-IV-TR as a provisional diagnosis requiring further study [30] but is likely to become a diagnosis in its own right in DSM-5. However, several questions regarding the validity of BED and its diagnostic criteria remain to be answered [31–33]. Individuals with BED report levels of shape and weight concerns that are comparable to those with AN and BN, and significantly higher than both normal-weight and overweight individuals without eating disorders [34–38]. In addition, overevaluation of shape and weight have been found to reliably predict elevated levels of psychosocial impairment [31, 39–42]. Goldschmidt and colleagues [43] found that overevaluation of shape and weight is a useful diagnostic specifier in BED, though they suggested that continued research is warranted to examine its predictive validity in natural-course and treatment-outcome studies.

Atypical disorders that usually present in childhood

None of the 'atypical' childhood-onset eating disorders have been well studied and their clinical features and nosological status are uncertain, although weight and shape concerns are not usually a feature of these disorders. What is known about these conditions is that there is dysfunctional behaviour around food, although the fundamental psychological disturbance is unclear. Using DSM-IV-TR criteria, children with atypical eating disorders would usually receive a diagnosis of EDNOS.

The criteria for EDNOS require some sort of dieting and/or purging behaviours, and the same sort of disturbance as required for AN or BN, but in an attenuated form. Indeed, Fairburn and Harrison [44] suggest that although most EDNOS cases resemble AN and BN in that the overevaluation of weight and shape is present, the focus in some cases is primarily on maintaining strict control over eating. However, it would appear that some atypical eating disorders of childhood onset differ qualitatively rather than quantitatively from the full-blown eating-disorder syndromes. Nicholls et al. [45] suggest that limiting the eating disorders to those for which dieting and/or purging are essential features would exclude a large number of children who have major eating difficulties. Bryant-Waugh and Lask [46] suggest that eating disorders of childhood could be conceptualised as 'a disorder of childhood in which there is an excessive preoccupation with weight or shape and/or food intake, and accompanied by grossly inadequate, irregular or chaotic food intake'. They go on to suggest syndrome-recognition guidelines more applicable to children, which have become known as the Great Ormond Street (GOS) criteria. Nicholls and colleagues [45] evaluated the reliability of the diagnostic classification systems for eating disorders when applied to children and young adolescents, and found that there were low inter-rater reliability values for both International Classification of Diseases 10 (ICD)-10 and DSM-IV criteria, while the GOS criteria proved to be much more reliable in this age group. The advantage of using the GOS criteria is that they allow for more homogeneous categories, and thus better-targeted treatment strategies [47].

Food-avoidance emotional disorder

FAED was originally thought to be a primary emotional disorder where food avoidance was a prominent feature [48]. More recently, a study investigating comorbidity in early-onset eating disorders found that only 15% of children with FAED fulfilled diagnostic criteria for an emotional disorder [49], suggesting that while there is some mood disturbance present, it is unlikely to constitute a primary affective disorder. Children with FAED present with symptoms similar to those seen in AN, in that they are usually significantly underweight and restrict their food intake. However, they do not have the same preoccupation with weight and shape, nor do they have the distorted view of their own body that is characteristic of AN. Higgs and colleagues [48] suggested that FAED may be an intermediate condition between AN and childhood emotional disorder (with no eating disorder): a partial syndrome of AN with an overall more favourable prognosis. This assertion is yet to be tested empirically.

The term 'non-fat-phobic anorexia nervosa' has been used to describe cultural variants of AN (e.g. [50]) and it is not clear at this time whether they would best be conceptualised as FAED [51].

There are no reports of the incidence, prevalence or sex ratio of FAED. However, Cooper and colleagues [15] reported that this was the most common diagnosis after AN in a consecutive series of 88 children presenting with childhood-onset eating disorder at two specialist clinics, with approximately 29% receiving a diagnosis of FAED. The ratio of girls to boys in this FAED group was 4 to 1.

Selective eating

Children who are selective eaters have typically eaten a very narrow range of foods for at least two years and are unwilling to try new foods. They do not have a distorted body image, nor the preoccupation with weight or shape characteristic of AN and BN. Growth and development in selective eaters does not appear to be affected by their eating habits, and they do not have a fear of choking or vomiting [52]. It has been suggested that selective eating may be a variant of normal eating behaviour, a stereotyped behaviour in developmental disorder or an emotional (phobic) disorder [52]. Preferred foods are often soft carbohydrate-based foods and it has been suggested that selective eaters may not have developed chewing skills or learned to use cutlery [51]. Eating is one of the areas that may be negatively affected by sensory sensitivity [53, 54] and difficulties in sensory integration may play a role in selective eating [55].

There are no reports of the incidence, prevalence or sex ratio of selective eating in the general population. However, Nicholls *et al.* [52] and Cooper *et al.* [15] both found a sex ratio of boys to girls of around 4 : 1 in recent studies, suggesting that boys are far more likely to present with selective eating than girls.

Functional dysphagia

The characteristic feature of functional dysphagia is a fear of swallowing, vomiting or choking, for which there is usually an easily identifiable precipitant, such as having choked on a piece of food, having had traumatic gastrointestinal investigations or having had experience of abuse that became associated with particular textures, tastes or types of food [25]. This makes the child anxious about and resistant to eating normally, resulting in a marked avoidance of food. These children do not have the characteristic weight and shape concerns seen in children with AN or BN. There has been very little reported about this disorder, and its incidence is unknown. Nicholls and Bryant-Waugh [51] suggest that functional dysphagia may be better considered as a symptom descriptor than a separate nosological entity, and it is found not only in isolation, but also in patients with FAED, selective eating and occasionally AN.

2.3 Comorbidity

Many studies have reported elevated rates of depressive disorders in individuals with eating disorders [56–58]. Major depression is common in those with AN, with reported lifetime prevalence rates ranging from 9.5 to 64.7% in those with restrictive AN and from 50 to 71.3% in those with AN binge–purge subtype [59]. A lifetime prevalence rate of 54% was reported for major depression in a rare study of males with eating disorders [60].

A high prevalence of anxiety disorders has been found in patients with eating disorders [56, 60–66]. Lifetime prevalence rates of at least one anxiety disorder range from 23 to 54% in those with AN and from 25 to 75% in those with BN [67]. In those with AN, social phobia has been reported to be the most common comorbid anxiety disorder [68–70]. Obsessive–compulsive disorder (OCD) has also been reported as having a high prevalence in those with AN [71, 72]. The findings in individuals with BN are more variable. For example, some studies report high prevalence rates of social phobia, simple phobia and OCD [68, 70], while others do not [73].

Few studies have investigated psychiatric comorbidity in BED, and most have been community studies [74–76]. Recently, however, a large-scale clinic study of 404 patients with BED, using semistructured diagnostic and clinical interviews to assess DSM-IV psychiatric disorders, found that almost half (43.1%) of participants had at least one current comorbid psychiatric disorder, with mood and anxiety disorders being the most common comorbid diagnoses [77]. Almost three quarters (73.8%) of participants in this study had at least one additional lifetime psychiatric disorder, with mood, anxiety and substance-use disorders being the most common comorbid lifetime psychiatric diagnoses [77].

There is some literature regarding the relationship between mood and anxiety disorders and eating disorders in children. For example, in their case series report of children with AN, Fosson and colleagues [7] suggested that about 50% of their cases were moderately to severely depressed. However, Gallelli and colleagues [78] found little depressive symptomatology in their sample of 15 children with premenarchal AN, but found that 26% of these children had a comorbid anxiety disorder. DiNicola et al. [79] have cautioned that in children, the relationship between eating and mood disorder is more complex than in the adult population, and suggested that the two types of disorder are even more likely to be intertwined. With regard to OCD, Shafran *et al.* [80] conducted a preliminary investigation into obsessive–compulsive symptoms in children with eating disorders and found that 11.5% of their sample of children with AN had obsessive–compulsive symptoms. This study is the only study to date that has looked at comorbidity in a sample of children who have a range of the childhood-onset eating disorders described above. A further study found that there were high rates of obsessive–compulsive symptoms in children and adolescents with a diagnosis of AN [81].

2.4   Epidemiology

Incidence and prevalence

The term 'incidence' refers to the number of new cases in a population in a given year, while the term 'prevalence' indicates the number of cases in a population at a given time.

Incidence

Although many studies of the incidence of AN have been conducted, different methodologies have been used and therefore published incidence rates vary widely. Some studies suggest the incidence is increasing [82–84], while others report stable rates [85–87]. The incidence rates in AN have been estimated at between 5 and 8 per 100 000 person years [88]. Meta-analyses have identified a small global increase throughout the twentieth century [89] and a stable European incidence since the 1970s [90]. Two studies that investigated new cases of AN in the UK, conducted over different time periods, using data drawn from primary care settings, reported similar rates of AN: 4.2 per 100 000 person years in 1993 [91] and 4.7 per 100 000 person years in 2000 [92]. However, Currin and colleagues [92] found that incidence rates varied enormously depending on gender. For females incidence was 8.6 per 100 000 person years and for males, 0.7 per 100 000 person years. This translates to a relative risk for females to males of 12 : 1. The highest rate, 34.6 per 100 000 person years, was found in females aged 10–19 years [92].

The incidence of eating disorders is highest in adolescents [93]. Incidence for AN is considerably higher for females aged 15–19, with reported rates in this age group ranging from 109 [94] to 270 [95] per 100 000 person years. This discrepancy in reported rates could be accounted for by the different sampling methods. The first sample was drawn from cases reported in primary care, while the latter was drawn from a community sample, suggesting that a significant number of community cases are not presenting for treatment.

With regard to AN in children and adolescents, an incidence rate of 17.5 per 100 000 person years has been reported in 10–19 year olds, and 0.3 per 100 000 person years in 0–9 year olds [91]. These figures included both males and females.

The incidence rates in BN have been estimated at between 11 and 13.5 per 100 000 person years [88]. Turnbull and colleagues [91] found that the rate for BN in UK primary care settings increased threefold between 1988 and 1993, but has since fallen [92]. More recently, the rate for BN using data from UK primary care settings was reported as 6.6 per 100 000 person years [92]. The rate for females was 12.4 per 100 000 person years and for males, 0.7 per 100 000 person years. This translated to a relative risk for females to males of 18 : 1. The highest rate, 35.8 per 100 000 person years, was found in females aged 10–19 years [92].

Prevalence

Recent large-scale, methodologically sound prevalence studies using DSM-IV criteria have found that 0.9–2.2% of women in Western countries suffer from AN during their lifetime, while prevalence rates of partial-syndrome AN (cases that fall below the diagnostic threshold) range between 2.4 and 4.3% [95–98]. All of these studies were conducted on nationally representative samples.

The prevalence rates of BN have been less well studied. Reported rates have varied between 0.1 and 1.4% for males, and between 0.3 and 9.4% of females [99]. Studies on time trends in the prevalence of BN have also yielded inconsistent results [100].

A recent review estimated the prevalence of BN to be 1% for women and 0.1% for men across Western Europe and the United States [90]. BN typically affects 1–3% of adolescent and young-adult women [90, 101].

There is a large and growing literature suggesting that BED and other forms of EDNOS are in fact much more common than AN and BN. In a recent Australian community survey [100] the prevalence for BED was 2.3% and for other EDNOS cases was 1.9%, significantly higher than the reported prevalence rates of AN (0.3%) and BN (0.9%) in the study population. A study in Portugal, which focused on females aged 12–23 years, found a prevalence of EDNOS over three times that of full-syndrome AN and BN combined – EDNOS 2.37%. 0.38% for AN and 0.30% for BN [102].

Age of onset

Epidemiological studies indicate that the peak age of onset of AN is between 15 and 19 years [103], while the median estimated age of onset of BN is 18.0 years [98]. There are no reported data for peak age of onset of EDNOS.

Mortality

A recent longitudinal study of mortality in eating disorders found that the crude mortality rates were 4.0% for AN, 3.9% for BN and 5.2% for EDNOS and that individuals with EDNOS had elevated mortality risks, similar to those found in AN [104].

Gender ratio

Eating disorders have a strong female preponderance, with an overall gender ratio of 10 : 1 [90]. This gender imbalance might be seen as a justification for research to focus on females. However, in adolescence, the female : male ratio is smaller, varying from 3 : 1 to 10 : 1 [105–107].

2.5   Aetiology and risk factors

Searching for a single cause for eating disorders is a fruitless task as they are varied, complex multifactorial disorders. It can be useful to consider aetiological factors under three broad categories: biological, psychological and sociocultural. It is also important to take into account that there are factors that are necessary preconditions for the development of an eating disorder (predisposing factors), factors that are more immediate to its emergence (precipitating factors) and factors that serve to maintain the disorder once it has arisen (perpetuating factors).

Sociocultural theories

Historically, AN has been considered as a sociocultural phenomenon [108]. Sociocultural theorists have pointed to the shift to thinness as a Western cultural norm during the twentieth century [109]. Although there does seem to be general agreement that Western cultures put pressure on women to be thin and that this contributes to the development of eating disorders [110, 111], Brumberg [112] points out that eating-disorder cases have been reported throughout medical history. Nevertheless, the possibility that sociocultural ideals may be a factor in play in the development of an eating disorder cannot be ignored. Indeed, in groups where thinness is deemed to be particularly important, for example in ballet dancers and models, there are high rates of AN [113, 114]. Children of migrant parents from non-Western cultures, where AN has not been reported, also present with eating disorders [115–117]. The emergence of eating disorders in these populations may relate to the adoption of Western values and subsequent intrapersonal and intrafamilial conflicts [24].

Many experimental studies have investigated the relationship between perceived pressure to be thin and factors associated with eating disorders. The majority have found significant relationships between perceived pressure to be thin and body dissatisfaction and dieting in adults [118], adolescents [119–122] and children [123]. However, some have not found this association [124, 125].

Groesz et al. [126], in their meta-analysis of the acute effects of media images of the thin ideal, found that such exposure resulted in immediate and significant increases in body dissatisfaction. They further reported that this effect was significantly stronger in women with an initial elevated body dissatisfaction in comparison to women who were satisfied with their bodies.

However, cross-cultural studies have yielded mixed findings. A number of studies have rejected weight and shape concerns as a defining feature of AN as high proportions of women in non-Western cultures who have been diagnosed with AN do not endorse weight or shape concerns [127–129]. Some studies have suggested that acculturation to Western values regarding weight and shape is implicated in the onset of AN. For example, Nasser [130] found that a higher proportion of Arab students in London met criteria for eating disorders than those in Cairo. Davis and Katzman [131] found that the Eating Disorder Inventory [132] scores of Chinese students living in the United States were correlated with the degree of acculturation to Western values. However, some studies disagree with this theory. For example, Haudek et al. [133] found no significant relationship between acculturation and eating-disorder psychopathology in Asian American women, and Hoek *et al.* [134] found that the prevalence rate of AN in Curacao was comparable to that in the West, despite the absence of a strong preoccupation with thinness. Thus, although cross-cultural research has been dominated by the assumption that Western values regarding thinness are responsible for the development of AN in non-Western contexts, the empirical research does not corroborate this assumption [135]. Indeed, some studies have even yielded the opposite effect: for example, Hill and Bhatti [136] found that high dietary restraint was associated with a more traditional, rather than Western, cultural orientation among pre-adolescent British Asian girls.

A recent meta-analytic review of risk factors for eating pathology highlighted the importance of factors associated with the 'dieting domain'. Family and personal history of obesity and critical comments from family members about weight, shape and eating were found to be risk factors for the development of BN, but not for the development of AN [137].

Although clearly relevant, sociocultural factors alone do not explain eating disorders, and thus it is important to consider both biological and psychological factors in order to work towards an integrated biopsychosocial understanding of aetiology.

Genetic factors

Support for genetic factors playing a role in the aetiology of eating disorders has come from a number of familial aggregation studies and twin studies.

Familial aggregation of eating disorders

There have been a number of controlled studies of the lifetime risk of eating disorder among the first-degree relatives of people with eating disorders. Some studies found no evidence of familial aggregation [138–140], but these all had methodological flaws. In the first two, the sample sizes were small, while in the third study, only the sufferers' parents were assessed.

A number of other studies have consistently found that there is a raised rate of AN and BN and their variants amongst the relatives of those who have either AN or BN. This suggests both family aggregation and a shared transmissible vulnerability to eating disorders [141–147]. For example, Strober and colleagues [145] found that the relative risks for AN were 11.3 in female relatives of those with AN and 12.3 in female relatives of those with BN. The relative risks for BN for female relatives of those with AN and BN were 4.2 and 4.4 respectively.

However, although these studies provide compelling evidence for a familial aggregation in both AN and BN, family studies do not provide evidence for a genetic transmission, and the degree to which this aggregation is accounted for by genetic versus environmental variation is unclear.

Twin studies

Twin studies have been conducted in an attempt to distinguish genetic from environmental contributions. These studies suggest heritabilities for a broad anorexia phenotype of 48–74% and for BN of 54–83% (see [148] for detailed review). A more recent twin study investigating the heritability of BED concluded that BED aggregates in families, and heritability was estimated as 57% [149].

Eating-disorder symptoms also appear to be heritable. The behavioural symptoms of dietary restraint, binge eating and self-induced vomiting have been found to have heritabilities ranging from 46 to 72% [150, 151], while the attitudinal symptoms of eating and weight concerns, weight preoccupation and body dissatisfaction have shown heritabilities of 32–72% [150, 152, 153]. More recent cross-sectional and longitudinal studies investigating the heritability of eating-disorder symptoms have identified developmental shifts in the aetiological influences across adolescence. Pre- and early adolescent twins showed lower heritability of eating-disorder symptoms when compared to twins in mid and late adolescence [154, 155]. Further studies analysing data from large-scale twin registers have suggested that puberty moderates genetic effects on eating-disorder symptoms, moving from no genetic influence in early puberty to significant genetic influence in mid- to post-puberty [156–158]. These findings help to refine hypotheses regarding regulators of genetic effects, such as ovarian hormones activating genes of potential aetiological significance during puberty [159] and potential candidate genes [160]. However, it is unclear whether the magnitude of genetic influence remains stable from late adolescence through to adulthood, as further longitudinal data are not yet available [161].

There are high levels of comorbidity between eating disorders and other psychiatric disorders and the question remains whether there is a unique genetic risk for the development of eating disorders or whether the genetic vulnerability may be shared with other disorders. Family and twin studies have found both shared and unique genetic influences on major depression and on both AN and BN [145, 147, 162–164].

Independent familial transmission of OCD and both AN and BN has been found, as well as an increased risk of obsessive–compulsive personality disorder (OCPD) in relatives of those with AN, whether or not the person with AN had comorbid OCPD [162].

Shared genetic transmission between BN and both phobia and panic disorder has also been found [165].

Neurobiology and molecular genetics

See Chapter 5 for a summary of knowledge on population and environmental genetics, followed by an overview of the findings from neurotransmitter and genetic studies exploring how abormality in brain chemistry could contribute to the development and maintenance of eating disorders.

Perinatal influences

Studies investigating perinatal influences as risk factors for the later development of eating disorders have consistently found an association. For example, Cnattingius and colleagues found that girls who were premature and small for gestational age and those born with cephalohematoma were at increased risk for developing AN [166]. These perinatal risk factors were independent of sociodemographic confounders and contributed a 3.6% risk for AN [167].

A more recent study found that several obstetric complications, including diabetes mellitus, hyporeactivity, maternal anaemia, preeclampsia, neonatal cardiac problems and placental infarction, were significant independent predictors of AN, and that the risk of developing AN increased with the total number of obstetric complications [168]. The same study found that placental infarction, early eating difficulties, neonatal hyporeactivity and a low birth weight for gestational age were significantly associated with BN. Being short for gestational age differentiated those with AN, BN and controls. The authors suggest that these obstetric complications may contribute to an impairment in neurodevelopment, which could be implicated in the pathogenesis of eating disorders [168].

Puberty

Connan and colleagues have presented a neurodevelopmental model of AN which includes consideration of both the biological changes and the psychosocial transitions faced by young people as they go through puberty. They suggest that, during puberty, the rigidity of those vulnerable to AN may be challenged by change, resulting in increased vulnerability to dysregulation in relevant biopsychosocial systems [169].

The onset of eating disorders is typically after puberty. Young people face many physical changes during pubertal development, such as a rise in the average proportion of body fat and in body weight. Girls in middle childhood have a mean proportion of body fat of 8% and this rises to 22% after puberty [170]. In addition, the period of maximum growth usually occurs between the ages of 11 and 13 years, during which time body weight rises by about 40% [170]. While boys also experience this weight gain, much of it is accounted for by an increase in muscle bulk. Both childhood obesity and early menarche, which are themselves often associated, are risk factors for the development of BN [171].

Puberty onset is also associated with profound changes in drives, motivations, psychology and social life, and these changes continue throughout adolescence. An increasing number of studies have investigated the developing brain through adolescence, although they tend to define development by chronological age rather than pubertal stage. The few neuroimaging studies that have associated brain development with pubertal stage provide tentative evidence to suggest that puberty might play an important role in some aspects of brain and cognitive development [172]. How this may pertain to the development of eating disorders is yet to be elucidated.

Psychodynamic theories

Early psychodynamic theories were based on Freud's [173] model of the mind. For example, one early theory for eating disorders was that self-starvation was a defence against the sexual fantasies of oral impregnation [174]. By the late 1950s, these early psychodynamic theories had become so widespread that upon review, Minuchin et al. [175] summarised that eating had been equated with gratification, impregnation, intercourse, performance, growing, castration, destroying, engulfing, killing and cannibalism, with food symbolising the breast, the genitals, faeces, poison, a parent or a sibling. However, as Goodsitt [176] pointed out, none of these theories accounted for the symptoms of AN, such as body-image distortion and a denial of emaciation. Nor were any of these theories conducive to empirical testing.

Palazzoli [177] suggested a developmental object-relations theory of how the infant progresses through stages in relating to her mother. She suggested that the future 'anorectic' has a confused ambivalent identification with her mother, due to unresolved problems in the oral incorporation stage of normal development, which in turn impedes the crucial stage of separation individuation. Self-starvation thus becomes an attempt by the girl with AN to end the feminisation of her body and to minimise her confused ambivalent identification with her mother. While this theory could potentially lead to testable hypotheses, no research has been conducted to date to test whether sufferers of AN confuse their bodies with those of their mothers.

Bruch [110] also suggested that the refusal to eat and fear of fatness have their roots in early mother–child interactions and proposed that food refusal represents a struggle for psychological autonomy and control [178]. She explained the symptoms of AN as a product of a failure by the mother to respond to her daughter's needs in infancy. Instead, she implied, the child becomes compliant with the mother's needs. As the child grows, she fails to develop a sense of herself as independent or entitled to take any initiative, and continues to gain maternal approval by absolute compliance. The consequence of this is a paralysing sense of ineffectiveness. The resulting lack of sense of self is aggravated by adolescence, with its demands on the individual to develop an identity separate from the parents. Bruch suggested that AN develops in this situation because, for these children, 'their own bodies become the arena for their only exercise of control' ([110], p. 58).

Family/systemic theories

Minuchin et al. [179] described the 'psychosomatic family'. They claimed that in these families, the child's 'psychosomatic symptoms' play an important role in maintaining the family's status quo and blocking change. They suggested that four key styles of interaction are characteristic of such families: enmeshment, overprotectiveness, rigidity and conflict avoidances. Strober and Humphrey [180] attempted to test these family styles of interaction experimentally. Their work showed that families with a child with AN tend to be out of touch with the child's emerging affective needs, are less than optimally expressive in the emotional domain, and may reinforce control and restraint at the expense of autonomous self-expression, but did not clearly validate the theory of a 'psychosomatic family'. Similarly, Kog et al. [181] attempted to validate this hypothesis by assessing the families of 55 female patients with AN on a number of domains related to the characteristics suggested by the model. They found that while some families appeared to be a 'close fit' to the model, others showed less extreme and even opposite kinds of family interaction. Thus the results of empirical testing of Minuchin et al.'s [179] model of the 'psychosomatic family' found no substantial support for this hypothesis. Eisler [182] points out that families in which someone has an eating disorder are a characteristically heterogeneous group. In recent years, there has been a shift away from an emphasis on a family aetiology of the eating disorder towards an understanding of the evolution of the family dynamics that may function as maintenance mechanisms in the context of the eating disorder [183, 184].

As Bryant-Waugh and Lask [24] have pointed out, more work needs to be done to clarify how much these family factors contribute to eating disorders, since not all families with communication problems include a child with AN.

Cognitive behavioural theory

Early behavioural theories of eating disorders suggested that fear of fatness and body-image disturbance were the primary motivational factors for behaviours related to restriction and compensation for weight gain associated with binge eating [23]. Garner and Bemis [185] proposed a cognitive behavioural model of AN, based on the principles of Beck's [186] cognitive theory of depression. They suggested that at some stage in the pathogenesis of the illness, causal factors converge and cause the sufferer to believe that it is absolutely essential to be thin. Maintenance of low weight and fear of loss of control over eating are then established as core beliefs, and the 'over-valued ideas' of the importance of weight and shape can account for the sufferer's behaviours. The typical behaviours associated with eating disorders, such as exercise, vomiting and using laxatives, serve as negative reinforcement to the removal of the aversive stimulus of fear of fatness [185].

Slade [187] suggested that a need for control is central to the development and maintenance of AN, and is manifested in dieting. The disorder is then perpetuated by the positive reinforcement the sufferer gets from succeeding in dieting, and the negative reinforcement gained through fear of weight gain and avoidance of other difficulties. This results in an intensification of the dieting coupled with further weight loss, which serves to maintain the disorder.

Further theories suggested that the primary motivational factors for binge eating were extreme dietary restraint [188] and escape from negative affect [189]. Cognitive theories of eating disorders suggested that there is an information-processing bias in those with eating disorders. For example, overestimation of body size is considered to be a cognitive bias that results from an easily activated (and readily accessible for retrieval from memory) self-schema that includes memory stores related to body size and eating [190–192].

Fairburn and colleagues [193] pointed out that the extreme need to control is a prominent feature of AN, and provides a solid principle that accounts for both the maintenance of the disorder and the influence of weight and shape concerns, as well as many other characteristics of the disorder, such as resistance to change and egosyntonicity. However, control over eating barely features in the theory of Garner and Bemis [185], and while control over eating is central to Slade's [187] theory, concerns about weight and shape do not play a prominent part. Thus, Fairburn and colleagues [193] proposed a cognitive behavioural theory (CBT) of the maintenance of AN, which suggests that a need for control is at the core of the disorder, but that concerns about weight and shape are an important maintaining factor.

This maintenance model proposes that attempts to restrict eating are reinforced through three main feedback mechanisms, with the result that the disorder becomes self-perpetuating. The first mechanism is that dietary restriction enhances the sense of being in control; that is, success in restricting food intake positively reinforces the sufferer's sense of being in control. The second mechanism is that aspects of starvation encourage further dietary restriction; that is, physiological and psychological changes can promote further dietary restriction by undermining the sufferer's sense of being in control. For example, increased feelings of hunger due to insufficient food intake may be perceived as a threat to the sufferer's control over eating [193]. Relevant to this theory, Fairburn and colleagues [193] suggest that the third mechanism is culturally specific and prominent in most cases seen in Western societies. It is that extreme concerns about weight and shape encourage dietary restriction; that is, failure to control body weight and shape, particularly in cultures where it is common for people to judge their self-worth in terms of weight and shape, leads to dietary restriction. The first two maintenance mechanisms could account for the heterogeneity noted in the early-onset case series [7–10], as they do not require extreme concerns about weight and shape.

This theory has a number of strengths, in that it both synthesises the views of previous theorists (Garner and Bemis [185] and Slade [187]), while also being an extension of the CBTs in that it provides a new framework and an integration of the component parts. It is also sufficiently specific to generate testable hypotheses.

More recently, Fairburn *et al.* [194] have proposed a 'transdiagnostic' theory of eating disorders. They suggest that AN, BN and EDNOS share the same distinctive psychopathology and, based on evidence from longitudinal outcome studies (e.g. [195, 196]), individuals with AN, BN and EDNOS move between diagnostic states over time. They further suggest that the maintenance of AN, BN and EDNOS in certain individuals is driven by one or more common mechanisms of 'clinical perfectionism' [197], core low self-esteem, mood intolerance and interpersonal difficulties.

Personality factors

Certain personality traits have consistently been associated with eating disorders and as such are thought to be risk factors. These personality traits are usually measured dimensionally. Correlational research suggests that AN and BN are both characterised by perfectionism, obsessive–compulsiveness, narcissism, sociotropy (concern with acceptance and approval from others) and autonomy (an orientation towards independence, control and achievement), whereas impulsivity and sensation-seeking are more typical of disorders characterised by bingeing, such as BN and BED [198].

Perfectionism is characterised by the tendency to set and pursue unrealistically high standards, despite the occurrence of adverse consequences (e.g. food and weight preoccupation, persistent hunger) [197]. Collectively, findings suggest that perfectionism may predict the onset of AN symptoms [199] and that it is a salient correlate of AN [200], BN [201, 202] and BED [202] in acutely ill women as well as after eating-disorder recovery [200, 201, 203–206]. However, certain elements of perfectionism, such as socially prescribed perfectionism, may diminish with eating-disorder remission [203]. While findings consistently support the association between perfectionism and eating disorders, it is uncertain whether perfectionism is associated specifically with disordered eating, or more generally with maladjustment [207].

Obsessive–compulsive traits, including doubting, checking and need for symmetry and exactness, have been associated with eating disorders [208, 209], are more common among individuals with eating disorders than psychiatric control groups [210] and persist after recovery from AN [204] and BN [211].

Impulsivity is characterised by a lack of forethought and a failure to contemplate risks and consequences before acting. Studies examining impulsivity in individuals with AN (restricting subtype) suggest that they are less impulsive than nonpsychiatric controls [212, 213]. In contrast, those with BN are more impulsive than individuals with AN (restricting subtype) and nonpsychiatric controls [209, 212, 214].

Sensation-seeking is characterised by a willingness to take physical and social risks in order to seek out varied, novel and complex sensations and experiences. Individuals with AN (binge–purge subtype), BN and BED usually score higher on measures of sensation-seeking than individuals with AN (restricting subtype) and controls [215, 216]. Individuals with AN (restricting subtype) score lower than community controls [215] but similar to psychiatric controls [216] on measures of sensation-seeking.

There have been few studies of narcissism in eating disorders. Narcissism is reported to be more characteristic of individuals with AN or BN than those with other psychiatric disturbances (anxiety, affective and adjustment disorders), suggesting that it may be a unique risk factor for eating disorders [216]. In addition, narcissism may persist after remission from BN, suggesting that it may be a trait characteristic [217].

Narduzzi and Jackson [218] suggest that eating disorders are associated with both sociotropy and autonomy in clinical samples. Heightened vulnerability for an eating disorder may be associated with a sociotropy–autonomy conflict in which individuals with eating disorders strive to maintain independence, but also rely on interpersonal relationships for validation and self-esteem [218].

Personality disorders are more common in patients with eating disorders than in patients with other axis 1 disorders [219]. In a recent meta-analysis of prevalence rates in adults diagnosed with eating disorders, avoidant personality disorder was found to be one of the most common personality disorders reported across all eating-disorder diagnoses. OCPD is one of the most common among adults with AN (restricting subtype) and adults with BED, dependent personality disorder is common among adults with AN (restricting subtype) and adults with BN, and borderline personality disorder is one of the most common among adults who engage in binge eating [198].

A major limitation of the research into the role of personality in the aetiology of eating disorders is the question of whether personality factors are causal, or whether they are correlates or consequences. Vitousek and Stumpf [220] have highlighted the possible transient effects of starvation or repeated binge–purge cycles on psychopathology, while Lilenfeld and colleagues [201] suggest that the personality traits of obsessionality and rigidity may be a result of, or exacerbated by, starvation. However, these traits persist after recovery from an eating disorder, which supports the idea that they may be predisposing risk factors for eating disorders [204]. Studies have found that personality-disorder symptoms often improve in tandem with an improvement in eating-disorder symptoms, which suggests that personality-disorder symptoms may not be causal factors of an eating disorder, but rather correlates or consequences of an eating disorder [221, 222]. However, personality-disorder diagnoses persist in some recovered individuals, particularly those with a history of AN (binge–purge subtype) [223].

In summary, both AN and BN are characterised by perfectionism, obsessive–compulsiveness, neuroticism, negative emotionality, harm-avoidance, low self-directedness, low cooperativeness and traits associated with avoidant personality disorder. However, further traits seen in AN (restricting subtype) (including high constraint and persistence and low novelty-seeking) and in BN (including high impulsivity, sensation-seeking and novelty-seeking) may influence symptomatic expression in eating disorders. It may be that high constraint and persistence predispose to dietary restriction while high impulsivity, sensation-seeking and novelty-seeking predispose to bingeing and purging behaviours [198].

2.6   Treatment

Adults

Anorexia nervosa

The evidence base for psychological therapies for AN is sparse and there have been only a limited number of randomised controlled trials (RCTs) of treatment, which are considered to be the gold standard for testing the efficacy or effectiveness of interventions. Patients with AN are hard to engage in treatment and motivational enhancement work can help them to complete a course of treatment [224]. In the UK, NICE (the National Institute for Health and Clinical Excellence) produces guidelines for the most appropriate treatment regimens for different illnesses [225]. These guidelines have been published following assessment of evidence-based treatments for the illness in question. The NICE guidelines suggest a range of psychological therapies for adults with AN, which include CBT, interpersonal psychotherapy (IPT), cognitive analytic therapy (CAT) and focal psychodynamic psychotherapy. For children and adolescents with AN, NICE recommends family interventions that directly target the eating disorder.

RCTs exploring the efficacy and effectiveness of treatment for AN show mixed results. For example, CBT has been found to offer better outcomes and longer time to relapse when compared to nutritional counselling. However, this finding appears not to apply to those patients who are acutely underweight [226]. In a further study, specialist supportive clinical management has been found to be more effective in the acute phase of illness than both CBT and IPT [227]. Another RCT compared three psychological therapies (CAT, focal psychoanalytic psychotherapy and family therapy) with a control condition of low-contact routine treatment. There was symptomatic reduction across the board, although more than two thirds of patients remained significantly underweight at the end of the treatment phase of the study. Nevertheless, the psychological therapies (as opposed to the control treatment) were more effective in producing weight gain, restoring the menstrual cycle and reducing bulimic symptoms [228].

An exciting advance in the treatment of AN, cognitive remediation therapy (CRT), developed by Tchanturia and colleagues, is discussed in more detail in Chapter 9.

Bulimia nervosa

The NICE guidelines [225] suggest that an evidence-based guided self-help (GSH) can be considered as a possible first step for treating BN. CBT specifically adapted for BN (CBT-BN) or IPT are recommended as face-to-face interventions and the guidelines add that if patients do not respond to or want CBT, other psychological therapies should be considered.

Due to their cost-effectiveness, self-help formats of treatment are appealing. Cooper and colleagues [229] conducted a small GSH treatment trial and found that at the end of the intervention, half the patients had stopped bingeing and vomiting, while most of the remainder had made significant improvements. Bara-Carril and colleagues [230] pointed out that it can be difficult for those with BN to access evidence-based treatments and thus investigated the feasibility and efficacy of a CD-ROM-based cognitive behavioural multimedia self-help intervention for the treatment of BN. They found that participants reported significant reductions in bingeing and compensatory behaviours. A further study investigated the efficacy of self-help based on CBT in combination with Internet support to treat BN and BED, and found that 46% of treatment completers were free of binge eating and purging at the end of treatment. This was maintained at six-month follow-up [231].

However, assessing the efficacy of self-help approaches in general is complicated by the wide variety of formats and delivery methods. For example, studies have compared GSH with group CBT [232], nonspecific self-help with CBT-based self-help [233], physician-based self-help with specialist self-help [234], and GSH with CBT [235]. This makes it very difficult to compare results and come to any conclusions about the efficacy of self-help approaches to treatment.

A comparison of CBT and IPT found that CBT produces greater decreases in binge eating, vomiting and restraint, coupled with a significantly greater probability of remission [236]. A further study also found greater decreases in vomiting and restraint in those receiving CBT than those receiving IPT, although these differences disappeared at one-year follow-up [237]. When delivered in a group format, CBT and IPT produced comparable results, and both interventions were superior to a waiting-list control condition in terms of a reduction in both the cognitive and behavioural symptoms of BN [238]. CBT has been found to be superior to nutritional counselling alone in reducing binge eating, vomiting, laxative use and body dissatisfaction [239]. On balance, although IPT produces similar results to CBT for BN at follow-up, symptomatic change appears to be more rapid with CBT [236, 237].

A randomised trial investigated whether a higher level of individualisation increased treatment efficacy in BN and found that more individualised CBT guided by logical functional analysis was slightly superior to manual-based CBT, with clinically significant differences found in eating concerns, body-shape dissatisfaction and abstinence from objective bulimic episodes [240].

In their meta-analysis of psychotherapy for BN, Thompson-Brenner and colleagues [241] found that only about 50% of patients make a complete recovery from BN.

EDNOS

Despite representing the largest proportion of patients with eating disorders, little treatment research has been conducted in this patient group, with the exception of studies investigating the effectiveness of treatments for BED, although those with BED make up less than half of those with EDNOS [242].

Much of the treatment research on BED has focused on CBT, although one treatment trial used dialectical behaviour therapy (DBT). Compared to waiting-list control subjects, patients who received CBT showed significant reductions in body mass index (BMI), the number of days that a binge occurred, disinhibition, hunger, depression and self-esteem, and they were more likely to be abstinent from binge eating at the end of treatment [243]. Compared to waiting-list control subjects, DBT led to greater reduction in binge episodes and in weight, shape and eating concerns, although no differences were observed between the two groups with regard to weight loss, depression or anxiety [244]. A comparison of CBT and IPT for BED, both delivered in a group format, found very little difference in the outcomes for patients in either group [245].

A study that compared self-help using a book (delivered with or without the help of a facilitator) with a waiting-list control condition found that both self-help approaches led to greater reductions in the mean number of days that a binge occurred and improvements in scores on the Eating Disorder Examination [246, 247]. Another self-help study comparing three methods of intervention delivery with a waiting-list control condition found that patients using self-help modalities in any of the three formats did better than control participants in reducing number of binge episodes and showed improvements in eating attitudes [248]. A further study by the same research group reported similar findings [249].

However, there are a number of methodological limitations in the literature pertaining to BED. A focus on reporting reduction of binge days and episodes does not give the full picture with regard to outcome. Small sample sizes and high drop-out rates, coupled with a rarity in performing intent-to-treat analyses to offset bias from differential drop-out across groups, mean that the strength of the research evidence for psychological interventions in BED remains only fair to moderate.

Transdiagnostic approach

More recently, Fairburn and colleagues [250, 251] developed an enhanced version of CBT for eating disorders (CBT-E). There are two forms of CBT-E: a focused form (CBT-Ef) that targets eating-disorder psychopathology and a broader form (CBT-Eb) that additionally targets common difficulties that appear to maintain eating disorders or complicate treatment – namely, mood intolerance, clinical perfectionism, low self-esteem and interpersonal difficulties [250]. The first study to investigate the efficacy of this treatment involved both patients with EDNOS and those with BN. A reduction in eating-disorder symptoms was observed following 20 weeks of treatment, and at 60-week follow-up, 51.3% of the sample had a level of eating-disorder features less than one standard deviation above the community mean. Diagnosis was not found to be a moderator of outcome either at end of treatment or at follow-up. However, over 40% of those eligible to participate in this study did not take part, and it is therefore unknown whether those patients would have responded to this treatment.

Children and adolescents

Anorexia nervosa

While the evidence base for treatment of children and adolescents with AN is strongest for family interventions, this is still somewhat limited. Five controlled trials for adolescent AN have been conducted, all of which involved family-based treatments. The first of these studies found that family therapy achieved better outcomes than individual therapy on measures of BMI and the Morgan Russell outcome scales [252]. Further family therapy was significantly more effective than individual therapy at follow-up, even after five years. Those who had received family therapy continued to do well while those who had received individual therapy were less likely to have made a full recovery [18]. However, while an improvement was reported in those with a short duration of illness, treatment was not effective for adolescents with longer duration. Indeed, at five-year follow-up, Eisler and colleagues [18] suggested that much of the improvement found could be attributed to the natural outcome of the illness. LeGrange and colleagues [253] compared two forms of family intervention: whole-family therapy, drawing on the models of Minuchin and Palazzoli, and a separated family intervention that offered support to the patient and guidance to the parents. The end-of-treatment effects of the two interventions were similar.

Robin and colleagues [254] compared behavioural family systems therapy (BFST) and ego-orientated individual therapy (EOIT). Both therapies were effective with relatively little difference at one-year follow-up, although the family intervention resulted in significantly greater weight gain and greater change in maternal positive and negative communication.

In a further study [255], adolescents with AN were randomly assigned to conjoint family therapy (CFT) or to separated family therapy (SFT). Considerable improvement in nutritional and psychological state occurred across both treatment groups. On global measure of outcome, the two forms of therapy were associated with equivalent end-of-treatment results. However, the participants in this study had a short history of AN and only 15 of 40 achieved what they described as their good outcome. Specifically, at the termination of treatment, patients with a 'good' outcome achieved only 87% of normal weight, and only 44% of the post-pubertal girls were menstruating. To illustrate the difficulty in treating seriously ill patients, 8 of 11 patients who had any previous treatment had a poor outcome. Moreover, the longer the patients had been ill, or the more emaciated they were, the less likely they were to improve. It is also quite striking that the improvements in the symptoms of AN among all the patients were accompanied by a significant increase in the symptoms of BN.

More recently, Lock and colleagues [256] compared short-term and longer-term courses of family therapy and reported improvements in both groups on outcome measures of AN. However, 20% dropped out of the study, which means that less than half of the participants improved substantially. In 2006, Lock and colleagues [256] reported the long-term outcome of these interventions. The results, however, are difficult to interpret because 67% of the patients had received psychological treatment during the period between the family therapy and the follow-up assessment, 53% had received medications and 15% had been hospitalised. Thus, while the patients may have been in partial remission from AN, their condition seems to have worsened in other respects. For example, at the time of admission, 14% received medication, but this number had increased to 35% at the time of follow-up. To describe the condition of the patients who had been treated with family therapy, Lock and colleagues [257] wrote 'even for those who do remit ... a substantial proportion have long-standing psychiatric disorders other than AN that will likely complicate their long-term prognosis in terms of overall mental health'.

While these studies provide the best evidence to date for the treatment of AN in adolescents, the sample sizes are very low, with two studies having only 18 and 21 participants [253, 254]. In addition, the mean age of the study participants ranges from 14.2 to 16.6 years, which means that the evidence base is for adolescents rather than for children.

Bulimia nervosa

Two studies have compared family-based therapy with individual interventions in adolescents with BN. Schmidt and colleagues [258] compared family therapy and CBT-guided self-care and found that CBT-guided self-care was superior in reduction of binge-eating behaviour. LeGrange and colleagues [259] compared family-based therapy and supportive psychotherapy (SPT) and found significantly greater early reductions in symptomatic behaviour for patients in family-based therapy. In addition, significantly more patients in family-based therapy remitted at end of treatment and at follow-up.

Limitations in the quality of the evidence base in child and adolescent eating disorders

Greater effort is needed in the field to improve the quality of treatment studies conducted in child and adolescent patients with eating disorders. Only two of the studies discussed above [256, 258] could be considered to be of the quality needed to provide a solid evidence base.

Studies have also been hampered by the use of nonmanualised treatments, less than state-of-the art diagnostic methods, poor description of inclusion and exclusion criteria, and incomplete reporting of data and analyses. While additional and larger clinical trials are currently being undertaken, they are exclusively studying AN and BN, and tend to focus on adolescents. One problem in evaluating treatment efficacy in children is the low base rate of DSM-IV AN and BN in children. Current eating-disorder definitions in both DSM and ICD classification systems fail to capture the majority of eating disorders that appear in children [45]. Much of this is because of the restriction of eating disorder 'types' to those that occur predominantly in late-adolescent and young-adult women. Thus, many diagnostic criteria are either inappropriate for prepubescent children, such as secondary amenorrhoea, or difficult to assess in children, such as the undue influence of weight or shape on self-evaluation. Nicholls and colleagues [45] recommended expansion of the classification to include syndromes that may be unique to children. These conditions include FAED, selective eating, functional dysphagia and pervasive refusal syndrome. There have been no controlled treatment studies of these conditions, which brings to mind the adage 'we study what we define' [260], and this may have a particularly deleterious effect on developing evidence-based treatments for eating disorders in children and adolescents.

Many controlled treatment studies exclude boys from participation, and boys represent a small proportion of patients in remaining studies. In contrast to their representation in controlled eating-disorder treatment studies, males comprise 10–15% of individuals who suffer from eating disorders [30], with some evidence that the male-to-female ratio may be higher in children [51]. However, the lower base rate of eating disorders in boys makes it difficult to recruit adequate numbers to establish gender differences in treatment efficacy. Because eating-disorder interventions have been designed, refined and tested predominantly in females, it remains unclear whether these treatments are useful in treating boys with eating disorders.

Most controlled treatment studies in adolescents provide no information concerning the ethnic/racial diversity of participants. In the studies that do describe ethnic/racial background, ethnic minority representation appears to be a function of the geographic locations in which research has been conducted, and analyses of differential treatment completion or response are not presented. Thus, the question of whether ethnicity/race serves as a moderator variable cannot be answered.

What about other treatment modalities? We risk ignoring potentially useful treatments in child and adolescent eating disorders by following only one line of enquiry: namely, family-based interventions. While the importance of family-based interventions cannot be ignored, it may be that individual or group therapies bring added value to the treatment of children and adolescents with eating disorders. CBT, DBT, IPT, psychodynamic psychotherapy, SPT, narrative therapy and acceptance and commitment therapy have all been used with adults with eating disorders. While there are varying levels of evidence for these therapies in adults, there is little or no evidence that they are effective in children and adolescents. We should not ignore the possibility that they may play a part in treating early-onset eating disorders, but we cannot simply extrapolate from the adult literature without considering developmental issues.

Future studies of treatment in eating disorders would benefit from examining the child and young-adolescent populations, increasing the ethnic and racial diversity of patient groups, including greater numbers of male patients, and investigating treatments for the full range of eating disorders that occur in the younger age group. Few studies examine the efficacy of treatments for individuals who fall outside the narrow diagnostic criteria set by various editions of the DSM. The majority of adolescents who suffer from clinically significant eating disorders do not fit the DSM categories; this is likely to explain the small number of studies of younger patients as well as the small sample sizes in the few studies that do exist.

In summary, the evidence base for psychosocial treatments for eating problems in children and adolescents is quite limited. As a consequence of the small number of studies and methodological limitations in existing studies, it is not possible to describe what treatments work for whom. Based on existing trends in treating AN in adolescent patients, family-based approaches represent a promising avenue for future treatment studies of other eating problems in children and adolescents.

2.7   Course and outcome

It is often difficult to generalise findings from studies of outcome of eating disorders as there is wide variation in the outcome parameters used across studies, and the following data should be considered in this context.

Keel and Brown [261] conducted a recent review on the course and outcome of eating disorders, focusing on studies conducted over the last five years. In general, they found that remission rates increased with longer duration of follow-up for all diagnoses.

Support for this assertion comes from a study of adolescents which found that remission from AN increased from 68 to 84% between 8- and 16-year follow-up [262]. Remission rates in AN also appear to vary depending on where the sample was drawn from. For example, relatively high rates of remission have been found in adolescent patients treated in the community at five-year follow-up (76%) and eight-year follow-up (82%), while relatively low rates of remission (29 and 48%) have been found for adult in-patient samples [263].

For BN, remission ranged from 27% at 1 year to 70% or more by 10 years [232, 264–266]. Rates of remission for BN do not appear to vary depending on where the sample was drawn from. For example, there appear to be no differences between rates of remission for adults and adolescents or for in-patients and those treated in the community. Remission rates for BN remain stable at around 70% or higher in samples followed up between 5 and 20 years after baseline assessment [261].

Remission rates at one-year follow-up for BED are generally higher than for AN and BN, and ranged from 25% [267] to 80% [268], while one study reported a remission rate at four-year follow-up of 82% [269].

Several outcome studies of EDNOS have looked at remission in the context of bulimic-type symptoms and have compared the outcome of those with EDNOS to those with BN. Remission rates for those with EDNOS appear to be consistently higher (67–69%) than for those with BN (28–37%) in studies of follow-up of less than five years in both adults [270] and adolescents [264]. However, remission rates for EDNOS and BN do not differ significantly at five-year follow-up, with both having remission rates of about 75% [271]. Similar rates of remission are found in EDNOS (75%) and BN (72%) at 20-year follow-up [266].

Those with AN who do not achieve remission over the course of follow-up often develop either BN or EDNOS. However, those with BN who do not achieve remission over the course of follow-up usually continue to meet full criteria for BN or transition to a diagnosis of EDNOS, including BED, and crossover to AN from BN is particularly rare [261].

2.8 Conclusion

This chapter has given a broad overview of the eating disorders, including clinical descriptions, comorbidity, epidemiology, aetiology and risk factors, psychological theories, treatment, and course and outcome, for both adult and child/adolescent eating disorders.

References

1. Bryant-Waugh, R. (2000) Overview, in *Anorexia Nervosa and Related Eating Disorders in Childhood and Adolescence* (eds B. Lask and R. Bryant-Waugh), Psychology Press, Hove.
2. Andersen, A. and Holman, J. (1997) Males with eating disorders: challenges for treatment and research. *Psychopharmacology Bulletin*, **33**, 391–397.
3. Bryant-Waugh, R. and Lask, B. (1995) Annotation: eating disorders in children. *Journal of Child Psychology and Psychiatry*, **36**, 191–202.
4. Fichter, M.M. and Daser, C. (1987) Symptomatology, psychosexual development and gender identity in 42 anorexic males. *Psychological Medicine*, **17**, 409–418.
5. Vandereycken, W. and Van den Brouke, S. (1984) Anorexia nervosa in males: a comparison study of 107 cases reported in the literature. *Acta Psychiatrica Scandinavica*, **70**, 447–454.

6. Gowers, S.G. and Crisp, A.H. (1990) Anorexia nervosa in an 80-year-old woman. *The British Journal of Psychiatry*, **157**, 754–757.
7. Fosson, A., Knibbs, J., Bryant-Waugh, R. and Lask, B. (1987) Early onset anorexia nervosa. *Archives of Disease in Childhood*, **621**, 114–118.
8. Gowers, S.G., Crisp, A.H., Joughin, N. and Bhat, A. (1991) Premenarcheal anorexia nervosa. *Journl of Child Psychology and Psychiatry*, **32**, 515–524.
9. Irwin, M. (1984) Early onset anorexia nervosa. *Southern Medical Journal*, **77**, 611–614.
10. Jacobs, B.W. and Isaacs, S. (1986) Pre-pubertal anorexia nervosa: a retrospective controlled study. *Journal of Child Psychology and Psychiatry*, **27**, 237–250.
11. American Psychiatric Association (1994) *Diagnostic and Statistical Manual of Mental Disorders (DSM-IV)*, 4th edn revised, American Psychiatric Association, Washington, DC.
12. World Health Organization (1992) The ICD-10 Classification of Mental and Behavioural Disorders: Clinical Descriptions and Diagnostic Guidelines, Author, Geneva.
13. Watson, T.L. and Andersen, A.E. (2003) A critical examination of the amenorrhea and weight criteria for diagnosing anorexia nervosa. *Acta Psychiatrica Scandinavica*, **108**, 175–182.
14. Gendall, K.A., Joyce, P.R., Carter, F.A. *et al.* (2006) The psychobiology and diagnostic significance of amenorrhea in patients with anorexia nervosa. *Fertility and Sterility*, **85**, 1531–1535.
15. Cooper, P.J., Watkins, B., Bryant-Waugh, R. and Lask, B. (2002) The nosological status of early onset anorexia nervosa. *Psychological Medicine*, **32**, 873–880.
16. Irwin, M. (1981) Diagnosis of anorexia nervosa in children and the validity of DSM-III. *American Journal of Psychiatry*, **138**, 1382–1383.
17. Rome, E.S., Ammerman, S., Rosen, D.S. *et al.* (2003) Children and adolescents with eating disorders: the state of the art. *Pediatrics*, **111**, e98–e108.
18. Eisler, I., Dare, C., Russell, G. *et al.* (1997) Family and individual therapy in anorexia nervosa. A 5-year follow-up. *Archives of General Psychiatry*, **54**, 1025–1030.
19. Matsumoto, H., Takei, N., Kawai, M. *et al.* (2001) Differences of symptoms and standardized weight index between patients with early onset and late onset anorexia nervosa. *Acta Psychiatrica Scandanavica*, **104**, 66–71.
20. Russell, G.F.M. (1985) Premanarchal anorexia nervosa and its sequelae. *Journal of Psychiatric Research*, **19**, 363–369.
21. Tanner, J.M. (1962) *Growth at Adolescence*, Blackwell Scientific Publications, Oxford.
22. Arnow, B., Sanders, M.J. and Steiner, H. (1999) Premenarcheal versus postmenarcheal anorexia nervosa: a comparative study. *Clinical Child Psychology and Psychiatry*, **4**, 403–414.
23. Russell, G. (1979) Bulimia nervosa: an ominous variant of anorexia nervosa. *Psychological Medicine*, **9**, 429–448.
24. Bryant-Waugh, R. and Lask, B. (1995) Eating disorders in children. *Journal of Child Psychology and Psychiatry*, **36**, 191–202.
25. Bryant-Waugh, R. and Lask, B. (2007) Overview of the eating disorders, in *Early Onset Eating Disorders* (eds B. Lask and R. Bryant-Waugh), John Wiley & Sons, Ltd, London.
26. Crow, S.J., Agras, W.S., Halmi, K. *et al.* (2002) Full syndromal versus subthreshold anorexia nervosa, bulimia nervosa, and binge eating disorder: a multicenter study. *International Journal of Eating Disorders*, **32**, 309–318.
27. Waller, G. (1993) Why do we diagnose different types of eating disorder? Arguments for a change in research and clinical practice. *Eating Disorders Review*, **1**, 74–89.
28. Walsh, B.T. and Garner, D.M. (1997) Diagnostic issues, in *Handbook of Treatment for Eating Disorders*, 2nd edn (eds D.M. Garner and P.E. Garfinkel), Guilford Press, New York, pp. 25–33.

29. Fairburn, C.G. and Bohn, K. (2005) Eating disorder NOS (EDNOS): an example of the troublesome 'not otherwise specified' (NOS) category in DSM-IV. *Behaviour Research and Therapy*, **43**, 691–701.

30. American Psychiatric Association (2000) *Diagnostic and Statistical Manual of Mental Disorders*, 4th edn, text revision. American Psychiatric Association, Washington, DC.

31. Latner, J.D. and Clyne, C. (2008) The diagnostic validity of the criteria for binge eating disorder. *International Journal of Eating Disorders*, **41**, 1–14.

32. Wilfley, D.E., Bishop, M.E., Wilson, G.T. and Agras, W.S. (2007) Classification of eating disorders: toward DSM-V. *International Journal of Eating Disorders Special Issue on Diagnosis and Classification*, **40**, S123–S129.

33. Wonderlich, S.A., Gordon, K.H., Mitchell, J.E. *et al.* (2009) The validity and clinical utility of binge eating disorder. *International Journal of Eating Disorders*, **42**, 687–705.

34. Masheb, R.M. and Grilo, C.M. (2000) Binge eating disorder: a need for additional diagnostic criteria. *Comprehnsive Psychiatry*, **41**, 159–162.

35. Striegel-Moore, R.H., Cachelin, F.M., Dohm, F.A. *et al.* (2001) Comparison of binge eating disorder and bulimia nervosa in a community sample. *International Journal of Eating Disorders*, **29**, 157–165.

36. Striegel-Moore, R.H., Dohm, F.A., Kraemer, H.C. *et al.* (2003) Eating disorders in white and black women. *American Journal of Psychiatry*, **160**, 1326–1331.

37. Striegel-Moore, R.H., Wilfley, D.E., Pike, K.M. *et al.* (2000) Recurrent binge eating in black American women. *Archives of Family Medicine*, **9**, 83–87.

38. Wilfley, D.E., Schwartz, M.B., Spurrell, E.B. and Fairburn, C.G. (1997) Assessing the specific psychopathology of binge eating disorder patients: interview or self-report? *Behaviour Research and Therapy*, **35**, 1151–1159.

39. Grilo, C.M., Hrabosky, J.I., White, M.A. *et al.* (2008) Overvaluation of shape and weight in binge eating disorder and overweight controls: refinement of BED as a diagnostic construct. *Journal of Abnormal Psychology*, **117**, 414–419.

40. Grilo, C.M., Masheb, R.M. and White, M.A. (2010) Significance of overevaluation of shape/weight in binge-eating disorder: comparative study with overweight and bulimia nervosa. *Obesity*, **18**, 499–504.

41. Hrabosky, J.I., Masheb, R.M., White, M.A. and Grilo, C.M. (2007) Overvaluation of shape and weight in binge eating disorder. *Journal of Consulting and Clinical Psychology*, **75**, 175–180.

42. Mond, J., Hay, P.J., Rodgers, B. and Owen, C. (2007) Recurrent binge eating with and without the 'undue influence of weight or shape on self-evaluationr': implications for the diagnosis of binge eating disorder. *Behavior Research and Therapy*, **45**, 929–938.

43. Goldschmidt, A.B., Hilbert, A., Manwaring, J.L. *et al.* (2010) The significance of overevaluation of weight and shape in binge eating disorder. *Behavior Research and Therapy*, **48**, 187–193.

44. Fairburn, C.G. and Harrison, P.J. (2003) Eating disorders. *The Lancet*, **361**, 407–416.

45. Nicholls, D., Chater, R. and Lask, B. (2000) Children into the DSM don't go: a comparison of classification systems for eating disorders in childhood and early adolescence. *International Journal of Eating Disorders*, **28**, 317–324.

46. Bryant-Waugh, R. and Lask, B. (2000) Overview of the eating disorders, in *Early Onset Eating Disorders* (eds B. Lask and R. Bryant-Waugh), John Wiley & Sons, Ltd, London.

47. Rosen, D.S. (2003) Eating disorders in children and young adolescents: etiology, classification, clinical features and treatment. *Adolescent Medicine*, **14**, 49–59.

48. Higgs, J.F., Goodyer, I.M. and Birch, J. (1989) Anorexia nervosa and food avoidance emotional disorder. *Archives of Disease in Childhood*, **64**, 346–351.

49. Watkins, B., Cooper, P., Lask, B. and Bryant-Waugh, R. (2003) Co-morbidity in early onset eating disturbance. Paper presented at the Eating Disorders Research Society 9th Annual Meeting, Ravello, Italy.

50. Tareen, A., Hodes, M. and Rangel, L. (2005) Non-fat-phobic anorexia nervosa in British South Asian adolescents. *International Journal of Eating Disorders*, **37**, 161–165.

51. Nicholls, D. and Bryant-Waugh, R. (2009) Eating disorders of infancy and childhood: definition, symptomatology, epidemiology, and comorbidity. *Child and Adolescent Psychiatric Clinics of North America*, **18**, 17–30.

52. Nicholls, D., Christie, D., Randall, L. and Lask, B. (2001) Selective eating: symptom, disorder or normal variant? *Clinical Child Psychology and Psychiatry*, **6**, 257–270.

53. Ayres, J. (1979) *Sensory Integration and the Child*, Western Psychological Services.

54. Dunn, W. (2007) Supporting children to participate successfully in every day life by using sensory processing knowledge. *Infants and young Children*, **20**, 84–101.

55. Cermak, S., Curtin, C. and Bandini, L.G. (2010) Food selectivity and sensory sensitivity in children with autism spectrum disorders. *Journal of the American Dietetic Association*, **110**, 238–246.

56. Blinder, B.J., Cumella, E.J. and Sanathara, V.A. (2006) Psychiatric comorbidities of female inpatients with eating disorders. *American Psychosomatic Society*, **68**, 454–462.

57. Courbasson, C.M.A., Smith, P.D. and Cleland, P.A. (2005) Substance use disorders, anorexia, bulimia and concurrent disorders. *Canadian Journal of Public Health*, **96**, 102–106.

58. Geist, R., Davis, R. and Heinmaa, M. (1998) Binge/purge symptoms and comorbidity in adolescents with eating disorders. *Canadian Journal of Psychiatry*, **43**, 507–512.

59. Godart, N., Perdereau, F., Rein, Z. *et al.* (2007) Comorbidity studies of eating disorders and mood disorders. Critical review of the literature. *Journal of Affective Disorders*, **97**, 37–49.

60. Carlat, D.J., Camargo, C.A. Jr and Herzog, D.B. (1997) Eating disorders in males: a report on 135 patients. *American Journal of Psychiatry*, **154**, 1127–1132.

61. Godart, N.T., Flament, M.F., Curt, F. *et al.* (2003) Anxiety disorders in subjects seeking treatment for eating disorders: a DSM-IV controlled study. *Psychiatry Research*, **117**, 245–258.

62. Hinrichsen, H., Wright, F., Waller, G. and Meyer, C. (2003) Social anxiety and coping strategies in eating disorders. *Eating Behaviours*, **4**, 117–126.

63. Hinrichsen, H., Waller, G. and van Gerko, K. (2004) Social anxiety and agoraphobia in the eating disorders: associations with eating attitudes and behaviours. *Eating Behaviors*, **5**, 285–290.

64. Iwasaki, Y., Matsunaga, H., Kiriike, N. *et al.* (2000) Comorbidity of axis I disorders among eating-disordered subjects in Japan. *Comprehensive Psychiatry*, **41**, 454–460.

65. Milos, G., Spindler, A., Schnyder, U. *et al.* (2004) Incidence of severe anorexia nervosa in Switzerland: 40 years of development. *International Journal of Eating Disorders*, **35**, 250–258.

66. Wonderlich, S.A. and Mitchell, J.E. (1997) Eating disorders and comorbidity: empirical, conceptual and clinical implications. *Psychopharmacology Bulletin*, **33**, 381–390.

67. Godart, N.T., Flament, M.F., Perdereau, F. and Jeammet, P. (2002) Comorbidity between eating disorders and anxiety disorders: a review. *International Journal of Eating Disorders*, **32**, 253–270.

68. Fornari, V., Kaplan, M., Sandberg, D.E. *et al.* (1992) Depressive and anxiety disorders in anorexia nervosa and bulimia nervosa. *International Journal of Eating Disorders*, **12**, 21–29.

69. Jordan, J., Joyce, P.R., Carter, F.A. *et al.* (2008) Specific and nonspecific comorbidity in anorexia nervosa. *International Journal of Eating Disorders*, **41**, 47–56.

70. Laessle, R.G., Wittchen, H.U., Fichter, M.M. and Pirke, K.M. (1989) The significance of subgroups of bulimia and anorexia nervosa: lifetime frequency of psychiatric disorders. *International Journal Eating Disorders*, **8**, 569–574.

71. Kaye, W.H., Bulik, C.M., Thornton, L. *et al.* (2004) Comorbidity of anxiety disorders with anorexia and bulimia nervosa. *American Journal of Psychiatry*, **161**, 2215–2221.

72. Thornton, C. and Russell, J. (1997) Obsessive compulsive comorbidity in the eating disorders. *International Journal of Eating Disorders*, **21**, 81–87.

73. Brewerton, T.D., Lydiard, R.B., Herzog, D.B. *et al.* (1995) Comorbidity of axis I psychiatric disorders in bulimia nervosa. *Journal of Clinical Psychiatry*, **56**, 77–80.

74. Dansky, B.S., Brewerton, T.D., O'Neil, P.M. and Kilpatrick, D.G. (1998) The nature and prevalence of binge eating disorder in a national sample of women, in *DSM-IV Sourcebook*, vol. **IV** (eds T.A. Widiger, A.J. Frances, H.A. Pincus *et al.*), American Psychiatric Association, Washington, DC, pp. 515–531.

75. Grucza, R.A., Przybeck, T.R. and Cloninger, C.R. (2007) Prevalence and correlates of binge eating disorder in a community sample. *Comprehensive Psychiatry*, **48**, 124–131.

76. Telch, C. and Stice, E. (1998) Psychiatric comorbidity in a non-clinical sample of women with binge eating disorder. *Journal of Consulting and Clinical Psychology*, **66**, 768–776.

77. Grilo, C., White, M. and Masheb, R. (2009) DSM-IV psychiatric disorder co-morbidity and its correlates in binge eating disorder. *International Journal of Eating Disorders*, **42**, 228–234.

78. Gallelli, K., Solanto, M., Hertz, S. and Golden, N. (1997) Eating-related and comorbid symptoms in premenarchal anorexia nervosa. *Eating Disorders: The Journal of Treatment and Prevention*, **5**, 309–324.

79. DiNicola, V., Roberts, N. and Oke, L. (1989) Eating and mood disorders in young children. *Psychiatric Clinics of North America*, **12**, 873–893.

80. Shafran, R., Bryant-Waugh, R., Lask, B. and Arscott, K. (1995) Obsessive–compulsive symptoms in children with eating disorders: a preliminary investigation. *Eating Disorders: Journal of Treatment and Prevention*, **3**, 304–310.

81. Serpell, L., Hirani, V., Willoughby, K. *et al.* (2006) Personality or pathology: obsessive–compulsive symptoms in children and adolescents with anorexia nervosa. *European Eating Disorders Review*, **14**, 404–413.

82. Eagles, J.M., Johnston, M.I., Hunter, D. *et al.* (1995) Increasing incidence of anorexia nervosa in the female population of northeast scotland. *American Journal of Psychiatry*, **152**, 1266–1271.

83. Møller-Madsen, S. and Nystrup, J. (1992) Incidence of anorexia nervosa in Denmark. *Acta Psychiatrica Scandinavica*, **86**, 197–200.

84. Milos, G., Spindler, A. and Schnyder, U. (2004) Psychiatric comorbidity and Eating Disorder Inventory (EDI) profiles in eating disorder patients. *Canadian Journal of Psychiatry*, **49**, 179–184.

85. Hall, A. and Hay, P.J. (1991) Eating disorder patient referrals from a population region 1977–1986. *Psychological Medicine*, **21**, 697–701.

86. Hoek, H.W., Bartelds, A.I.M., Bosveld, J.J.F. *et al.* (1995) Impact of urbanization on detection rates of eating disorders. *American Journal of Psychiatry*, **152**, 1272–1278.

87. Nielsen, S. (1990) The epidemiology of anorexia nervosa in Denmark from 1973 to 1987: a nationwide register study of psychiatric admissions. *Acta Psychiatrica Scandinavica*, **81**, 507–514.

88. Hoek, H.W. (2002) The distribution of eating disorders, in *Eating Disorders and Obesity: A Comprehensive Handbook* (eds C.G. Fairburn and K.D. Brownell), Guilford Press, New York, pp. 233–237.

89. Keel, P.K. and Klump, K.L. (2003) Are eating disorders culture-bound syndromes? Implications for conceptualizing their etiology. *Psychological Bulletin*, **129**, 747–769.

90. Hoek, H. and van Hoeken, D. (2003) Review of the prevalence and incidence of eating disorders. *International Journal of Eating Disorders*, **34**, 383–396.
91. Turnbull, S., Ward, A., Treasure, J. *et al.* (1996) The demand for eating disorder care. An epidemiological study using the General Practice Research Database. *British Journal of Psychiatry*, **169**, 705–712.
92. Currin, L., Schmidt, U., Treasure, J. and Jick, H. (2005) Time trends in eating disorder incidence. *British Journal of Psychiatry*, **186**, 132–135.
93. Lewinsohn, P.M., Striegel-Moore, R.H. and Seeley, J.R. (2000) Epidemiology and natural course of eating disorders in young women from adolescence to young adulthood. *Child and Adolescent Psychiatry*, **39**, 1284–1292.
94. van Son, G.E., van Hoeken, D., Bartelds, A.I. *et al.* (2006) Time trends in the incidence of eating disorders: a primary care study in the Netherlands. *International Journal of Eating Disorders*, **39**, 565–569.
95. Keski-Rahkonen, A., Hoek, H.W., Susser, E.S. *et al.* (2007) Epidemiology and course of anorexia nervosa in the community. *American Journal of Psychiatry*, **164**, 1259–1265.
96. Bulik, C.M., Sullivan, P.F., Tozzi, F. *et al.* (2006) Prevalence, heritability, and prospective risk factors for anorexia nervosa. *Archives of General Psychiatry*, **63**, 305–312.
97. Wade, T.D., Bergin, J.L., Tiggemann, M. *et al.* (2006) Prevalence and long-term course of lifetime eating disorders in an adult Australian twin cohort. *Australian and New Zealand Journal of Psychiatry*, **40**, 121–128.
98. Hudson, J.I., Hiripi, E., Pope, H.G. Jr and Kessler, R.C. (2007) The prevalence and correlates of eating disorders in the National Comorbidity Survey Replication. *Biological Psychiatry*, **61**, 348–358.
99. Makino, M., Tsuboi, K. and Dennerstein, L. (2004) Prevalence of eating disorders: a comparison of Western and non-Western countries. *Medscape General Medicine*, **6**, 49.
100. Hay, P.J., Mond, J., Buttner, P. and Darby, A. (2008) Eating disorder behaviors are increasing: findings from two sequential community surveys in South Australia. *PLoS ONE*, **3**, 1541.
101. Keel, P.K., Heatherton, T.H., Dorer, D.J. *et al.* (2006) Point prevalence of bulimia nervosa in 1982, 1992, and 2002. *Psychological Medicine*, **36**, 119–127.
102. Machado, P.P., Machado, B.C., Goncalves, S. and Hoek, H.W. (2007) The prevalence of eating disorders not otherwise specified. *International Journal of Eating Disorders*, **40**, 212–217.
103. Lucas, A.R., Beard, C.M., O'Fallon, W.M. and Kurland, L.T. (1991) 50-year trends in the incidence of anorexia nervosa in Rochester, Minn.: a population-based study. *American Journal of Psychiatry*, **148**, 917–922.
104. Crow, S.J., Peterson, C.B., Swanson, S.A. *et al.* (2009) Increased mortality in bulimia nervosa and other eating disorders. *American Journal of Psychiatry*, **166**, 1342–1346.
105. Morande, G., Celada, J. and Casas, J.J. (1999) Prevalence of eating disorders in a Spanish school-age population. *Journal of Adolescent Health*, **24**, 212–219.
106. Patton, Gc., Selzer, R., Coffey, C. *et al.* (1999) Onset of adolescent eating disorders: population based cohort study over three years. *British Medical Journal*, **318**, 765–768.
107. Kjelsas, E., Bjornstrom, C. and Gotestam, K.G. (2004) Prevalence of eating disorders in female and male adolescents (14–15 years). *Eating Behaviors*, **5**, 13–25.
108. Nasser, M., Katzman, M.A. and Gordon, R. (2001) *Eating Disorders and Cultures in Transition*, Routledge Press, London.
109. Garner, A. and Garfinkel, P. (1980) Sociocultural factors in the development of anorexia nervosa. *Psychological Medicine*, **10**, 647–656.
110. Bruch, H. (1974) *Eating Disorders: Obesity, Anorexia Nervosa and the Person Within*, Routledge & Kegan Paul, London.

111. Crisp, A.H. (1983) Anorexia nervosa. *British Medical Journal*, **287**, 855–858.

112. Brumberg, J.J. (1988) *Fasting Girls*, Harvard University Press, Cambridge, MA.

113. Garfinkel, P. and Garner, D. (1982) *Anorexia Nervosa: A Multi-dimensional Perspective*, Basic Books, New York.

114. Szmukler, G., McCance, C., McCrone, L. and Hunter, D. (1986) Anorexia nervosa: a psychiatric case register study from Aberdeen. *Psychological Medicine*, **16**, 49–58.

115. Bhadrinath, B.R. (1990) Anorexia nervosa in adolescents of Asian extraction. *British Journal of Psychiatry*, **156**, 565–568.

116. Bryant-Waugh, R. and Lask, B. (1991) Anorexia nervosa in a group of Asian children living in Britain. *British Journal of Psychiatry*, **158**, 229–233.

117. Hsu, L.K.G. (1987) Are the eating disorders becoming more common in blacks? *International Journal of Eating Disorders*, **6**, 113–124.

118. Vogeltanz-Holm, N., Wonderlich, S., Lewis, B. *et al.* (2000) Longitudinal predictors of binge-eating, intense dieting, and weight concerns in a national sample of women. *Behaviour Therapy*, **31**, 221–235.

119. Cattarin, J. and Thompson, J. (1994) A three year longitudinal study of body image, eating disturbance and general psychological functioning in adolescent females. *Eating Disorders*, **2**, 114–125.

120. Patton, G., Johnson-Sabine, E., Wood, K. *et al.* (1990) Abnormal eating attitudes in London schoolgirls – a prospective epidemiological study: outcome at twelve month follow-up. *Psychological Medicine*, **20**, 383–394.

121. Stice, E., Mazotti, L., Krebs, M. and Martin, S. (1998) Predictors of adolescent dieting behaviors: a longitudinal study. *Psychology of Addictive Behaviors*, **12**, 195–205.

122. Stice, E. and Whitenton, K. (2002) Risk factors for body dissatisfaction in adolescent girls: a longitudinal investigation. *Developmental Psychology*, **38**, 669–678.

123. Field, A., Camargo, C., Taylor, C. *et al.* (2001) Peer, parent and media influences on the development of weight concerns and frequent dieting among preadolescent and adolescent girls and boys. *Pediatrics*, **107**, 54–60.

124. Byely, L., Archibald, A., Graber, J. and Brooks-Gunn, J. (2000) A prospective study of familial and social influences on girls' body image and dieting. *International Journal of Eating Disorders*, **28**, 155–164.

125. Cooley, E. and Toray, T. (2001) Disordered eating in college freshman women: a prospective study. *Journal of American College Health*, **49**, 229–235.

126. Groesz, L.M., Levine, M.P. and Murnen, S.K. (2002) The effect of experimental presentation of thin media images on body satisfaction: a meta-analytic review. *International Journal of Eating Disorders*, **31**, 1–16.

127. Lee, S., Ho, P. and Hsu, L. (1993) Fat phobic and non-fat phobic anorexia nervosa: a comparative study of 70 Chinese patients in Hong Kong. *Psychological Medicine*, **23**, 999–1017.

128. Neumarker, U., Dudek, U., Volrath, M. *et al.* (1992) Eating attitudes among adolescent anorexia nervosa patients and normal subjects in former East and West Berlin: a transcultural comparison. *International Journal of Eating Disorders*, **12**, 281–289.

129. Steinhausen, H.C. (1984) Transcultural comparison of eating attitudes in young females and anorectic patients. *European Archives of Psychiatry and Neurological Science*, **234**, 198–201.

130. Nasser, M. (1986) Comparative study of the prevalence of abnormal eating attitudes among Arab female students of both London and Cairo universities. *Psychological Medicine*, **16**, 621–625.

131. Davis, C. and Katzman, M. (1999) Perfection as acculturation: psychological correlates of eating problems in Chinese male and female students living in the United States. *International Journal of Eating Disorders*, **25**, 65–70.

132. Garner, D.M., Olmsted, M.P. and Polivy, J. (1983) Development and validation of a multidimensional eating disorder inventory for anorexia nervosa and bulimia. *International Journal of Eating Disorders*, **2**, 15–34.

133. Haudek, C., Rorty, M. and Henker, B. (1999) The role of ethnicity and parental bonding in the eating and weight concerns of Asian-American and Caucasian college women. *International Journal of Eating Disorders*, **25**, 425–433.

134. Hoek, H.W., van Harten, P.N., van Hoeken, D. and Susser, E. (1998) Lack of relation between culture and anorexia nervosa: results of an incidence study on Curaçao. *New England Journal of Medicine*, **338**, 1231–1232.

135. Rieger, E., Touyz, S., Swain, T. and Beumont, P. (2000) Cross-cultural research on anorexia nervosa: assumptions regarding the role of body weight. *International Journal of Eating Disorders*, **29**, 205–215.

136. Hill, A.J. and Bhatti, R. (1995) Body shape perception and dieting in preadolescent British Asian Girls: links with eating disorders. *International Journal of Eating Disorders*, **17**, 175–183.

137. Stice, E. (2002) Risk and maintenance factors for eating pathology: a meta-analytic review. *Psychological Bulletin*, **128**, 825–848.

138. Halmi, K.A., Eckert, E., Marchi, M. *et al.* (1991) Co-morbidity of psychiatric diagnoses in anorexia nervosa. *Archives of General Psychiatry*, **48**, 712–718.

139. Logue, C.M., Crowe, Rr. and Bean, J.A. (1989) A family study of anorexia nervosa and bulimia. *British Journal of Psychiatry*, **30**, 179–188.

140. Stern, S., Dixon, K., Sansone, R. *et al.* (1992) Psychoactive substance use disorder in relatives of patients with anorexia nervosa. *Comprehensive Psychiatry*, **33**, 207–212.

141. Gershon, E.S., Schreiber, J.L., Hamovit, J.R. *et al.* (1984) Clinical findings in patients with anorexia nervosa and affective illness in their relatives. *American Journal of Psychiatry*, **141**, 1419–1422.

142. Hudson, J.I., Pope, H.G. Jr, Jonas, J.M. *et al.* (1987a) A controlled family history study of bulimia. *Psychological Medicine*, **17**, 883–890.

143. Kassett, J., Gershon, E., Maxwell, M. *et al.* (1989) Psychiatric disorders in the relatives of probands with bulimia nervosa. *American Journal of Psychiatry*, **146**, 1468–1471.

144. Lilenfeld, L.R. and Kaye, W.H. (1998) Genetic studies of anorexia nervosa and bulimia nervosa. *Neurobiology in the Treatment of Eating Disorders*, **7**, 171–193.

145. Strober, M., Freeman, R., Lampert, C. *et al.* (2000) Controlled family study of anorexia and bulimia nervosa: evidence of shared liability and transmission of partial syndromes. *American Journal of Psychiatry*, **157**, 393–401.

146. Strober, M., Freeman, R., Lampert, C. *et al.* (2001) Males with anorexia nervosa: a controlled study of eating disorders in first-degree relatives. *International Journal of Eating Disorders*, **29**, 263–269.

147. Strober, M., Lampert, C., Morrell, W. *et al.* (1990) A controlled family study of anorexia nervosa: evidence of familial aggregation and lack of shared transmission with affective disorders. *International Journal of Eating Disorders*, **9**, 239–253.

148. Bulik, C.M., Sullivan, P.F., Wade, T. and Kendler, K.S. (2000) Twin studies of eating disorders: a review. *International Journal of Eating Disorders*, **27**, 1–20.

149. Javaras, K.N., Laird, N.M., Reichborn-Kjennerud, T. *et al.* (2008) Familiality and heritability of binge eating disorder: results of a case-control family study and a twin study. *International Journal of Eating Disorders*, **41**, 174–179.

150. Klump, K.L., McGue, M. and Iacono, W.G. (2000) Age differences in genetic and environmental influences on eating attitudes and behaviors in preadolescent and adolescent female twins. *Journal of Abnormal Psychology*, **109**, 239–251.

151. Sullivan, P.F., Bulik, C.M. and Kendler, K.S. (1998) Genetic epidemiology of binging and vomiting. *The British Journal of Psychiatry*, **173**, 75–79.

152. Rutherford, J., McGuffin, P., Katz, R.J. and Murray, R.M. (1993) Genetic influences on eating attitudes in a normal female twin pair population. *Psychological Medicine*, **23**, 425–436.

153. Wade, T., Neale, M.C., Lake, R.I.E. and Martin, N.G. (1999) A genetic analysis of the eating and attitudes associated with bulimia nervosa: dealing with the problem of ascertainment. *Behavior Genetics*, **29**, 1–10.

154. Klump, K.L., Burt, S.A., McGue, M. and Iacono, W.G. (2007) Changes in genetic and environmental influences on disordered eating across adolescence. *Archives of General Psychiatry*, **64**, 1409–1415.

155. Silberg, J.L. and Bulik, C.M. (2005) The developmental association between eating disorders symptoms and symptoms of depression and anxiety in juvenile twin girls. *Journal of Child Psychology and Psychiatry*, **46**, 1317–1326.

156. Culbert, K.M., Burt, S.A., McGue, M. *et al.* (2009) Puberty and the genetic diathesis of disordered eating. *Journal of Abnormal Psychology*, **118** (4), 788–796.

157. Klump, K.L., McGue, M. and Iacono, W.G. (2003) Differential heritability of eating attitudes and behaviors in prepubertal and pubertal twins. *International Journal of Eating Disorders*, **33**, 287–292.

158. Klump, K.L., Perkins, P.S., Burt, S.A. *et al.* (2007) Puberty moderates genetic influences on disordered eating. *Psychological Medicine*, **37**, 627–634.

159. Klump, K.L., Culbert, K.M., Edler, C. and Keel, P.K. (2008) Ovarian hormones and binge eating: exploring associations in community samples. *Psychological Medicine*, **38** (12), 1749–1757.

160. Klump, K.L. and Culbert, K.M. (2007) Molecular genetic studies of eating disorders: current status and future directions. *Current Directions in Psychological Science*, **16**, 37–41.

161. Klump, K.L., Burt, S.A., Spanos, A. *et al.* (2010) Age differences in genetic and environmental influences on weight and shape concerns. *International Journal of Eating Disorders*, **43**, 679–688.

162. Lilenfeld, L.R., Kaye, W.H., Greeno, C.G. *et al.* (1998) A controlled family study of anorexia nervosa and bulimia nervosa: psychiatric disorders in first-degree relatives and effects of proband comorbidity. *Archives of General Psychiatry*, **55**, 603–610.

163. Wade, T.D., Bulik, C.M., Neale, M. and Kendler, K.S. (2000) Anorexia nervosa and major depression: shared genetic and environmental risk factors. *American Journal of Psychiatry*, **157**, 469–471.

164. Walters, E.E., Neale, M.C., Heath, A.C. *et al.* (1992) Bulimia nervosa and major depression: a study of common genetic and environmental factors. *Psychological Medicine*, **22**, 617–622.

165. Kendler, K.S., MacLean, C., Neale, M. *et al.* (1991) The genetic epidemiology of bulimia nervosa. *American Journal of Psychiatry*, **148**, 1627–1637.

166. Cnattingius, S., Hultman, C., Dahl, M. and Sparen, P. (1999) Very preterm birth, birth trauma, and the risk of anorexia nervosa among girls. *Archives of General Psychiatry*, **56**, 634.

167. Lindberg, L. and Hjern, A. (2003) Risk factors for anorexia nervosa: a national cohort study. *International Journal of Eating Disorders*, **34**, 397.

168. Favaro, A., Tenconi, E. and Santonastaso, P. (2006) Perinatal factors and the risk of developing anorexia nervosa and bulimia nervosa. *Archives of General Psychiatry*, **63**, 82–88.

169. Connan, F., Campbell, I.C., Katzman, M. *et al.* (2003) A neurodevelopmental model for anorexia nervosa. *Physiology and Behaviour*, **79**, 13–24.

170. Tanner, J.M. (1989) *Foetus into Man: Physical Growth from Conception to Maturity*, 2nd edn, Castlemead Ware.

171. Fairburn, C.G., Welch, S.L., Doll, H.A. *et al.* (1997) Risk factors for bulimia nervosa. A community based case-control study. *Archives of General Psychiatry*, **54**, 509–517.

172. Blakemore, S., Burnett, S. and Dahl, R. (2010) The role of puberty in the developing adolescent brain. *Human Brain Mapping*, **31**, 926–933.

173. Freud, S. (1961) The ego and the id, in *The Standard Edition of the Complete Psychological Works of Sigmund Freud*, vol. **19** (ed. J. Strachey), The Hogarth Press, London, pp. 3–66 (Originally published in 1923).

174. Waller, J.V., Kaufman, R.M. and Deutsch, F. (1940) Anorexia nervosa: a psychosomatic entity. *Psychosomatic Medicine*, **2**, 3–16.

175. Minuchin, S., Rosman, B.L. and Baker, L. (1978) *Psychosomatic Families: Anorexia Nervosa in Context*, Harvard University Press, Cambridge, MA.

176. Goodsitt, A. (1985) Self-psychology and the treatment of anorexia nervosa, in *Handbook of Psychotherapy for Anorexia Nervosa and Bulimia* (eds D.M. Garner and P.E. Garfinkel), The Guilford Press, New York, pp. 55–82.

177. Palazzoli, M.S. (1974) *Self Starvation*, Chancer, London.

178. Bruch, H. (1973) *Eating Disorders*, Basic Books, New York.

179. Minuchin, S., Baker, L., Rosman, B.L. *et al.* (1975) A conceptual model of psychosomatic illness in children. *Archives of General Psychiatry*, **32**, 1031–1038.

180. Strober, M. and Humphrey, L.L. (1987) Familial contributions to the etiology and course of anorexia nervosa and bulimia. *Journal of Consulting and Clinical Psychology*, **55**, 654–659.

181. Kog, E., Vertommen, H. and Vandereycken, W. (1987) Minuchin's pychosomatic family model revised: a concept validation study using a multitrait–multimethod approach. *Family Process*, **26**, 235–253.

182. Eisler, I. (1995) Family models of eating disorders, in *Handbook of Eating Disorders: Theory, Treatment and Research* (eds G.I. Szmukler, C. Dare and J. Treasure), John Wiley & Sons, Ltd, London.

183. Eisler, I. (2005) The empirical and theoretical base of family therapy and multiple family day therapy for adolescent anorexia nervosa. *Journal of Family Therapy*, **27**, 104–131.

184. Schmidt, U. and Treasure, J. (2006) Anorexia nervosa: valued and visable. A cognitive interpersonal maintenance model and its implications for research and practice. *British Journal of Clinical Psychology*, **45**, 343–366.

185. Garner, D.M. and Bemis, K.M. (1982) A cognitive-behavioural approach to anorexia nervosa. *Cognitive Therapy and Research*, **6**, 123–150.

186. Beck, A.T. (1975) *Cognitive Therapy and the Emotional Disorders*, International Universities Press.

187. Slade, P. (1982) Towards a functional analysis of anorexia nervosa and bulimia nervosa. *British Journal of Clinical Psychology*, **21**, 167–179.

188. Polivy, J. and Herman, C.P. (1985) Dieting and binging: a causal analysis. *American Psychologist*, **40**, 193–201.

189. Heatherton, T.F. and Baumeister, R.F. (1991) Binge eating as escape from self-awareness. *Psychological Bulletin*, **110**, 86–108.

190. Fairburn, C.G. (1997) Eating disorders, in *Science and Practice of Cognitive Behaviour Therapy* (eds D.M. Clark and C.G. Fairburn), Oxford University Press, Oxford.

191. Vitousek, K. and Hollon, S.D. (1990) The investigation of schematic content and processing in eating disorders. *Cognitive Therapy and Research*, **14**, 191–214.

192. Williamson, D. (1996) Body image disturbance in eating disorders: a form of cognitive bias? *Eating Disorders The Journal of Treatment and Prevention*, **4**, 47–58.

193. Fairburn, C., Shafran, R. and Cooper, Z. (1999) A cognitive behavioural theory of anorexia nervosa. *Behavioural Research and Therapy*, **37**, 1–13.

194. Fairburn, C.G., Cooper, Z. and Shafran, R. (2003) Cognitive behaviour therapy for eating disorders: a 'transdiagnostic' theory and treatment. *Behaviour Research and Therapy*, **41**, 509–528.

195. Fairburn, C.G., Norman, P.A., Welch, S.L. *et al.* (1995) A prospective study of outcome in bulimia nervosa and the long-term effects of three psychological treatments. *Archives of General Psychiatry*, **52**, 304–312.

196. Sullivan, P., Bulik, C., Fear, J. and Pickering, A. (1998) Outcome of anorexia nervosa: a case-control study. *American Journal of Psychiatry*, **155**, 939–946.

197. Shafran, R., Cooper, Z. and Fairburn, C.G. (2002) Clinical perfectionism: a cognitive-behavioural analysis. *Behaviour Research and Therapy*, **40**, 773–791.

198. Cassin, S.E. and von Ranson, K.M. (2005) Personality and eating disorders: a decade in review. *Clinical Psychology Review*, **25**, 895–916.

199. Tyrka, A.R., Waldron, I., Graber, J.A. and Brooks-Gunn, J. (2002) Prospective predictors of the onset of anorexic and bulimic syndromes. *International Journal of Eating Disorders*, **32**, 282–290.

200. Halmi, K.A., Sunday, S.R., Strober, M. *et al.* (2000) Perfectionism in anorexia nervosa: variation by clinical subtype, obsessionality, and pathological eating behavior. *American Journal of Psychiatry*, **157**, 1799–1805.

201. Lilenfeld, L.R., Stein, D., Bulik, C.M. *et al.* (2000) Personality traits among currently eating disordered, recovered, and never ill first degree relatives of bulimic and control women. *Psychological Medicine*, **30**, 1399–1410.

202. Pratt, E.M., Telch, C.F., Labouvie, E.W. *et al.* (2001) Perfectionism in women with binge eating disorder. *International Journal of Eating Disorders*, **29**, 177–186.

203. Bastiani, A.M., Rao, R., Weltzin, T. and Kaye, W.H. (1995) Perfectionism in anorexia nervosa. *International Journal of Eating Disorders*, **17**, 147–152.

204. Srinivasagam, N.M., Kaye, W.H., Plotnicov, K.H. *et al.* (1995) Persistent perfectionism, symmetry, and exactness after long-term recovery from anorexia nervosa. *American Journal of Psychiatry*, **152**, 1630–1634.

205. Stein, D., Kaye, W.H., Matsunaga, H. *et al.* (2002) Eating-related concerns, mood, and personality traits in recovered bulimia nervosa subjects: a replication study. *International Journal of Eating Disorders*, **32**, 225–229.

206. Sutandar-Pinnock, K., Woodside, D.B., Carter, J.C. *et al.* (2003) Perfectionism in anorexia nervosa: a 6–24-month follow up study. *International Journal of Eating Disorders*, **33**, 225–229.

207. Steiger, H. and Bruce, K. (2004) Personality traits and disorders in anorexia nervosa, bulimia nervosa, and binge eating disorder, in *Clinical Handbook of EATING Disorders: An Integrated Approach* (ed. T.D. Brewerton), Marcel Dekker, Inc., New York, pp. 209–230.

208. Anderluh, M.B., Tchanturia, K., Rabe-Hesketh, S. and Treasure, J. (2003) Childhood obsessive–compulsive personality traits in adult women with eating disorders: defining a broader eating disorder phenotype. *American Journal of Psychiatry*, **160**, 242–247.

209. Newton, J.R., Freeman, C.P. and Munro, J. (1993) Impulsivity and dyscontrol in bulimia nervosa: is impulsivity an independent phenomenon or a marker of severity? *Acta Psychiatrica Scandinavica*, **87**, 389–394.

210. Cassidy, E., Allsopp, M. and Williams, T. (1999) Obsessive compulsive symptoms at initial presentation of adolescent eating disorders. *European Child and Adolescent Psychiatry*, **8**, 193–199.

211. von Ranson, K.M., Kaye, W., Weltzin, T.E. *et al.* (1999) Obsessive compulsive disorder symptoms before and after recovery from bulimia nervosa. *American Journal of Psychiatry*, **156**, 1703–1708.

212. Claes, L., Vandereycken, W. and Vertommen, H. (2002) Impulsive and compulsive traits in eating disordered patients compared with controls. *Personality and Individual Differences*, **32**, 707–714.

213. Fahy, T. and Eisler, I. (1993) Impulsivity and eating disorders. *British Journal of Psychiatry*, **162**, 193–197.

214. Diaz-Marsa, M., Carrasco, J.L. and Saiz, J. (2000) A study of temperament and personality in anorexia nervosa and bulimia nervosa. *Journal of Personality Disorders*, **14**, 352–359.

215. Rossier, V., Bolognini, M., Plancherel, B. and Halfon, O. (2000) Sensation seeking: a personality trait characteristic of adolescent girls and young women with eating disorders. *European Eating Disorders Review*, **8**, 245–252.

216. Steiger, H., Jabalpurwala, S., Champagne, J. and Stotland, S. (1997) A controlled study of trait narcissism in anorexia and bulimia nervosa. *International Journal of Eating Disorders*, **22**, 173–178.

217. Lehoux, P.M., Steiger, H. and Jabalpurlawa, S. (2000) State/trait distinctions in bulimic syndromes. *International Journal of Eating Disorders*, **27**, 36–42.

218. Narduzzi, K.J. and Jackson, T. (2000) Personality differences between eating disordered women and a nonclinical comparison sample: a discriminant classification analysis. *Journal of Clinical Psychology*, **56**, 699–710.

219. Grilo, C.M., Sanislow, C.A., Skodol, A.E. *et al.* (2003) Do eating disorders co-occur with personality disorders? Comparison groups matter. *International Journal of Eating Disorders*, **33**, 155–164.

220. Vitousek, K.M. and Stumpf, R.E. (2005) Difficulties in the assessment of personality traits and disorders in eating-disordered individuals. *Eating Disorders*, **13**, 37–60.

221. Bornstein, R.F. (2001) A meta-analysis of the dependency–eating-disorders relationship: strength, specificity, and temporal stability. *Journal of Psychopathology and Behavioral Assessment*, **23**, 151–162.

222. Garner, D.M., Olmsted, M.P., Davis, R. *et al.* (1990) The association between bulimic symptoms and reported psychopathology. *International Journal of Eating Disorders*, **9**, 1–15.

223. Matsunaga, H., Kaye, W.H., McConaha, C. *et al.* (2000) Personality disorders among subjects recovered from eating disorders. *International Journal of Eating Disorders*, **27**, 353–357.

224. Treasure, J. and Bauer, B. (2003) Assessment and motivation, in *Handbook of Eating Disorders*, 2nd edn (eds J. Treasure, U. Shmidt and E. VanFurth), John Wiley & Sons, Ltd, Chichester, pp. 219–231.

225. NICE (2004) *Eating Disorders, Core Interventions in the Treatment and Management of Anorexia Nervosa, Bulimia Nervosa and other Related Eating Disorders*, National Clinical Practice Guideline Number CG9, British Psychological Society.

226. Pike, K.M., Walsh, B.T., Vitousek, K. *et al.* (2003) Cognitive behavior therapy in the posthospitalization treatment of anorexia nervosa. *American Journal of Psychiatry*, **160**, 2046–2049.

227. McIntosh, V.V., Jordan, J., Carter, F.A. *et al.* (2005) Three psychotherapies for anorexia nervosa: a randomized, controlled trial. *American Journal of Psychiatry*, **162**, 741–747.

228. Dare, C., Eisler, I., Russell, G. *et al.* (2001) Psychological therapies for adults with anorexia nervosa: randomised controlled trial of out patient treatments. *British Journal of Psychiatry*, **178**, 216–221.

229. Cooper, P.J., Coker, S. and Fleming, C. (1994) Self-help for bulimia nervosa: a preliminary report. *International Journal of Eating Disorders*, **16**, 401–404.

230. Bara-Carril, N., Williams, C., Pombo-Carril, M. *et al.* (2004) A preliminary investigation into the feasibility and efficacy of a CD-ROM-based cognitive-behavioral self-help intervention for bulimia nervosa. *International Journal of Eating Disorders*, **35**, 538–548.

231. Ljotsson, B., Lundin, C., Mitsell, K. *et al.* (2007) Remote treatment of bulimia nervosa and binge eating disorder: a randomized trial of Internet-assisted cognitive behavioural therapy. *Behavior Research and Therapy*, **45**, 649–661.

232. Bailer, U., de Zwaan, M., Leisch, F. *et al.* (2004) Guided self-help versus cognitive-behavioral group therapy in the treatment of bulimia nervosa. *International Journal of Eating Disorders*, **35**, 522–537.

233. Carter, J.C., Olmstead, M.P., Kaplan, A.S. *et al.* (2003) Self-help for bulimia nervosa: a randomized controlled trial. *American Journal of Psychiatry*, **160**, 973–978.

234. Durand, A. and King, M. (2003) Specialist treatment versus self-help for bulimia nervosa: a randomized controlled trial in general practice. *British Journal of General Practice*, **53**, 371–377.

235. Thiels, C., Schmidt, U., Treasure, J.L. *et al.* (1998) Guided self change for bulimia nervosa incorporating a self-care manual. *American Journal of Psychiatry*, **155**, 947–953.

236. Agras, W.S., Walsh, B.T., Fairburn, C.G. *et al.* (2000) A multicenter comparison of cognitive-behavioral therapy and interpersonal therapy for bulimia nervosa. *Archives of General Psychiatry*, **57**, 459–466.

237. Fairburn, C.G., Jones, R., Peveler, R.C. *et al.* (1991) Three psychological treatments for bulimia nervosa. A comparative trial. *Archives of General Psychiatry*, **48**, 463–469.

238. Wilfley, D.E., Agras, W.S., Telch, C.F. *et al.* (1993) Group cognitive-behavioral therapy and group interpersonal psychotherapy for the nonpurging bulimic individual: a controlled comparison. *Journal of Consulting and Clinical Psychology*, **61**, 296–305.

239. Wolk, S.L. and Devlin, M.J. (2001) Stage of change as a predictor of response to psychotherapy of bulimia nervosa. *International Journal of Eating Disorders*, **30**, 96–100.

240. Ghaderi, A. (2006) Psychometric properties of the Swedish version of Self-Concept Questionnaire. *European Journal of Psychological Assessment*, **21**, 139–146.

241. Thompson-Brenner, H., Glass, S. and Westen, D. (2003) A multidimensional meta-analysis of psychotherapy for bulimia nervosa. *Clinical Psychology*, **10**, 269–287.

242. Fairburn, C.G., Cooper, Z., Bohn, K. *et al.* (2007) The severity and status of eating disorder NOS: implications for DSM-V. *Behaviour Research and Therapy*, **45**, 1705–1715.

243. Gorin, A., Le Grange, D. and Stone, A. (2003) Effectiveness of spouse involvement in cognitive behavioral therapy for binge eating disorder. *International Journal of Eating Disorders*, **33**, 421–433.

244. Telch, C.F., Agras, W.S. and Linehan, M.M. (2001) Dialectical behavior therapy for binge eating disorder. *Journal of Consulting and Clinical Psychology*, **69**, 1061–1065.

245. Wilfley, D.E., Welch, R.R., Stein, R.I. *et al.* (2002) A randomized comparison of group cognitive-behavioral therapy and group interpersonal psychotherapy for the treatment of overweight individuals with binge-eating disorder. *Archives of General Psychiatry*, **59**, 713–721.

246. Fairburn, C. and Cooper, Z. (1993) The eating disorder examination, in *Binge Eating: Nature, Assessment and Treatment*, 12th edn (eds C. Fairburn and G.T. Wilson), Guilford, New York, pp. 317–331.

247. Carter, J.C. and Fairburn, C.G. (1998) Cognitive-behavioral self-help for binge eating disorder: a controlled effectiveness study. *Journal of Consulting and Clinical Psychology*, **66**, 616–623.

248. Peterson, C.B., Mitchell, J.E., Engbloom, S. *et al.* (1998) Group cognitive-behavioral treatment of binge eating disorder: a comparison of therapist-led versus self-help formats. *International Journal of Eating Disorders*, **24**, 125–136.

249. Peterson, C.B., Mitchell, J.E., Engbloom, S. *et al.* (2001) Self-help versus therapist-led group cognitive-behavioral treatment of binge eating disorder at follow-up. *International Journal of Eating Disorders*, **30**, 363–374.

250. Fairburn, C.G., Cooper, Z. and Shafran, R. (2008) Enhanced cognitive behavior therapy for eating disorders ('CBT-E'): an overview, in *Cognitive Behavior Therapy and Eating Disorders* (ed. C.G. Fairburn), Guilford, New York.

251. Fairburn, C.G., Cooper, Z., Doll, H.A. *et al.* (2008) Transdiagnostic cognitive-behavioral therapy for patients with eating disorders: a two-site trial with 60-week follow-up. *American Journal of Psychiatry*, **166**, 311–319.

252. Russell, G.F.M., Szmukler, G.I., Dare, C. and Eisler, I. (1987) An evaluation of family therapy in anorexia and bulimia nervosa. *Archives of General Psychiatry*, **44**, 1047–1056.

253. Le Grange, D., Eisler, I., Dare, C. and Russell, G.F.M. (1992) Evaluation of family therapy in anorexia nervosa: a pilot study. *International Journal of Eating Disorder*, **12**, 347–357.

254. Robin, A., Siegel, P., Koepke, T. *et al.* (1994) Family therapy versus individual therapy for adolescent females with anorexia nervosa. *Journal of Developmental and Behavioural Pediatrics*, **15**, 111–116.

255. Eisler, I., Dare, C., Hodes, M. *et al.* (2000) Family therapy for adolescent anorexia nervosa: the results of a controlled comparison of two family interventions. *Journal of Child Psychology and Psychiatry*, **41**, 727–736.

256. Lock, J., Agras, W.S., Bryson, S. and Kraemer, H.C. (2005) A comparison of short- and long-term family therapy for adolescent anorexia nervosa. *Journal of the American Academy of Child and Adolescent Psychiatry*, **44**, 632–639.

257. Lock, J., Couturier, J. and Agras, W.S. (2006) Comparison of longterm outcomes in adolescents with anorexia nervosa treated with family therapy. *Journal of the American Academy of Child and Adolescent Psychiatry*, **45**, 666–672.

258. Schmidt, U., Lee, S., Beecham, J. *et al.* (2007) A randomized controlled trial of family therapy and cognitive behavioral therapy guided self-care for adolescents with bulimia nervosa and related disorders. *American Journal of Psychiatry*, **164**, 591–598.

259. LeGrange, D., Crosby, R.D., Rathouz, P.J. and Leventhal, B.L. (2007) A randomized controlled comparison of family based treatment and supportive psychotherapy for adolescent bulimia nervosa. *Archives of General Psychiatry*, **64**, 1049–1056.

260. Walsh, B.T. and Kahn, C.B. (1997) Diagnostic criteria for eating disorders: current concerns and future directions. *Psychopharmacology Bulletin*, **33**, 369–372.

261. Keel, P.K. and Brown, T.A. (2010) Update on course and outcome in eating disorders. *International Journal of Eating Disorders*, **43**, 195–204.

262. Nilsson, K. and Hagglof, B. (2005) Long-term follow-up of adolescent onset anorexia nervosa in northern Sweden. *European Eating Disorders Review*, **13**, 89–100.

263. Fichter, M.M., Quadflieg, N. and Hedlund, S. (2006) Twelve-year course and outcome predictors of anorexia nervosa. *International Journal of Eating Disorders*, **39**, 87–100.

264. Schmidt, U., Lee, S., Perkins, S. *et al.* (2008) Do adolescents with eating disorder not otherwise specified or full-syndrome bulimia nervosa differ in clinical severity, comorbidity, risk factors, treatment outcome or cost? *International Journal of Eating Disorders*, **41**, 498–504.

265. Fichter, M.M. and Quadflieg, N. (2004) Twelve-year course and outcome of bulimia nervosa. *Psychological Medicine*, **34**, 395–1406.

266. Keel, P.K., Gravener, J.A., Joiner, T.E. Jr and Haedt, A.A. (2010) Twenty-year follow-up of bulimia nervosa and related eating disorders not otherwise specified. *International Journal of Eating Disorders*, **43**, 492–497.

267. Schlup, B., Munsch, S., Meyer, A.H. *et al.* (2009) The efficacy of a short version of a cognitive-behavioral treatment followed by booster sessions for binge eating disorder. *Behaviour Research and Therapy*, **47**, 628–635.

268. Dingemans, A.E., Spinhoven, P. and van Furth, E.F. (2007) Predictors and mediators of treatment outcome in patients with binge eating disorder. *Behaviour Research and Therapy*, **45**, 2551–2562.

269. Agras, W.S., Crow, S., Mitchell, J.E. *et al.* (2009) A 4-year prospective study of eating disorder NOS compared with full eating disorder syndromes. *International Journal of Eating Disorders*, **42**, 565–570.

270. Clausen, L. (2008) Time to remission for eating disorder patients: a 2(1/2)-year follow-up study of outcome and predictors. *Nordic Journal of Psychiatry*, **62**, 151–159.

271. Grilo, C.M., Pagano, M.E., Skodol, A.E. *et al.* (2007) Natural course of bulimia nervosa and of eating disorder not otherwise specified: 5-year prospective study of remissions, relapses, and the effects of personality disorder psychopathology. *Journal of Clinical Psychiatry*, **68**, 738–746.

3 Neuroimaging

Tone Seim Fuglset[1] and Ian Frampton[2]

[1]*Regional Eating Disorders Service, Oslo University Hospital, Oslo, Norway*
[2]*College of Life and Environmental Sciences, University of Exeter, UK*

3.1 Introduction

Neuroscientists have developed a wide variety of techniques to obtain brain images. Some, such as computerised tomography (CT) and magnetic resonance imaging (MRI), provide 'snapshot' information about the structure of the brain. Others, such as functional magnetic resonance imaging (fMRI), positron emission tomography (PET) and single-photon emission computed tomography (SPECT) measure the brain's function. All these methods can be used to explore how eating disorders affect the brain and sometimes to test theories about the causes or consequences of disordered eating. In the future they could even be used as an outcome measure for specific treatments, although this science is still in its early stages of development. In this chapter the different imaging techniques will be outlined, along with recent findings within eating disorders using each of these techniques. Finally, the clinical and theoretical implications will be discussed. Studies referred to in this chapter are summarised in Table 3.1.

3.2 Structural imaging

Why study the structure of the brain in eating disorders? One of the major tenets of a neuroscience approach to eating disorders is that starving the body will also starve the brain. It could be that many of the clinical characteristics we see in patients with restrictive eating disorders are caused by changes in brain structure secondary to starvation. In particular, starvation reduces body composition of fats, since fat stores are converted to energy to sustain life, in preference to converting the protein in muscles, which is preferentially preserved. In the brain, fat is predominantly stored in the myelin sheath surrounding the long axon projection of neurons. Myelin improves the conductivity of the axon, and thus increases the speed at which electrical signals can pass.

Eating Disorders and the Brain. Edited by Bryan Lask and Ian Frampton.
© 2011 John Wiley & Sons, Ltd. Published 2011 by John Wiley & Sons, Ltd.

Table 3.1 Neuroimaging studies in eating disorders.

Method	Authors	Sample	Aim	Results	Discussion/conclusion
CT	Heinz et al. [63]	AN: n = 1 Cushing syndrome: n = 1	An observation of two cases with 'reversible' cerebral atrophy.	Both patients showed cerebral atrophy. Several months later, CT showed total return to normality.	Mechanisms responsible for atrophic changes may be related to protein loss or fluid retention, or both.
CT	Kohlmeyer et al. [7]	AN: n = 23	To confirm the observations of other authors on so-called reversible cerebral atrophy.	Enlargement of cortical sulci and interhemispheric fissures was found in 21 of 23 cases, which was reversed in 11 cases after weight gain. Psychological tests were carried out at the same time as the CT to correlate the changes in the brain tissue with brain function. The differences were significant.	The results indicate that AN is not only a psychodynamic problem, but also one in which an organic brain lesion plays an important role during the course of the illness.
CT	Artmann et al. [2]	AN: n = 35	To investigate whether cerebral dystrophic changes correlate with weight loss in patients with AN.	Cerebral dystrophic changes correlated with weight loss and the reversibility of these changes also correlated with the normalisation of body weight. The most numerous and pronounced enlargements were of the cortical sulci and the interhemispheric fissure. Moderate widening affected the ventricles. The rarest and most insignificant changes were found in the cerebellum.	The high incidence of early acquired minimal brain disease in patients with AN is discussed as a nonspecific predisposing factor. There is no explanation of the aetiology of the reversible enlargement of the CSF in AN and the changes resemble those in alcoholics. The mechanisms of brain changes in alcoholism seem to throw light on the probable mechanism of reversible dystrophic brain changes in AN.

(Continued)

Table 3.1 (*Continued*)

Method	Authors	Sample	Aim	Results	Discussion/conclusion
CT	Dolan *et al.* [3]	AN: n = 25 Controls: n = 17	To investigate further the cerebral structural appearance in patients with AN by comparison with a healthy normal control group and to ascertain the stability in the CT appearance on repeat scanning following the attainment of normal body weight.	Patients displayed significantly greater ventricular and sulcal enlargement compared to controls. No correlation was found between CT scan appearance and illness severity or weight loss. After body-weight restoration there were no signs of ventricular changes, but there was significantly less sulcal widening.	The finding of both ventricular and sulcal enlargement in a proportion of patients with AN is consistent with previous reports in the literature. The improvement in sulcal widening on refeeding is also in agreement with previous findings and would appear to indicate a reversible pathological process.
CT	Krieg *et al.* [9]	BN: n = 50 AN: n = 50 Controls: n = 50	To determine whether ventricular dilation and enlarged external CSF spaces are as common in BN as in AN.	Patients with BN had enlarged ventricles and/or sulcal widening, but to a lesser degree and frequency than in AN. In both BN and AN patients, ventricular size was inversely correlated with the plasma levels of triiodothyronine, a low concentration which is an indicator of starvation.	As the BN patients were of normal body weight, the CT abnormalities cannot be attributed to emaciation, which has often been suggested as the cause of abnormalities found in AN. Since many bulimic patients attempt to lose weight by going on restrictive diets, the morphological brain alterations may reflect the endocrine and metabolic reactions to extreme dieting.
CT	Laessle *et al.* [10]	AN: n = 17 BN: n = 22 Controls: n = 22	To clarify the relationship between cerebral atrophy and cognitive performance in AN and BN.	Patients performed poorly on cognitive tasks. Twenty patients (16 BN, 4 AN) had normal VBR values. 19 patients (6 BN, 13 AN) had abnormal VBR	As expected, patients with abnormal VBR values had a significantly lower BMI than patients in the normal VBR group. The results

				values. 19 patients (6 BN, 13 AN) had abnormal VBR values. Patients with ventricular dilatation did not perform worse on the cognitive tests than patients with normal-sized ventricles. Symptom severity and duration of illness were not correlated with ventricular size.	support the interpretation that cerebral atrophy does not have severe consequences for neuropsychological or psychopathological status in eating-disorder patients.
CT	Kiriike et al. [8]	BN: n = 17 Controls: n = 21	Previous MRI studies on VBR in BN patients are conflicting. Therefore, VBR was measured in BN patients using CT and compared with controls.	VBR was significantly greater in the BN group compared to controls. There was no correlation between VBR and clinical variables, or endocrine or metabolic parameters.	VBR was significantly greater in normal-weight bulimic patients than in controls. The mechanism for development of enlarged lateral ventricles in BN remains unclear. Further longitudinal studies of BN patients using serial CT scans and monitoring of endocrine and biochemical parameters are needed.
CT	Palazidou et al. [6]	AN: n = 17 Controls: n = 10	To investigate CT scan brain appearances and assess cognitive function.	AN patients had enlarged external CSF spaces compared to controls. There were no differences in ventricular size and X-ray absorption-density measurements. No differences were found in performance on neuropsychological tests between patients and controls. Significant negative correlation was found between performance on symbol digit test and CT scan changes.	Confirms the presence of enlargement of external CSF spaces in patients with AN, which are most likely related to the illness itself. These changes are not associated with abnormalities in brain-tissue absorption density for X-rays, and although cognitive testing showed no difference in mean scores between patients and controls, evidence of cognitive impairment on one test was significantly related to the scan abnormalities.

(Continued)

Table 3.1 (*Continued*)

Method	Authors	Sample	Aim	Results	Discussion/conclusion
CT and MRI	Kormreich *et al.* [4]	AN: MRI: n = 13, AN: CT: n = 11, Controls: n = 15	To evaluate the contribution of MRI to the investigation of brain abnormalities in AN, and to assess its ability to detect neoplastic or dystrophic changes not yet revealed by CT studies.	CT detected sulcal and ventricular enlargement in 5 of 11 AN patients. On the MR images, enlarged sulci were seen in 10 of 13 patients and dilated ventricles in 5 of 13. Overall, the patients had larger ventricles than the control group, but the difference was not significant. The number of visible cortical sulci was greater in the AN group, indicating peripheral volume loss in AN.	The CT findings of CSF-space enlargement in AN patients corroborate previous reports. MRI seems more sensitive than CT in detecting sulcal enlargement. No clear relationship was found between weight loss, duration of illness and amount of brain atrophy.
MRI	Hoffman *et al.* [17]	BN: n = 8 Controls: n = 8	To study cerebral atrophy in a group of bulimics with no previous anorectic history.	Sagittal cerebral : cranial ratio was significantly lower in the BN group than controls. Ventricle : brain ratio was not significantly different between groups.	The results show significant cerebral atrophy in normal-weight bulimic women, without any history of AN. Malnutrition seems unlikely as an explanation for the brain atrophy.
MRI	Doraiswamy *et al.* [19]	BN: n = 12 AN: n = 14 Controls: n = 14	To confirm preliminary MRI findings in an expanded sample of patients and to test the hypothesis that pituitary size and shape might be altered in patients with eating disorders.	Patients with eating disorders had significantly smaller pituitary glands than controls.	This study confirms previous MRI findings and provides further evidence of pituitary abnormalities in eating-disorder patients.

Modality	Study	Sample	Aim	Results	Conclusions
MRI	Husain et al. [18]	AN: n = 12 BN: n = 12 Controls: n = 11	To assess changes in midline subcortical structures and brainstem in patients with eating disorders.	AN patients showed smaller thalamus and midbrain area than BN patients and controls. Bulimics did not differ from controls. Ratios of thalamus : cerebral hemisphere and midbrain : cerebral hemisphere were different between AN patients and controls.	This study suggests it is possible that neuronal circuits involved in AN and BN may be different. The role of the midbrain is unclear. It may be that dopamine neurons in the midbrain are affected in AN, but further research is needed. Focal brain abnormalities may be involved in the aetiology or manifestation of AN.
MRI	Golden et al. [11]	AN: n = 12 Controls: n = 12	To determine the reversibility of the loss of brain parenchyma and ventricular enlargement in patients with AN after refeeding.	Total ventricular volume decreased after weight gain. The degree of enlargement of the third ventricle was larger than that of the lateral ventricles. There was a significant inverse relationship between BMI and total ventricular volume.	In AN, the cause of the structural changes remains unclear. Cerebral ventricular enlargement correlates with the degree of malnutrition and is reversible with weight gain during long-term follow-up.
MRI	Katzman et al. [12]	AN: n = 13 Controls: n = 8	To determine whether the increased CSF volumes found in AN are the results of differences in grey-matter or white-matter volume, or both.	AN patients had larger total CSF volume in association with deficits in both total grey-matter and total white-matter volume. Lowest reported BMI was inversely correlated with total CSF volume and positively correlated with total grey-matter volume.	The results support the view that the brain abnormalities found in AN are in large part the result of the effects of the illness. The extent to which the differences in grey-matter and white-matter volume are reversible with recovery remains to be established.

(Continued)

Table 3.1 (*Continued*)

Method	Authors	Sample	Aim	Results	Discussion/conclusion
MRI	Kingston et al. [13]	AN: n = 46 Controls: n = 41	To clarify the nature of the cognitive impairment exhibited by emaciated patients with AN. Also, to investigate brain morphology before and after weight gain and to explore the relationship between neuropsychological functioning and brain morphology against weight loss and duration of illness.	The AN group performed worse on attention, visuospatial ability and memory. There were no group differences in flexibility and learning. Following treatment and at least 10% weight gain, the AN group improved on attention tasks. AN patients had larger lateral ventricles and dilated sulci on both cortical and cerebellar surfaces, but no dilation was evident for the third and fourth ventricular measures.	Improvements were found after treatment, but on some of the radiological measures, many differences remained. Relationships between morphological brain changes and cognitive impairments are weak. Lower weight, but not duration of illness, is associated with poorer performance in tasks assessing flexibility/inhibition and memory, and with greater MRI ventricular size.
MRI	Swayze et al. [14]	Underweight AN patients: n = 8 BN: n = 1 EDNOS: n = 1 Controls: n = 10	(i) To demonstrate that automated methods reduce measurement errors in MRI. (ii) To quantify changes in brain and ventricular volume with greater precision and reliability. (iii) To measure both ventricular and brain volume in patients with eating disorders, at two time points.	AN patients had larger ventricles compared with controls, but did not differ in total brain volume. At follow-up scan after weight gain, ventricular volume decreased and total brain volume increased. The analyses showed that ventricular and total brain volumes derived from the initial/rescan pair were nearly identical, but that follow-up ventricular volume decreased significantly and total brain volume increased significantly after weight gain.	Provides clear evidence that nearly all patients with AN show some reversibility towards normal brain and ventricular volumes upon weight normalisation. Further studies are needed to clarify the mechanisms that lead to these brain changes and their functional significance in this psychiatric disorder.

MRI	Katzman *et al.* [15]	AN: n = 6 Controls: n = 16	To assess whether grey- and white-matter volume deficits described in patients with AN are fully reversible with weight rehabilitation.	White-matter and ventricular CSF volume changed significantly on weight-recovery from AN. Weight-recovered patients had grey-matter volume deficits and elevated CSF volumes compared to controls. They no longer had white-matter volume deficits.	The finding of persistent grey-matter volume deficits in weight-recovered patients suggests an irreversible component to structural brain changes associated with AN.
MRI	Lambe *et al.* [16]	AN weight-recovered: n = 12 AN low-weight: n = 13 Controls: n = 18	To test the hypothesis that subjects who are weight-recovered from AN will show elevated CSF volumes and reduced grey-matter volumes compared with controls.	The weight-recovered group had greater CSF volumes and smaller grey-matter volumes than controls. Compared with low-weight patients, weight-recovered subjects had smaller CSF volumes and larger grey- and white-matter volumes. In the weight-recovered group, neither CSF elevations nor grey-matter deficits were correlated with the length of time since weight recovery.	The persistent grey-matter volume deficits in weight-recovered subjects suggest that there may be an irreversible component to the brain changes associated with the illness.
MRI	Sieg *et al.* [64]	AN: n = 2	To observe previously unreported MRI alterations in two cases of AN.	The MRI brain scans revealed evidence of subcortical hyperintense changes on T2-weightened images.	No previous reports of these findings have been described in the literature on AN to date.

(Continued)

Table 3.1 (Continued)

Method	Authors	Sample	Aim	Results	Discussion/conclusion
MRI	Ellison et al. [34]	AN: n = 6 Controls: n = 6	To test whether patients with AN experiencing calorie fear would show a neural response similar to patients with simple phobias confronting their feared object, involving the anterior cingulate and left insula.	Results showed that calorie fear in AN is associated with activation in a limbic and paralimbic network.	The left amygdala hippocampal region may mediate conditioned fear to high-calorie foods, whereas the insula and anterior cingulate may be involved in autonomic arousal and attentional processes. Abnormal activity in the limbic/paralimbic system has also been associated with OCD and depressive symptoms, and may contribute to the increased rate of these symptoms in AN.
MRI	Giordano et al. [20]	AN: n = 20 Controls: n = 20	To evaluate the volume of the HAF in patients with AN, given this structure is a crucial target for the glucocorticoid action in the adaptive stress response.	AN patients showed a reduction of total (right + left) HAF volume compared with controls. There were no significant difference between left and right HAF in either AN or controls. In AN, there were no differences between HAF and hormononal parameters or BMI, while there was a trend towards an effect of duration of illness.	–
MRI	Wagner et al. [38]	AN: n = 13 Controls: n = 10	To replicate a previous pilot study with a larger sample, and examine distorted body image in patients with AN,	Subjects were presented with their own digitally distorted body images. AN patients showed a greater activation in the prefrontal cortex and the inferior	AN patients showed only a specific increase in activation to their own pictures compared to others, indicating different visuospatial

			with the hypothesis that there would be activation of the fear network and the attention network.	parietal lobule – including the anterior intraparietal sulcus – than controls.	processing, while controls did not differentiate.
MRI	McCormick et al. [65]	AN: n = 18 Controls: n = 18	To determine whether ACC volume is affected by starvation in active AN and if so, whether this had any clinical significance.	Right dorsal ACC volume was significantly reduced in active AN patients versus controls and was correlated with lower performance IQ. While ACC normalisation occurred with weight restoration, smaller change in right dorsal ACC volume prospectively predicted relapse after treatment.	Reduced right dorsal ACC volume during active AN relates to deficits in perceptual organisation and conceptual reasoning. The degree of right dorsal ACC normalisation during treatment is related to outcome.
MRI	Castro-Fornieles et al. [66]	AN: n = 12 Controls: n = 9	To examine whether cerebral volumes are reduced, and in what regions, in adolescents with AN, and to study changes after nutritional recovery.	The groups showed differences in grey-matter and CSF but not in white-matter volume. In AN patients, grey-matter volumes correlated negatively with the copy time from REY. In the regional study, several temporal and parietal grey-matter regions were reduced. During follow-up there was a greater global increase in grey matter and decrease in CSF in AN patients. The increase in grey matter correlated with a decrease in cortisol. At follow-up there were no differences in global grey-matter, white-matter or CSF volumes between the two groups. There were still some smaller areas, in the right temporal and both supplementary motor areas, showing differences between them in the regional study.	In adolescent AN patients, grey matter is more affected than white matter, mainly involving the posterior regions of the brain. Overall grey matter alterations are reversible after nutritional recovery.

(Continued)

Neuroimaging

Table 3.1 (*Continued*)

Method	Authors	Sample	Aim	Results	Discussion/conclusion
PET	Herholz et al. [67]	Female AN: n = 5 Male controls: n = 15	To measure regional cerebral glucose metabolism in patients with AN, during the anorectic state and after weight gain.	In AN patients, caudate hypermetabolism was found bilaterally, but not after weight gain or in controls. There were no differences between AN patients after improvements and normals.	Interpretation of the results remains speculative. To overcome problems of the multiplicity of tests and small sample size, the finding of caudate hypermetabolism needs to be confirmed in another patient series.
PET	Hagman et al. [68]	BN: n = 8 Major affective disorder: n = 8 Controls: n = 8	To compare brain metabolism in patients with BN, major depressive disorder and controls.	Controls had higher right than left cortical metabolic rates and active basal ganglia. BN patients lost the normal right activation in some areas, but maintained basal ganglia activity. Patients with major affective disorder retained right hemisphere activation, but had decreased metabolism in basal ganglia.	The results suggest that although women with BN frequently present with symptoms of depression, the pathophysiological changes associated with BN differ from those in major affective disorder.
PET	Wu et al. [51]	BN: n = 8 Controls: n = 8	To address the possibility of abnormalities of functional brain metabolism in BN while avoiding the possible artefacts of concurrent starvation.	Controls had higher metabolic rate in the right hemisphere than in the left. BN patients did not have this asymmetry.	Other studies have found lower metabolic rates in the basal ganglia in depressed subjects and higher rates in AN subjects, but this was not found in this study. The results suggest that BN is a diagnostic grouping distinct from these disorders.

PET	Krieg et al. [47]	BN: n = 9 AN: n = 7	To investigate whether patients with BN show increased glucose metabolism in the caudate nuclei as an abnormality characteristic of both AN and BN.	Relative caudate glucose metabolism was significantly higher in AN patients than in BN patients.	The results suggest that caudate hyperactivity is characteristic of the anorexic state. Whether it is a consequence of AN behaviour or directly involved in the pathogenesis of AN is still to be clarified.
PET	Andreason et al. [52]	BN: n = 11 Controls: n = 18	To further delineate the character of cerebral metabolism in BN and to determine whether functional links exist between regional cerebral metabolism and the symptoms of depression, OCD and BN.	BN patients showed correlation between lower left anterolateral prefrontal regional cerebral glucose metabolism and greater depressive symptoms. Orbitofrontal regional cerebral glucose metabolism in patients was not greater than in controls. High orbitofrontal metabolism was not correlated with greater OCD symptoms.	Left anterior lateral prefrontal cortex hypometabolism seems to vary with the depressive symptoms observed in BN. Temporal lobe hypermetabolism and asymmetries appear to be independent of mood state.
PET	Delvenne et al. [48]	AN: n = 20 Controls: n = 10	To investigate CMRglu in the basal ganglia and cortical areas in a large group of patients with AN. In addition, to evaluate the correlation with different clinical aspects such as weight loss, depression scores, anxiety and duration of illness.	Compared to controls, patients with AN showed hypometabolism globally and in cortical regions, with most significant differences found in the frontal and parietal cortices. There were no correlations between rCMRGlu and BMI, anxiety scores or Hamilton scores of depression.	Different factors might explain the reduction of glucose metabolism in AN. The authors suggest it may be the consequence of neuropsychological or morphological aspects of AN and/or the result of associated symptoms such as anxiety or depression. Supported by cognitive studies, they also hypothesise a primary corticocerebral dysfunction in AN.

(Continued)

Table 3.1 (*Continued*)

Method	Authors	Sample	Aim	Results	Discussion/conclusion
PET	Delvenne *et al.* [49]	AN: n = 10 Controls: n = 10	To evaluate the reversibility of brain glucose metabolism in AN patients in their underweight state and after weight gain.	In absolute values, AN patients showed global and regional hypometabolism of glucose, which normalised after weigh gain. In relative values, there were no global differences between the groups. But there was a trend towards parietal and superior frontal cortex hypometabolism associated with a relative hypermetabolism in the caudate nuclei and the inferior frontal cortex. After weight gain, all regions normalised for absolute and relative values, although there was a trend in AN of relative parietal hypometabolism and inferior frontal cortex hypermetabolism.	Absolute brain glucose metabolism might result from neuroendocrinological or morphological aspects of AN or from altered neurotransmission following deficient nutritional state. Some differences persist after weight gain, which could support potential abnormal cerebral functioning, different reactions to starvation within several regions of the brain or different restoration rates according to the region.
PET	Delvenne *et al.* [53]	BN: n = 11 Controls: n = 11	To evaluate, at rest, brain glucose metabolism in BN patients.	In absolute values, BN patients showed global and regional hypometabolism of glucose. In relative values, parietal cortex metabolism was lower in BN. There was no correlation within groups between absolute or relative cerebral glucose metabolic rates and BMI, anxiety scores or Hamilton scores of depression.	These observations may be a consequence of neurobiological perturbations following nutritional deficiencies or a particular cerebral dysfunction in eating disorders.

	Delvenne et al. [50]	AN: n = 10 Underweight, depressed, without AN: n = 10 Controls: n = 10	To evaluate the impact of weight loss on cerebral glucose metabolism evaluated by PET.	In absolute values, global and regional glucose activity was significantly lower in AN and low-weight depressed patients than in controls. In relative values, AN showed lower metabolism of glucose in parietal cortex compared to controls.	Absolute hypometabolism of glucose seems to be a consequence of low weight, while there is a positive correlation between absolute metabolism of glucose and BMI.
PET	Delvenne et al. [69]	BN: n = 10 AN: n = 10	To compare brain glucose metabolism at rest in patients with AN and BN.	Absolute global cortical glucose activity was lower in AN patients compared to BN patients and controls. AN compared to controls showed higher relative cerebral glucose metabolism in the inferior parietal cortex and basal ganglia, and putamen and caudate relative hypermetabolism compared with BN. Both AN and BN had low relative parietal values of glucose.	While absolute global metabolism seems to be related to weight loss, the authors hypothesise either a common parietal cortex dysfunction in eating disorders or a particular sensitivity of this cortex to consequences of eating disturbances.
PET	Gordon et al. [70]	AN: n = 8 Controls: n = 8	To delineate functional brain abnormalities associated with AN.	Subjects were exposed to three types of stimulus: high- and low-calorie foods and nonfood items. In the high-calorie condition: controls reported desire to eat, AN patients reported elevated anxiety and exhibited increased heart rate. AN patients also showed elevated bilateral medial temporal lobe rCBF compared with control subjects.	Elevated rCBF in bilateral medial temporal lobes is similar to results in patients with psychotic disorder and may be related to body-image distortion in AN.

(Continued)

Table 3.1 (*Continued*)

Method	Authors	Sample	Aim	Results	Discussion/conclusion
PET	Kaye *et al.* [57]	BN recovered: n = 9 Controls: n = 12	To confirm that 5-HT alterations are present in patients who have recovered from BN.	Controls had an age-related decline in 5-HT2A binding. Patients recovered from BN had a reduction of medial orbital frontal cortex 5-HT2A binding.	The lack of age-related changes in 5-HT activity is further evidence of 5-HT alterations in subjects recovered from BN. Vulnerabilities for eating disorders including impulse dyscontrol and mood disturbances may involve 5-HT and frontal lobe activity.
PET	Frank *et al.* [54]	AN recovered: n = 16 Controls: n = 11	To investigate 5-HT2A, which could contribute to disturbances of appetite and behaviour in AN.	Patients who had recovered from AN had significantly reduced (F18) altanserin-binding relative to controls in mesial temporal (amygdala and hippocampus) as well as cingulate cortical regions.	Altered 5-HT neuronal system activity persists after recovery from AN, and may be related to disturbances of mesial temporal lobe function.
PET	Bailer *et al.* [55]	BN recovered: n = 10 Controls: n = 16	To investigate 5-HT2A, which could contribute to disturbances of appetite and behaviour in AN.	Patients recovered from BN had significantly reduced (^{18}F) altanserin-binding potential relative to controls in the left subgenual cingulate, left parietal cortex and right occipital cortex. (^{18}F) altanserin-binding potential was positively related to harm-avoidance and negatively correlated to novelty-seeking in cingulate and temporal regions in patients recovered from BN. Patients	This study suggests that altered 5-HT neuronal system activity persists after recovery from BN, particularly in subgenual cingulate regions. Altered 5-HT neurotransmission after recovery supports that this might be a trait-related disturbance that contributes to the pathophysiology of eating disorders.

PET	Tiihonen et al. [59]	BN: n = 8 Controls: n = 10	To measure brain 5-HT1A receptor binding among nonmedicated patients with BN.	The binding potential value of 5-HT1A was greater in patients than in controls in all brain regions studied. The most robust differences were observed in the angular gyrus, the medial prefrontal cortex and the posterior cingulate cortex.	recovered from BN had a negative relationship between (¹⁸F) altanserin-binding potential and drive for thinness in several cortical regions. The results suggest that brain 5-HT1A receptor binding is increased in several cortical areas in BN patients during their state of impulsive binge eating. This widespread increase in cortical areas might reflect dysregulation of the overall 5-HT1A activity and might be associated with impaired impulse control during the state of impulsive binge eating, rather than specifically due to BN per se.
PET	Bailer et al. [58]	AN recovered: n = 13 BAN recovered: n = 12 Controls: n = 18	To characterise the 5-HT1A system in AN.	Patients recovered from BAN had increased binding potential in cingulate, lateral and mesial temporal, temporal and medial orbital frontal, parietal and prefrontal cortical regions and the dorsal raphe compared to controls. For patients recovered from AN, postsynaptic receptor binding in mesial temporal and subgenual cingulated regions was positively correlated to harm-avoidance.	The results led to the conclusion that increased 5HT1A receptor binding was observed in patients recovered from BAN but not those recovered from AN. However, 5HT1A receptor binding was associated with a measure of anxiety in women recovered from AN. Altered serotonergic function and anxiety symptoms persist after recovery from AN. These alterations might be trait-related and may contribute to the pathogenesis of AN.

(Continued)

Table 3.1 (*Continued*)

Method	Authors	Sample	Aim	Results	Discussion/conclusion
PET	Frank *et al.* [60]	AN recovered: n = 10 Controls: n = 12	To assess DA D2/D3 receptor function in AN.	Patients recovered from AN had higher raclopide binding potential in the antero ventral striatum than controls. For patients recovered from AN, raclopide-binding potential was positively related to harm-avoidance in the dorsal caudate and dorsal putamen.	The results support the possibility that intrasynaptic DA concentration or increased D2/D3 receptor density or affinity is associated with AN and might contribute to the characteristic harm-avoidance or increased physical activity found in AN. It is also possible that AN patients might have a DA-related disturbance of reward mechanisms in contributing to altered hedonics of feeding behaviour and their ascetic, anhedonic temperament.
PET	Bailer *et al.* [71]	AN recovered: n = 11 BAN recovered: n = 7 BN recovered: n = 9 Controls: n = 10	To use PET to determine whether alterations of 5-HT persist after recovery from BN and AN. A secondary aim was to examine the possible effects of the functional polymorphism in the promoter region of the 5-HT transporter genes on in vivo expression of 5-HT in controls and patients recovered from eating disorders.	PET was used to assess the 5-HT transporters. Results showed significant differences between the four groups in the dorsal raphe and anteroventral striatum. Patients recovered from AN had significantly increased (11C) McN5652 BP compared to patients recovered from BAN in these regions.	Divergent 5-HT activity in subtypes of eating-disorder subjects may provide important insights as to why these groups have differences in affective regulation and impulse control.

PET	Bailer et al. [72]	AN: n = 15 Controls: n = 29	To characterise the 5-HT1A and 5-HT2A receptors in patients with AN.	Patients with AN had increases in (11C)WAY100635 BP prefrontal and lateral orbital frontal regions, mesial and lateral temporal lobes, parietal cortex and dorsal raphe nuclei compared with controls. The (^{18}F) altanserin BP was normal in AN but was positively and significantly related to harm avoidance in suprapragenual cingulate, frontal and parietal regions.	Increased 5-HT1A receptor activity may help explain poor response to 5-HT medication in ill AN patients. This study extends data suggesting that 5-HT function, and specifically the 5-HT2A receptor, is related to anxiety in AN.
PET	Frank et al. [73]	AN recovered: n = 10 AN recovered with bingeing history: n = 8 BN recovered: n = 9 Controls: n = 18	To investigate rCBF in long-term recovered BN and AN patients.	Partial volume corrected rCBF values in cortical and subcortical regions were similar between groups. Neither current BMI nor age correlated with rCBF values.	The results indicate that rCBF normalises with long-term recovery.
PET	Galusca et al. [74]	AN: n = 8 AN recovered: n = 9 Controls: n = 7	To evaluate the hypothesis of particular (^{18}F) MPPF-binding in subjects with AN.	AN had increased MPFF binding in a selective area of the right cortex, including part of the superior temporal gyrus, inferior frontal gyrus, parietal operculum and temporoparietal junction. Regional similarities of increased MPFF binding were found in recovered AN patients. Most psychiatric scores were increased in AN. Elevated perfectionism and interpersonal distrust scores were noticed in recovered AN patients.	The persistent increased 5-HT1A receptor binding in the frontotemporal region of recovered AN patients concomitant with specific psychopathological traits supports the hypothesis of an organic dysfunction of this area and corroborates previous literature reports of AN cases induced by temporal lesions.

(Continued)

Table 3.1 (*Continued*)

Method	Authors	Sample	Aim	Results	Discussion/conclusion
SPECT	Krieg *et al.* [9]	AN: n = 12	To find out whether there could be some functional correlate to structural brain alterations.	The majority of the patients displayed ventricular dilation and/or sulcal widening. rCBF was measured at admission and after weight gain. There was an inverse relationship between the size of the CSF spaces and the CBF in AN. A decrease in ventricular space after weight gain was associated with an increase in CBF in this area.	These findings must be interpreted with caution, as partial volume effects render the flow rates ambiguous in brain areas, which, in addition to neuronal tissue, also include ventricular and sulcal structures. SPECT yields no suggestion that there is any reduced functioning in certain brain areas in patients with AN.
SPECT	Nozoe *et al.* [28]	BN: n = 5 AN: n = 8 Controls: n = 9	To examine the characteristics of rCBF in patients with BN, AN and controls.	BN patients showed signs of higher R (corrected ratio for rCBF) before (food-intake stimulus) values in the bilateral inferior frontal and left temporal regions. AN patients showed lower before values in the left parietal region than controls. There were no differences in R after food-intake stimulus among the three groups.	The findings indicate that differences in cerebral function of BN and AN can be characterised through SPECT imaging.
SPECT	Kuruoglu *et al.* [23]	AN: n = 2	To investigate CBF of two patients with AN, both at the time of diagnosis and after remission of symptoms.	Pre-treatment there was a diffuse bilateral hypoperfusion in frontal, parietal and frontotemporal areas, which was more prominent in the left hemisphere. Post-treatment (obtained	This technique may be used to follow up the effect of treatment and predict the clinical response to therapy in patients with eating disorders. However, further research

		Sample	Aim	Results	
				after a clinical remission period of three months) both patients had normal brain perfusion.	is needed to clarify the relationship between the psychopathological features of these disorders and the neurophysiological cerebral cortex.
SPECT	Naruo et al. [24]	AN: n = 7 Binge–purge AN: n = 7 Controls: n = 7	To investigate the effect of imaging food on the rCBF of AN patients with and without habitual binge–purge behaviour.	Patients with binge–purge AN had greater changes in inferior, superior, prefrontal and parietal regions of the right brain than patients with AN and controls.	Specific activation in cortical regions suggests an association between habitual binge–purge behaviour and the food-recognition process linked to anxiety in AN patients.
SPECT	Naruo et al. [75]	Restricting AN: n = 7 BAN: n = 7 Controls: n = 7	To investigate localised differences of brain blood flow in AN patients in an attempt to link brain blood-flow patterns to neurophysiological characteristics.	The blood flow of frontal area mainly containing bilateral ACC was significantly decreased in the AN group compared to the BAN and control groups.	These findings suggest that some localised functions of the ACC may be relevant to the psychopathological aspects of AN.
SPECT	Rastam et al. [25]	AN: n = 21, 19/21 weight-restored Controls: n = 9	To compare rCBF in a group of individuals with AN to a group of individuals free from eating disorders and neurological disorders.	Former patients with AN showed marked hypoperfusion of temporal, parietal, occipital and orbitofrontal lobes compared to controls. rCBF was not correlated to BMI.	The results suggest that AN may be associated with moderate to severe CBF hypoperfusion in the temporoparietal region and the orbitofrontal region.
SPECT	Takano et al. [26]	AN: n = 14 Controls: n = 14	To compare cerebral perfusion in patients with AN and healthy volunteers.	AN showed hypoperfusion in medial prefrontal cortex and the anterior cingulate gyrus, and hyperperfusion in the thalamus and the amygdala–hippocampus complex.	The results suggest that a dysfunction in neuronal circuitry may be related to AN.

(Continued)

Table 3.1 (*Continued*)

Method	Authors	Sample	Aim	Results	Discussion/conclusion
SPECT	Tauscher *et al.* [76]	BN: n = 10 Controls: n = 10	To investigate the in vivo availability of brain serotonin transporters and dopamine transporters in BN patients.	BN patients showed 17% reduced brain serotonin transporter availability in the hypothalamus and thalamus compared to controls, and a similar reduction in striatal dopamine transporter availability. There was a negative correlation of illness duration and serotonin transporter availability and a strong positive correlation between hypothalamic/thalamic and striatal transporter availability.	The results suggest that there is a reduced hypothalamic and thalamic serotonin transporter availability in BN, which is more pronounced with longer duration of illness.
SPECT	Audenaert *et al.* [77]	AN: n = 15 Controls: n = 11	To evaluate the 5-HT2a BI in patients with AN.	AN patients had signs of reduced 5-HT2a binding index in the left frontal cortex, the left and right parietal cortex and the left and right occipital cortex. A significant left–right asymmetry (left < right) was noted in the frontal cortex.	The results are in accordance with diminished metabolic activity and perfusion of frontal and parietal cortices reported in recent neuroimaging studies, and imply localised serotonergic function.
SPECT	Chowdhury *et al.* [32]	AN: n = 15	To understand the pathophysiology of the brain in early-onset AN, and attempt to validate findings from an earlier study of	Eleven patients had asymmetry (hypoperfusion) of blood flow in at least one area. These regions included temporal, parietal and frontal lobe, thalamus and the caudate nuclei.	Most patients had abnormal rCBF, predominantly affecting the temporal lobe. These results support earlier suggestions of imbalance of neuronal pathways

SPECT			rCBF and correlate abnormalities in blood flow with eating-disorder psychopathology.	Patients with hypoperfusion had higher median EDE score than those without, although not statistically significant.	or circuits, possible within the limbic system.
SPECT	Key et al [27]	AN = 11 Controls = 11	To determine whether consistent functional abnormalities of the brain exist in a homogeneous sample of women with AN.	Hypoperfusion was demonstrated in the anterior temporal lobe and/or caudate nuclei in 8 of 11 patients. No hypoperfusion was identified in the control group.	The findings in this adult cohort were very similar to those in studies of children and adolescents with AN and significantly different from controls. Cortical involvement in the pathogenesis of AN is postulated and further research requirements are outlined.
SPECT	Yonezawa et al. [30]	Restricting AN: n = 13 Binge–purge AN: n = 13 Controls: n = 10	To investigate the differences in CBF in restricting AN, binge–purge AN and controls.	The results showed bilateral decreased perfusion of the SCG, midbrain and PCG in both restricting AN and binge–purge AN compared to controls. There were no signs of differences in CBF between restricting AN and binge–purge AN.	Analyses of the resting SPECT images found no sign of differences between patients with restricting AN and binge–purge AN. Abnormalities of the neuronal circuits containing the SCG, midbrain and PCG may be relevant to trait-related AN.
SPECT	Beato-Fernandez et al. [29]	AN: n = 9 BN: n = 13 Controls: n = 12	To investigate the relationship between perceptual distortion and cognitive-evaluation components of body-image disturbances to brain activity.	AN patients showed a hyperactivation of the right temporal and right occipital areas. Changes in BSQ were associated with changes in the right inferior frontal and right temporal rCBF, whereas changes in body distortion were related to the left parietal lobe.	The activation of the right temporal lobe after own-body-image exposure may be in accordance with the aversive-events response. Functional abnormalities in AN may be related to the storage of a distorted prototypical image of the body in the left parietal lobe.

(Continued)

Table 3.1 (*Continued*)

Method	Authors	Sample	Aim	Results	Discussion/conclusion
fMRI	Ellison *et al.* [34]	AN: n = 6 Controls: 6	To test the hypothesis that AN patients experiencing calorie fear will show a neural response similar to patients with simple phobias confronting their feared object, involving the anterior cingulate and left insula.	The results provided evidence that calorie fear in people with AN is associated with activation in a limbic and paralimbic network.	The left amygdala hippocampal region may mediate conditioned fear to high-calorie foods, whereas the insula and anterior cingulate may be involved in autonomic arousal and attentional processes. Abnormal activity in the limbic/paralimbic system has also been associated with obsessive–compulsive and depressive symptoms, and may therefore contribute to the increased rate of these symptoms in AN.
fMRI	Uher *et al.* [35]	AN long-term recovered: n = 9 AN chronically ill: n = 8 Controls: n = 9	To identify functional neural correlates associated with differential outcomes.	Brain reaction to food and visual stimuli was measured. In recovered AN patients there was an increase in medial and prefrontal and anterior cingulate activation, as well as lack of activity in the parietal lobule, compared to controls. Recovered AN patients differed from chronically ill subjects in their increased activation of the right lateral prefrontal, apical prefrontal and dorsal ACC.	Separate neural correlates underlie trait and state characteristics of AN. The medial prefrontal response to disease-specific stimuli may be related to trait vulnerability.

| fMRI | Uher et al. [36] | BN: n = 10 AN: n = 16 Controls: n = 19 | To identify neural correlates of eating disorders in order to contribute to the debate on the genesis and classification of eating disorders and provide endophenotypes for genetic research. | Subjects were presented with food and aversive emotional images. Women with AN and BN identified the food stimuli as threatening and disgusting. They had greater activation in the left medial orbitofrontal and anterior cingulate cortices and less activation in the lateral prefrontal cortex, inferior parietal lobule and cerebellum, relative to controls. BN patients had less activation in the lateral and apical prefrontal cortex. | A medial prefrontal response to symptom-provoking stimuli was identified as a common feature of AN and BN. This finding supports that eating disorders are transdiagnostic at a neural level. An abnormal propepensity to activate medial prefrontal circuits in response to inappropriate stimuli is common to eating, obsessive–compulsive and addictive disorders and may account for the compulsive features of behaviour in these conditions. |
| fMRI | Uher et al. [78] | BN: n = 9 AN: n = 13 Controls: n = 18 | To measure brain responses to line drawings of underweight, normal-weight and overweight female bodies, while participants rated the stimuli for fear and disgust. | In all three groups, the lateral fusiform gyrus, inferior parietal cortex and lateral prefrontal cortex were activated in response to body shapes compared to control condition (drawings of houses). Responses in lateral fusiform gyrus and the parietal cortex were less strong in patients with eating disorders than in controls. Patients rated the body shapes in all weight categories as more aversive than did controls. The aversion ratings correlated positive with activity in the right medial apical prefrontal cortex. | Processing of female body shapes engages a distributed neural network, parts of which are underactive in women with eating disorders. The variability in subjective emotional reaction to body shapes in patients with eating disorders is associated with activity in the right medial apical prefrontal cortex. |

(Continued)

Table 3.1 (*Continued*)

Method	Authors	Sample	Aim	Results	Discussion/conclusion
fMRI	Frank *et al.* [45]	BN recovered: n = 10 Controls: n = 6	To find out whether BN patients have alterations in the physiological response to the blind administration of glucose.	Recovered BN patients had lower activation in the right ACC and in the left cuneus when glucose was administered compared with artificial saliva.	The ACC plays a role in the anticipation of reward. Recovered BN patients may have a reduced reward response to nutrients, and thus be vulnerable to overeating.
fMRI	Santel *et al.* [37]	AN: n = 13 Controls: n = 10	To explore the neural correlates of AN-specific cognitions to food by investigating the differential impact of hunger and satiety in two separate sessions.	When satiated, AN patients showed decreased activation in left inferior parietal cortex relative to controls. When hungry, AN patients displayed weaker activation of the right visual occipital cortex than controls. Food stimuli during satiety compared with hunger were associated with stronger right occipital activation in patients and with stronger activation in left lateral orbitofrontal cortex, the middle portion of the right anterior cingulate and left middle temporal gyrus in controls.	Differences in the fMRI activation to food pictures point to decreased food-related somatosensory processing in AN during satiety and to attentional mechanisms during hunger that might facilitate restricted eating in AN.
fMRI	Uher *et al.* [79]	Healthy nonsmokers: n = 18; 10 men, 8 women	To examine the neural circuitry responsible for integration of internal and external determinants of human eating behaviour, by	When fasted, subjects reported more hunger, nervousness and worse mood, and rated the visual food-related stimuli as more pleasant. The effect of fasting on hunger was stronger in	The results led to the conclusion that food reactivity in modality-specific sensory cortical areas is modulated by internal motivational states. The stronger

			measuring brain responses to visual and complex gustatory food-related stimuli using fMRI. Subjects were tested after eating and after 24 hours of fasting.	women than in men. No circuitry was identified as differentially responsive in fasting compared to satiety to both visual and gustatory food-related stimuli. The left insula response to the gustatory stimuli was stronger during fasting.	reactivity to external food-related stimuli in women may be explored as a marker of gender-related susceptibility to eating disorders.
fMRI	Wagner et al. [40]	Restricting AN recovered: n = 13 Controls: n = 13	To assess the response of the anterior ventral striatum to reward and loss in this disorder.	Recovered AN patients showed greater hemodynamic activation in the caudate than controls. Recovered AN patients showed a positive relationship between trait anxiety and the percentage change in the hemodynamic signal in the caudate during both wins and losses in the reward task. In the anterior ventral striatum, controls distinguished positive and negative feedback whereas recovered AN patients had similar responses.	Recovered AN patients might have difficulties in differentiating positive and negative feedback. The authors hypothesise that AN patients have an imbalance in information processing.
fMRI	Redgrave et al. [42]	AN: n = 6 Controls: n = 6	To measure brain activation in patients with AN and controls performing a novel emotional Stroop task using fat, thin and neutral words and words made of XXXXs.	Reaction times increased in the patient group in thin and fat conditions. In the thin–XXXX contrast, patients showed greater activation than controls at the junction of left insula, frontal and temporal lobes and in left middle and medial frontal gyri. In the fat–XXXX contrast, controls showed greater activation in left dorsalateral prefrontal cortex and right parietal areas.	Mechanisms underlying attentional bias in AN likely differ under conditions of positive and negative valence. This paradigm is a promising tool to examine neural mediation of emotional response in AN.

(Continued)

Table 3.1 (Continued)

Method	Authors	Sample	Aim	Results	Discussion/conclusion
fMRI	Sachdev et al. [39]	AN: n = 10 Controls: n = 10	To examine whether brain processing of an image of self is different in the brains of AN patients.	Processing of nonself images by control subjects activated the inferior and middle frontal gyri, superior and inferior parietal lobules, posterior lobe of the cerebellum and the thalamus. Patients had a similar pattern of activation, with greater activation in the medial frontal gyrus. When the two groups were contrasted for the differential activation with self- versus nonself-images, control subjects had greater activation than patients in the middle frontal gyri, insula, precuneus and occipital regions, while the patients did not have greater activation in any region. AN patients had no significant regions of activation with self-images compared to baseline.	The results led to the conclusion that AN patients process nonself-images similarly to control subjects, but their processing of self-images is quite discrepant, with a lack of activation of the attentional system in the insula. Such discrepant emotional and perceptual processing may underlie the distortion of self-images by AN patients.
fMRI	Wagner et al. [41]	AN recovered: n = 16 Controls: n = 16	To examine whether there is a primary disturbance of taste processing and experience of pleasure using a sucrose/water task in conjunction with fMRI.	Neural activation was tested in primary and secondary taste cortical regions after sucrose and water administration using ROI-based fMRI. Recovered AN patients showed lower activation in the insula, including the primary cortical taste region, and ventral and dorsal striatum to both sucrose and water.	Patients with AN process taste stimuli differently than controls, based on differences in neural activation patterns.

fMRI	Zastrow et al. [43]	AN: n = 15 Controls: n = 15	To investigate the neural correlates of cognitive-behavioural flexibility in executive functioning in AN, by using a target-detection task. This task distinguishes between shifts in behavioural response and shifts in cognitive set.	AN patients showed significantly higher error rate in shifting behavioural response, including reduced activation in the left and right thalamus, ventral striatum, anterior cingulate cortex, sensorimotor brain regions and the cerebellum.	Impaired behavioural response shifting in AN seems to be associated with hypoactivation in the ventral anterior cingulate–striato–thalamic loop that is involved in motivation-related behaviour. In contrast, AN patients showed predominant activation of frontoparietal networks, which is indicative of effortful and supervisory cognitive control during task performance.
fMRI	Mohr et al. [80]	AN: n = 16 Controls: n = 16	To investigate the neural correlates of two parts of the own-body-image using fMRI: satisfaction rating and size estimation for distorted own-body photographs in patients with AN and controls.	AN patients were less satisfied with their current body shape than controls. Patients demonstrated stronger activation of the insula and lateral prefrontal cortex during the satisfaction rating of thin self-images. This indicated a stronger emotional involvement when patients were presented with distorted images close to their own ideal body size. Patients also overestimated their own body size. There were complex differential modulations in activation of the precuneus during body-size estimation in control and AN patients. It could be speculated that a deficit in the retrieval of a multimodal coded body schema in precuneus/posterior parietal cortex is related to body-size overestimation.	Specific behavioural responses and neural-activation patterns for two parts of body image in AN and healthy controls were found. The results underline the importance of developing research and therapeutic strategies that target the two different aspects of body image separately.

(Continued)

Table 3.1 (*Continued*)

Method	Authors	Sample	Aim	Results	Discussion/conclusion
fMRI	Wagner *et al.* [46]	BN recovered: n = 10 Controls: n = 10	To test the hypothesis that disturbances in reward systems may contribute to vulnerability to development of an eating disorder.	For the AVS, which is known to be activated by a monetary-reward task, controls distinguished positive and negative feedback. Recovered BN patients had similar responses to both conditions.	Previous findings show that recovered AN patients also have altered striatal responses and difficulties in differentiating positive and negative feedback. AN and BN may share a difficulty in discriminating the emotional significance of a stimulus.
MRS	Roser *et al.* [81]	AN and BN: n = 20 Controls: n = 15	To investigate the brains of patients with AN and BN by localised proton magnetic resonance spectroscopy (1H-MRS) and to look for metabolic alterations.	There were signs of decrease of both myo-inositol and lipid compounds within the frontal white matter in patients compared to controls. The concentration of these compounds was reduced with decreasing BMI. Reduced lipid signals were also found in the occipital grey matter. In the cerebellum, the concentration of all metabolites, except lipids, was increased.	The metabolic changes seem to be a consequence of nutritional deficiency. It has to be further investigated whether these findings have any relevance for brain function. 1H-MRS might serve as a valuable investigation tool to observe eating disorders and to follow the success of therapy.

| MRS | Schlemmer et al. [82] | AN: n = 12 Controls: n = 17 | To investigate potential alterations in localised proton magnetic resonance (1H-MR) spectra of patients with AN immediately after an interval of excessive weight loss. | Significantly higher signal-intensity ratios of choline-containing compounds relative to total creatine as well as lower ratios of N-acetyl-aspartate relative to choline-containing compounds were found in the white-matter region. | The results may indicate an abnormal starvation-associated membrane turnover, which predominantly takes place in the white matter. |

CT = computed tomography; MRI = magnetic resonance imaging; MRS = magnetic resonance spectroscopy; PET = positron emission tomography; SPECT = single-photon emission computed tomography; fMRI = functional magnetic resonance imaging; AN = anorexia nervosa; AVS = anterior ventral striatum; BAN = bulimia-type AN; BI = binding index; BMI = body mass index; BN = bulimia nervosa; BSQ = Body Shape Questionnaire; CBF = cerebral blood flow; CMRglu = cerebral glucose metabolic rates; CSF = cerebrospinal fluid; DA = dopamine; EDE = eating disorder examination; HAF = hippocampus–amygdala formation; MPFF = methoxyphenyl ligand; PCG = posterior cingulated gyrus; PMRS = proton magnetic resonance spectroscopy; rCBF = regional cerebral blood flow; REY = Rey Complex Figure; SCG = subcallosal gyrus; VBR = ventricular brain ratio.

Structural neuroimaging techniques can reveal the extent to which myelin-rich areas of the brain containing bundles of axons (the white matter) are reduced as a result of starvation and, importantly, how well they recover following weight restoration. These techniques can also be used to explore how parts of the brain with dense connections between neuronal cell bodies (the grey matter) are affected. Studies of brain structure have therefore explored the relationship between the amount of change in the brain and overall body weight, and looked for links between brain structure and the characteristic cognitive and behavioural features of eating disorders.

Computerised tomography

One of the first methods developed for structural brain imaging was CT, a medical imaging X-ray method employing tomography (imaging by sections created by computer processing). Digital geometric processing is used to generate a three-dimensional image of the inside of an object from a large series of two-dimensional X-ray images. Characteristics of the internal structure of the object such as its dimensions, shape, internal defects and density are readily available from CT images. These images are helpful in allowing clinicians to assess damage to soft-tissue structures and to identify areas of brain-tissue damage (infarction), solid space-occupying lesions (tumours) and blood-supply damage (haemorrhage). In the study of eating disorders, CT scans have been used to investigate overall brain structure and total brain volume.

Because a CT scan is built up from a number of individual X-ray images, there is a radiation risk associated with its use. It has been calculated that CT scans come with a small but measurable additional risk of cancer, especially for children (the lifetime risk of fatal cancer for a North American child younger than 15 years has been calculated to increase from a baseline of approximately 700 in 3000 to about 701 in 3000 after undergoing a CT examination as an infant; [1]). Because of this non-negligible risk, CT scans are less commonly used today than other structural scanning approaches not requiring radiation.

CT research findings

Studies using CT have consistently reported abnormal findings in the ventricles and the sulci of patients with eating disorders. The ventricular system is a set of four fluid-filled cavities in the brain that contain cerebrospinal fluid (CSF). Compared to healthy controls, patients with anorexia nervosa (AN) often have dilated ventricles [2–6]. The sulci are deep fissures, or furrows, located on the cortical surface of the brain. Like the ventricles, the sulci are often enlarged in patients with AN [2–5, 7]. Similar results have also been reported in patients with bulimia nervosa (BN), but to a lesser degree and frequency than in patients with AN [8, 9].

In addition to ventricular and sulcal dilatation, significant enlargement of the interhemispheric fissure has been observed in AN [2, 7]. This is one of the major fissures in the brain, leading down as far as the corpus callosum (the band of fibres that connects the left and right hemispheres) and effectively dividing it into two halves through the midline in the sagittal plane.

All these related findings (dilated ventricles, enlarged sulci and enlarged interhemispheric fissure) are indicators of an overall reduction in brain volume. As the brain shrinks due to lack of nutrition, the fluid-filled ventricles and sulcal gaps between folds of the cortex enlarge to take up the additional space. Structural imaging studies using CT have enabled identification of the specific anatomical features of such 'brain shrinkage' or cerebral atrophy in patients with AN compared to healthy subjects. CT imaging reveals a loss of neuronal cell bodies (grey matter) and a reduction in the density of the synaptic connections between them (white matter).

Are these changes a result of weight loss, and do they reverse with nutritional restoration? In one of the first reported CT studies by Artmann *et al.* [2], these characteristic cerebral changes were correlated with weight loss in 35 patients with AN and were fully reversed with normalisation of body weight. In another study [7], enlargement of both cortical sulci and the interhemispheric fissure was reversed in about half of 21 patients after weight gain.

In a study of 25 patients with AN, Dolan *et al.* [3] found significantly greater ventricular and sulcal enlargement compared to 17 matched controls. However, there was no correlation between CT scan appearance and illness severity or weight loss. After the patients had regained their premorbid body weight, the ventricular changes had resolved, but significant differences between groups in the extent of sulcal widening persisted.

Krieg *et al.* [5] found a correlation between ventricular size and body weight in 70% of 50 patients with AN compared to controls with personality or adjustment disorders, but no relationship with duration of illness. In a further study including a group of 50 patients with BN, they also found enlarged ventricles and/or sulcal widening, but to a lesser degree and frequency than in AN. In both BN and AN, ventricular size was inversely correlated with plasma levels of triiodothyronine, an endocrine marker of starvation. They concluded that in eating disorders, morphological brain alteration may reflect the endocrine and metabolic reactions to starvation.

To explore whether such changes in brain tissue identified by CT scanning are related to changes in brain function, Laessle *et al.* [10] compared patients with AN and BN to healthy controls. They divided their clinical groups into 20 patients with normal ventricular : brain ratios (VBRs), of whom 4 had AN and 16 BN, and 19 patients with abnormal VBR values (13 AN, 6 BN). There were no differences between the groups in performance on a range of cognitive tests. Laessle *et al.* concluded that cerebral atrophy does not have severe consequences for the neuropsychological or psychopathological status of patients with eating disorders.

Finally, Palzidou *et al.* [6] compared the CT scans of 17 patients with AN and 10 controls. They found that the patients had significantly enlarged external CSF spaces compared to controls, but there were no differences in ventricular size or X-ray absorption density measurements. They also found a significant negative correlation between performance on the digit symbol test (a measure of brain processing speed) and their documented CT scan changes, suggesting that there was a link between changes in brain structure and functioning.

Summary

Studies using CT scanning have frequently reported enlargement of the ventricles, sulci and interhemispheric fissure in patients with AN (and to a lesser extent, BN), which seems to reverse with weight restoration in the majority of cases. Concomitant cerebral atrophy in white and grey matter observed in patients with AN also reverses with weight gain in most cases. No correlation has been reported between the extent of ventricular enlargement and duration of illness or performance on cognitive tests.

Magnetic resonance imaging

MRI is a medical imaging technique that can be used to visualise the internal structures of the body by using strong magnetic fields to create images of biological tissue and fluid (see Figure 3.1). One of the major advantages of MRI over CT scanning is that no radiation is used. MRI scanners contain powerful electromagnets that are super-cooled to produce large static magnetic fields (the M in MRI) into which a second fluctuating-radiofrequency electromagnetic field is introduced at a specific frequency to *resonate* with a particular tissue type or fluid (the R in MRI). This 'pulse' causes protons in the tissue or fluid to flip to a high-energy state; when the pulse is removed, this energy is emitted, detected by the scanner and processed to produce an *image* of the tissue or fluid (the I in MRI). MRI scanning makes use of the fact that different types of biological substrate (grey matter, white matter and CSF, for example) respond at unique resonant frequencies to produce *weighted images* that selectively focus on them alone.

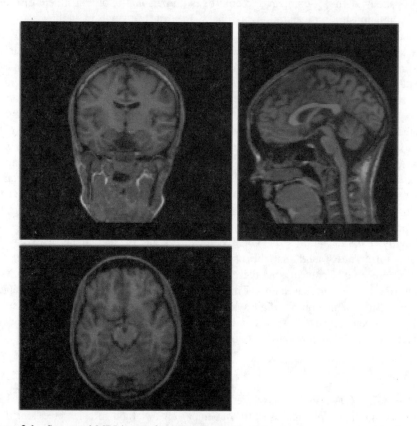

Figure 3.1   Structural MRI image from a patient with AN.

MRI has significant advantages over earlier neuroimaging techniques. It can construct very high-resolution images of the structural characteristics of the brain in any plane, without any risk associated with ionising radiation, and so enables us to explore brain structure in much greater detail than CT. However, the engineering, mathematics and physics required to capture and process tiny energy emissions from protons are complex and challenging. Although the fundamental theoretical basis for MRI was largely defined by 1977, it took a further 25 years before Paul Lauterbur and Peter Mansfield were jointly awarded the Nobel Prize in 2003 for their work on techniques capable of producing clinically and experimentally useful images.

MRI research findings

In the late 1990s, developments in MRI technology led to a flurry of studies confirming the previous CT findings that patients with low-weight AN had significantly larger ventricles and sulci on both cortical and cerebellar surfaces compared to controls [11–14]. The increased resolution of the new technology permitted an exploration of the consequences of subsequent weight-restoration treatment. A subset of 6 of Katzman's original 13 patients continued to have significant grey-matter volume reduction and increased CSF volumes compared to controls following weight restoration at one-year follow-up [15]. They no longer had significantly reduced white-matter volumes, suggesting that the acute demyelination effects of starvation are reversible.

Reporting in the same year, Lambe *et al.* [16] also found that a group of 12 weight-recovered patients with AN continued to have significantly greater CSF volumes and smaller grey-matter volumes than controls. Compared with current low-weight patients, these weight-recovered subjects also had significantly smaller CSF volumes and significantly larger grey- and white-matter volumes. In their weight-recovered group, neither CSF elevations nor grey-matter deficits were correlated with the length of time since weight recovery. Both groups of authors concluded that their findings of persistent grey-matter-volume deficits in weight-recovered patients suggested an irreversible component to structural brain changes associated with AN.

In the case of BN, Hoffman *et al.* [17] identified a significantly reduced MRI cerebral : cranial ratio in eight normal-weight patients compared to controls, though there were no differences between the groups in relative ventricular volumes. Conversely, Hussain *et al.* [18] found that 12 patients with AN showed smaller thalamus and midbrain area than controls but that there was no difference between 12 patients with BN and controls.

Finally, early MRI studies of specific brain structures showed that patients with both AN and BN had smaller pituitary glands (an endocrine organ that secretes homeostasis-regulating hormones) than controls [19]. Patients with low-weight AN have also been shown to have a reduction of total (left + right) hippocampus–amygdala formation (HAF) volume than controls, through this was not related to differences in hormonal levels [20].

Clinical implications of structural studies

CT scanning technologies have helped to clarify that measurable changes in brain structure occur in patients with low-weight eating disorders, probably as a direct consequence of the effect of starvation on the brain. From a purely clinical perspective, it is not clear whether routine CT scanning adds any information to the clinician in practice, since, in a study of 397 consecutive CT brain scans of patients presenting with a range of psychiatric conditions including eating disorders, specific abnormalities were identified in only 5%, and none of these were considered to be clinically related to the patients' psychiatric conditions [21].

Whole-brain MRI studies in AN have consistently identified structural changes in ventricular and sulcal volumes that do not fully resolve following treatment. Grey-matter reductions in AN do not seem to return to pre-illness levels in the short term, though it is encouraging that white-matter changes do appear to resolve. It does seem to be the case from these studies that absolute lowest weight rather than illness duration is the most important factor in determining structural brain outcome following weight-restoration treatment, which may have important implications for treatment and refeeding regimens. However, longer-term outcome studies will be needed to explore the effect of starvation on brain structure over the lifespan.

3.3   Functional imaging

Why image brain function? Clearly, the ability to look into the internal working of the brain has enormous potential for researchers interested in the neuroscience of eating disorders.

It is central to current thinking in neuroscience that the brain is built up by complex interconnected systems, such that any given brain region may support more than one function, and each function may be supported by multiple brain regions. Furthermore, the effects of a brain lesion can change over time, such that injured regions heal and may once again be able to support processing, or other regions may take over the function originally served by the damaged area. Particularly in children, such neuroplastic factors mean that damage occurring in early development may not become apparent until later in life [22].

Single-photon emission computed tomography

SPECT is a nuclear medicine tomographic imaging technique that uses gamma rays (see Figure 3.2). This technique, one of the first developed for functional imaging, enables visualisation of brain function by measuring the rate of blood flow (or perfusion) in different parts of the brain: regional cerebral blood flow (rCBF). The methodology is based on the premise that more active parts of the brain will require more oxygen and therefore an increased perfusion rate in order to fuel the more active neurons. The technique requires injection of a gamma-emitting marker radioisotope, usually the gamma-emitting tracer 99mTc-hexamethylpropyleneamine oxime (HMPAO), which is preferentially distributed to regions of high brain blood flow. The distribution of the isotope in the brain is detected using an imaging camera that constructs 2D or 3D images with a pixel or voxel resolution of up to 1 cm.

SPECT research findings

Some studies of rCBF in AN have used resting-state measures of perfusion, rather than functional response to specific stimuli. In an early study of two patients with

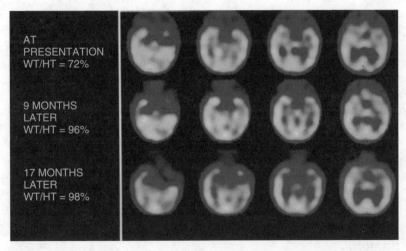

Figure 3.2   SPECT image of regional cerebral blood flow in a patient with AN, at initial presentation and then following weight restoration. (See Plate 1 for colour figure.)

AN, Kuruoglu *et al.* [23] found diffuse bilateral hypoperfusion in frontal, parietal and frontotemporal areas, more prominent in the left hemisphere before treatment, which was no longer evident in either hemisphere three months post-treatment. They suggested that this technique might be useful in following up the effect of treatment and predicting the clinical response to therapy in patients with eating disorders.

Naruo *et al.* [24] assessed seven patients with restricting AN, seven with binge–purge AN and seven controls using SPECT, before and after imagining food. Those patients with the AN binge–purge subtype had a significantly greater change in inferior, superior, prefrontal and parietal regions of the right brain than those with restricting AN and the controls, suggesting an association between habitual binge–purge behaviour and the food-recognition process linked to anxiety in these patients.

In 2001, Rastam *et al.* [25] reported on the long-term follow-up of a group of 21 patients previously treated for early-onset AN in their cohort study. Nineteen of these patients were weight-restored. Compared to a small control group, two thirds of the former patients showed marked hypoperfusion of temporal, parietal, occipital and orbital frontal lobes, though these changes in rCBF were not correlated with weight or body mass index (BMI). In the same year, Tokano *et al.* [26] showed hypoperfusion in medial prefrontal cortex and the anterior cingulate gyrus, and hyperperfusion in the thalamus and the amygdala–hippocampus complex in 14 patients with AN, as compared with controls. They suggested that their results pointed towards a dysfunction in neuronal circuitry related to AN. Finally, Key *et al.* [27] demonstrated hypoperfusion in the medial temporal region in 11 patients with AN but normal perfusion in 11 matched controls.

In BN, an early study by Nozoe *et al.* [28] comparing patients with AN, BN and controls found significantly reduced blood flow in the frontal area, mainly containing bilateral anterior cingulate gyrus, in the AN group compared to the BN and control groups, suggesting that this neurophysiological characteristic may be specific to AN.

Subsequent studies [29, 30] have confirmed this finding, indicating that rCBF changes may be specific to AN, or that this methodology may not be sufficiently sensitive to detect changes in BN. With the development of fMRI, it is now possible to explore more subtle aspects of brain function in both AN and BN.

Very few neuroimaging studies using SPECT have been conducted in children with early-onset AN, and none in BN, partly because of the relative rarity of these disorders in this age group, and partly because of the ethical issues raised by using this technique with children. Gordon *et al.* [31] demonstrated hypoperfusion in at least one brain region, primarily temporal, in 13 of 15 patients with early-onset AN. These findings were replicated by the same group in a new sample, in which 11 of 15 patients with AN showed similar degrees of hypoperfusion, again primarily in the temporal region [32]. This abnormality appears not to reverse with weight restoration [33].

Functional MRI

As well as producing high-resolution images of brain structure, MRI technology also enables us to explore how different parts of the brain function together. As if structural MRI were not computationally complex enough (requiring complex mathematical Fourier transformation of spatial MR data into virtual k-space images), techniques have been developed to overlay the resultant images with a representation of the amount of *functional* activity occurring at each location at a given point in time (see Figure 3.3).

These techniques rely on the rapid reduction in blood oxygenation levels in areas of the brain that are functionally active. As blood passing through the network of arteries and capillaries in the brain comes into contact with oxygen-demanding active tissue, it gives up its oxygen (contained in oxyhaemoglobin) to be metabolised. Detection of these changes in blood oxygen levels is made possible by modelling the characteristic changes in the time series of MR images consistent with the blood oxygen level detection (BOLD) effect in a series of images acquired while the research participant completes a functional task (such as watching some still or moving images, responding to questions or playing a computer game) in the scanner.

fMRI research findings

The first studies using these newly-developed fMRI technologies explored brain activation associated with the core symptoms of eating disorders. Ellison *et al.* [34] showed a series of pictures of high-calorie foods to six patients and six controls while collecting functional MR images. They confirmed the hypothesis that patients experiencing 'calorie fear' would show a neural response similar to that in patients with simple phobias when confronting their feared object, involving increased activation of anterior cingulate and left insula regions. They also found that calorie fear in people with AN was associated with increased activation of the left Hippocampal-Amygdala Formation (HAF), which may therefore mediate conditioned fear to high-calorie foods. They noted that abnormal activation of this limbic/paralimbic system has also been associated with obsessive–compulsive and depressive symptoms and speculated that this could explain the increased rate of these symptoms in AN.

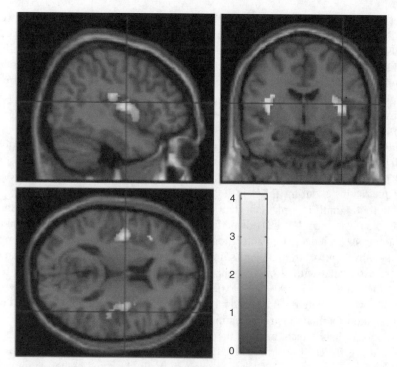

Figure 3.3 Composite fMRI image comparing brain activation in response to a mental rotation task in a group of patients with AN versus matched control participants. (See Plate 2 for colour figure.)

Uher *et al.* [35] compared women who had long-term recovered from restricting AN with a group of chronically ill patients with restricting AN and a healthy control group, showing them pictures of food and nonfood items in the scanner. They found that compared to the chronically ill patients, the recovered women had increased activation of a range of brain regions, including the right lateral prefrontal, apical prefrontal and anterior cingulate cortices (ACCs). Compared to the controls, the recovered women also had increased medial, prefrontal and anterior cingulate activation, as well as reduced activation of the parietal lobe. Their results suggest that food-image-related brain activity in women recovered from AN is a combination of responses seen in currently ill patients and those recorded in healthy women. These results indicate that there may be different neural substrates for the acute low-weight phase in AN, and an underlying *trait* vulnerability that is still apparent following weight-restoration treatment.

Developing this work in a creative if macabre direction, Uher *et al.* [36] showed pictures of foods and disgusting images (of severed limbs and mutilated bodies) to patients with BN and AN and healthy controls (presumably following robust negotiations with their local research ethics committee!). The women with AN and those with BN both rated the food stimuli as threatening and disgusting. Their neural responses to these stimuli included greater activation of left medial and orbitofrontal cortices and ACCs than controls. There was also less activation in the lateral prefrontal cortex, inferior parietal lobule and cerebellum relative to the control group. In addition, women with BN had less activation in the lateral and apical prefrontal cortex compared to controls. The similarities in neural response between the AN and BN group in prefrontal activation led the authors to speculate that both disorders may share a common underlying 'transdiagnostic' factor. They also proposed that an abnormal activation of medial prefrontal circuits in response to inappropriate stimuli is common to eating, obsessive–compulsive and addictive disorders and may therefore account for the shared compulsive features of behaviour in these conditions.

It has been questioned whether patients with eating disorders process visual food stimuli differently when they are hungry and when they are full. In a study by Santel *et al.* [37], patients with AN and controls rated visual food and nonfood stimuli for pleasantness during fMRI in both a hungry and a satiated state. AN patients rated the food simuli less pleasant than controls. When satiated, AN patients showed decreased activation in left inferior parietal cortex relative to controls. When hungry, AN patients showed decreased activation of the right visual occipital cortex compared to the healthy control group. Food stimuli presented when satiated rather than hungry were associated with stronger right occipital activation in patients. These results suggest that patients with AN may experience decreased food-related somatosensory processing when satiated and attentional processing biases when hungry, which might in combination facilitate restricted eating in AN.

Body-image disturbance, perhaps the single most pathognomic feature of AN, was explored using fMRI by Wagner *et al.* [38] in a study of 13 current patients with AN using pictures of their own and other people's digitally distorted bodies. Compared to controls, the patients with AN showed increased activation of prefrontal and inferior parietal lobe when presented with distorted versions of their own bodies, but not those of others. This suggests that patients use a different visuospatial system to process images of their own bodies, which could help us to understand more about this beguiling aspect of AN.

Exploring the same theme, Sachdev and colleagues conducted an elegant experiment in 2008 [39] to examine whether the brain processing of an image of self is different in AN compared with matched controls. They showed that although patients with AN process nonself-images similarly to control subjects, their processing of self-images is quite discrepant, with a lack of activation of the attentional systems and in the insula. They concluded that such discrepant emotional and perceptual processing may underlie the distortion of self-images by patients with AN.

More recently, researchers using fMRI have moved on from studying the core symptoms of eating disorders (body image and response to food stimuli) to exploring more subtle biological and psychological features. Thus, imaging studies have been used to investigate how risk and reward tasks are processed in women who have recovered from restricting AN, using event-related fMRI [40]. The recovered women showed increased activation in the caudate nucleus compared to the healthy control group in response to both wins and losses on a reward task. In the anterior ventral striatum (AVS), the healthy controls distinguished between positive and negative feedback, while the former patients had similar responses to both conditions. Based on these results, it appears individuals who have recovered from AN may have difficulties in differentiating positive and negative feedback, and thus an impaired ability to identify the emotional significance of a stimulus.

Exploring more basic biological processes, Wagner *et al.* [41] also used fMRI to test whether patients with eating disorders process taste stimuli differently than healthy subjects, using a region of interest (ROI) approach to focus on a specific area of the brain, rather than conducting whole-brain analyses. The aim of the study was to test neural activation in primary and secondary taste cortical regions after sucrose and water administrations. The results showed that patients recovered from AN had significantly lower activation in the insula – including the primary cortical taste region – and ventral and dorsal striatum in response to both sucrose and water. This suggests that recovered AN patients may process taste stimuli differently than controls, based on differences in neural activation patterns.

Redgrave and colleagues [42] reported on an innovative study using fMRI to measure brain activation in patients with AN and control participants performing a novel emotional Stroop task using fat, thin and neutral words, and control nonwords. They showed that reaction times increased in the patient group in thin and fat conditions. In the thin versus nonword contrast, patients showed greater activation than controls at the junction of left insula, frontal and temporal lobes and in left middle and medial frontal gyri. In the fat versus nonword contrast, controls showed greater activation in left dorsalateral prefrontal cortex and right parietal areas. These results suggest that the mechanisms underlying attentional bias in AN may differ under conditions of positive and negative valence. This paradigm is a promising tool to examine neural mediation of emotional response in AN.

Zastrow *et al.* [43] have explored set-shifting in AN using fMRI. That it is characteristic for patients with AN to have difficulties with cognitive flexibility has been well documented in 'offline' neuropsychological tasks conducted outside of the scanner; with the advent of fMRI it is now possible to explore the neural correlates. Fifteen patients with AN in this study made significantly more errors than controls in set-shifting, accompanied by reduced activation in the left and right thalamus, ventral striatum, ACC, sensorimotor brain regions and cerebellum. Impaired set-shifting in AN seems to be associated with reduced activation in the ventral anterior cingulate–striato–thalamic loop (the CSPT network), which has been implicated in motivation-related behaviour in a range of disorders [44].

Studies using fMRI have now reached the level of sophistication where it becomes possible to use this technique to test specific hypotheses, rather than mere collecting further sets of images comparing patients and control participants without any underlying theoretical basis. A good example of this sort of study was reported by Wagner *et al.* [46], who set out to test their hypothesis that disturbances in reward systems may contribute to vulnerability to development of an eating disorder. Focusing on the AVS, which is known to be activated by a monetary reward task, they supported their hypothesis that control participants would show different activation patterns to positive and negative feedback, whereas former patients recovered from BN would have similar responses to both conditions. Given previous findings showing that former patients recovered from AN also had altered striatal responses and difficulties in differentiating positive and negative feedback, these results suggest that both disorders may share a common underlying difficulty in discriminating the emotional significance of a stimulus.

Other studies of BN using fMRI have explored the functional response to glucose in recovered patients [45]. The recovered patients had reduced activation in the right

ACC and in the left precuneus for glucose versus artificial saliva compared to controls. Since the ACC is thought to play a role in the anticipation of reward, it may be that former patients continue to show an underlying trait for reduced reward response to nutritients, which makes them vulnerable to overeating and hence bingeing.

Summary

Functional imaging techniques using MRI have significantly enhanced the neuroscience of eating disorders. However, there is a risk that simply cataloguing the parts of the brain activated by specific functional tasks becomes a sort of 'internal phrenology' whereby 'lumps and bumps' on the inside of the brain rather than the surface of the skull are linked to behaviours. On the other hand, exploratory empirical studies using fMRI have enabled us to identify reliable differences in activation between patients (current and recovered) compared to well-matched healthy controls. At this stage in the neuroscience, these findings can help us to explore differences in neural processing associated with acute-state and long-term trait vulnerabilities in eating disorders, which can help in developing and testing future theories.

Studies in fMRI have shown that patients with AN process visual food stimuli differently both when hungry and when satiated, and that this may be linked to reduced reward valency of food and to experiencing these stimuli as disgusting and threatening. Taste stimuli are also processed differently by current and former patients, who have a different response to their own body image than to images of others. Studies of risk and reward processing in AN and BN suggest that both disorders are characterised by difficulties in evaluating the emotional significance of a stimulus. In the case of BN, reduced reward activation to glucose may confer an increased risk of overeating.

These functional findings have been reliably linked to specific brain structures, including the limbic, visuospatial, reward and response motivation systems, in a series of studies conducted over the past 10 years. As the neuroscience progresses, we should be able to refine our understanding of the relationship between these structural systems and the functional implications in eating disorders.

Positron emission tomography

An additional method developed to study the function of the brain is PET, which is used to examine the relationship between energy consumption and neuronal activity based on the movement of injected radioactive material. To produce a PET scan image, a radioactive isotope attached to a form of glucose (fluorodeoxyglucose, FDG) is injected into the bloodstream and travels to metabolically active areas, including the brain. Once in the brain, FDG levels are concentrated in the most active regions, which require the highest levels of energy. As the radioisotope attached to the FDG decays, it emits a positron, which interacts with an electron in an encounter that annihilates both of them, producing a pair of gamma photons. The two photons travel in opposite directions, leaving the brain, and are detected by the scanner. It is possible to build up a three-dimensional image of active brain areas by calculating the origin of pairs of photons arriving on opposite points of the scanner at the same point in time.

PET research findings

In an early study, Krieg and colleagues [47] compared regional cerebral glucose metabolism in seven patients with AN to that in nine patients with BN, showing that relative levels were significantly higher in the former in the caudate region. They concluded that caudate hyperactivity could be a characteristic feature of AN, but did not explore whether these differences persisted following weight restoration.

Delvenne and colleagues in 1995 [48] explored cerebral glucose metabolism in 20 patients with AN compared with 10 controls. They found that the AN patients had a global hypometabolism, with significant regional differences in the frontal and parietal cortices. There were no significant correlations between metabolic activity level and BMI, anxiety or depression scores. The authors suggested that the observed hypometabolism could be a consequence of neuropsychological or morphological aspects of AN and/or the result of associated symptoms such as anxiety or depression. Supported by additional cognitive studies, they suggested that their results implicated a primary corticocerebral dysfunction in AN.

In a further study exploring the effect of weight restoration on brain glucose metabolism, Delvenne *et al.* [49] replicated their findings in a different group of 10 patients with AN by showing that they had global and regional hypometabolism of glucose compared to controls. There was a trend towards parietal and superior frontal cortex hypometabolism and relative hypermetabolism in the caudate nuclei and the inferior frontal cortex in the patients compared to the controls. After weight gain, all regions normalised for absolute and relative values, although a trend remained in patients with AN for relative parietal hypometabolism and inferior frontal cortex hypermetabolism. The authors concluded that the observed reduction in brain glucose metabolism might result from neuroendocrinological or morphological aspects of AN, or be secondary to altered neurotransmitter activity associated with a deficient nutritional state.

To explore whether these findings were related specifically to AN or simply to the effect of low weight, the same group compared 10 patients with AN to a matched group of underweight and depressed women without AN, and to healthy controls [50]. In absolute values, global and regional glucose activity were significantly lower in patients with AN and in low-weight depressed patients than in controls. Relative values showed that patients with AN compared to controls showed lower metabolism of glucose in parietal cortex. The group concluded that absolute hypometabolism of glucose seems to be a consequence of low weight rather than being specifically associated with a diagnosis of AN.

In the case of BN, Wu *et al.* [51] compared cerebral metabolic rates in eight patients with matched controls. They found that the control group had a higher metabolic rate in the right hemisphere than the left, an asymmetry that was not present in the patients. They noted that previous studies had found lower metabolic rates in the basal ganglia in patients with depression and higher rates in patients with AN, neither of which was found in their study, suggesting that BN as a diagnostic grouping is distinct from these disorders.

In 1992, Andreason and colleagues [52] aimed to further delineate the character of cerebral metabolism in BN and to determine whether functional links could be established between regional cerebral metabolism and the symptoms of depression and obsessive–compulsive disorder (OCD) in 11 patients and 18 controls. In the patient group there was a correlation between increased left prefrontal regional cerebral glucose hypometabolism and greater depressive symptoms; no group differences were found between glucose metabolism and OCD symptoms. These findings suggest that the observed changes in brain function were associated with depression, but not with obsessive or compulsive features.

Repeating the design of their earlier study in AN, Delvenne *et al.* [53] set out to evaluate, at rest, brain glucose metabolism in 11 patients with BN compared to matched controls. In absolute values, the patients with BN showed global and regional hypometabolism of glucose; in relative values, parietal cortex metabolism was lower in the BN group compared to other brain regions. There were no correlations within groups between cerebral glucose metabolic rates and BMI, anxiety or depression scores, suggesting that the observed brain activation differences could not be accounted for by weight or psychological functioning.

As well as imaging brain function or activity by tracing the update of labelled glucose, PET scanning also allows exploration of how other brain chemicals are processed. These technologies can help discover potential differences in neurotransmitter functioning between patients and healthy controls. For example, in the case of AN, Frank *et al.* [54] used PET to explore altanserin binding in a group of 16 weight-recovered patients compared with 11 controls (since malnutrition itself produces changes in neuroendocrine function, such studies tend to be conducted with weight-recovered participants, to avoid this confounding effect). Altanserin is a compound that binds to the serotonin 2A-type receptor on the 'receiver' end of the synapse. It can be 'labelled' with a radioactive isotope of fluorine (^{18}F) so that its uptake can be monitored using PET. In this study, the former patients had significantly reduced ^{18}F-labelled altanserin binding potential (a combined measure of neuroreceptor density and affinity for a given neurotransmitter) relative to controls in medial temporal (amygdala and hippocampus) as well as in cingulate cortical regions. This suggests that altered serotonin activity persists following weight recovery in AN and may be related to disturbance of medial temporal lobe function.

In a similar study, Bailer *et al.* [55] showed that a group of 10 recovered patients with BN had significantly reduced altanserin binding potential compared with 16 control participants in the left subgenual cingulate gyrus, left parietal cortex and right occipital cortex. They also showed that altanserin binding potential was positively related to harm-avoidance and negatively correlated to novelty-seeking in cingulate and temporal regions in the recovered patients. The recovered patients also had a negative relationship between altanserin binding potential and drive for thinness in several cortical regions.

Harm-avoidance is a multifaceted temperament trait that contains elements of anxiety, inhibition and inflexibility and has been extensively explored in relation to eating disorders [56]. PET imaging using altanserin enables exploration of the relationship between postsynaptic serotonin uptake and temperament and so can help begin to make connections between neurochemical and psychological functioning. The findings of Bailer *et al.*'s [55] study suggest that reduced serotonin binding potential means that more serotonin is produced presynaptically by the brain in an attempt to 'get the message through', which in turn contributes to increased harm-avoidance. For novelty-seeking, the process works the other way round, with a reduction in willingness to try new things and an increased tendency to rigidity and fixed routines.

This research group had previously shown reduced serotonin 2A receptor binding potential in medial orbital frontal cortex in 9 women recovered from BN compared with 12 control participants, again suggesting long-term changes in serotonin processing [57]. They also found that the healthy control women, but not the recovered patients, had an age-related decline in receptor binding. They argued that this lack of age-related changes in serotonin activity lends further support for its importance as a trait marker in BN.

As well as imaging the activity of the serotonin 2A receptor, PET scanning has been used to explore the activity of the 1A receptor. This receptor has an inhibitory effect, such that the more serotonin it receives across the synapse, the more it tends to prevent the release of an action potential – and hence 'signal' transmission – in the postsynaptic neuron (in neurotransmission, as in many biological systems, evolution has operated to produce a balanced system of inhibition and excitation). In PET imaging, the activity of the postsynaptic serotonin 1A receptor can be explored using a drug called WAY-100635 labelled with a radioactive isotope of carbon [11]C. Using this isotope, Bailer *et al.* [58] found significantly increased inhibitory binding potential in cingulate, lateral and mesial temporal, temporal and medial orbital frontal, parietal and prefrontal cortical regions and the dorsal raphe nucleus in 12 women recovered from binge–purge AN compared to 18 control participants. There were no differences between the controls and a group of 13 women recovered from restricting AN, suggesting that different eating disorder subtypes might experience different patterns of altered neurotransmitter activity.

Another study of serotonin 1A receptor activity in 8 patients with BN showed increased binding potential values compared to 10 control participants in all brain regions studied, suggesting that this is a widely distributed characteristic of the disorder [59]. The most robust differences were observed in the angular gyrus, the medial prefrontal cortex and the posterior cingulate cortex.

Finally, PET imaging has also been used to explore the activity of the dopamine neurotransmitter system using an ^{11}C-labelled compound of raclopride [60]. In this study, 10 women recovered from AN had higher raclopride binding potential in the anteroventral striatum than 12 control participants. In addition, raclopride binding potential was positively related to harm-avoidance in the dorsal caudate and dorsal putamen. These findings are important because dopamine neurotransmitter dysfunction, particularly in striatal circuits, might contribute to altered reward-processing, decision-making and executive control, as well as stereotypic motor movements and decreased food ingestion, in people with AN [56].

Summary

PET has contributed to our understanding of changes in regional brain activity in eating disorders, by measuring regional glucose metabolism. However, its dependence on high-energy gamma radiation presents problems for human studies. Radiation exposure in human research is carefully regulated, and individuals can participate in only a few PET scans each. In any case, the spatial resolution of PET is limited by the distance the positron travels after being released from the labelled molecule before it collides with an electron and emits a signal. Since the signal originates from the point of collision rather than the original breakdown of the molecule, there is inherent 'noise' in the resulting activation map. For example, a positron emitted by ^{18}F-labelled glucose might travel up to 2.6 mm before encountering an electron; the resulting activation map will show this electron's location rather than the original metabolic process.

Even more limiting is the very poor temporal resolution of PET imaging. Because many emissions must be detected before an image with sufficient signal-to-noise ratio can be produced, PET studies must collect data over a long period of time. For example, an image of glucose metabolism using ^{18}F may take 30–40 minutes to acquire. These acquisition times severely limit the temporal resolution of PET imaging and restrict the types of experimental design that can be used.

Despite these limitations, PET imaging techniques have been extremely helpful in furthering our understanding of the role of neurotransmitters in eating disorders, both in the low-weight state during acute illness and as long-term trait markers following weight recovery. Taken together, studies using PET have established that altered serotonin and dopamine functioning are central to AN and BN. Individuals who are vulnerable to developing an eating disorder might have a trait for increased extracellular serotonin concentrations and an imbalance in postsynaptic 1A and 2A receptor activity, which together might contribute to increased satiety and an anxious, harm-avoidant temperament [56]. This *predisposing* vulnerability might be triggered by the challenges of adolescence to *precipitate* an eating disorder. An altered reward response to food and dieting modulated by the dopamine system could then *perpetuate* the eating disorder. Since eating disorders have a complex aetiology, in which genetic, biological, psychological and sociocultural factors seem to contribute, PET scanning, despite its limitations, has uniquely contributed to our understanding of the neurochemistry.

Clinical implications of functional studies

The clinical implications of fMRI findings have yet to be fully realised. Caria *et al.* [61] have suggested that differential emotional responses to food stimuli and risk/reward decisions may be treatable in the future through 'online' biofeedback approaches in the scanner. The same may apply to the treatment of body-image disturbance. In the more immediate future, increased understanding of these subtle yet persistent deficits may help to guide the development of new treatment approaches such as cognitive remediation therapy for set-shifting difficulties, mentalisation-based therapy for emotional-awareness deficits and motivational approaches to risk/reward decisions around eating.

The neurotransmitter imaging capabilities of PET also have important clinical implications. For example, evidence of reduced serotonin activity in the synapse in patients with acute AN accounts for the ineffectiveness of specific serotonin reuptake inhibitor (SSRI) medication. Since there is already reduced activity and a depleted supply in the synapse as a result of malnutrition, preventing the presynaptic uptake of serotonin will not help. On the other hand, a recent preliminary study has shown that olanzapine (and potentially other atypical antipsychotics), which has effects on both dopamine and serotonin receptors, might be useful for increasing weight gain and reducing anxiety and obsessionality in AN [62]. PET imaging will continue to be a vital tool in our understanding of the underlying pharmacological mechanisms.

3.4 Conclusion

Neuroimaging technology has revolutionised the neuroscience of eating disorders. New techniques have increased our understanding of brain structure, neurochemistry and function in patients, both during the acute illness and following treatment. We can visualise the effect of starvation on the developing brain and explore in detail its long-term consequences. New paradigms have enabled us to explore concepts as diverse as visuospatial functioning, reward sensitivity and neurobiofeedback, and to understand more about brain chemistry. Such studies have required collaborative efforts between clinicians, researchers, nuclear physicists and image analysts, along with the selfless contribution of research participants who are willing to tolerate long periods in the noisy and claustrophobic scanner environment. Their willingness to take part in our studies, knowing that the benefits for treatment innovation may not be realised for many years, is remarkable.

References

1. Brenner, D., Elliston, C., Hall, E. and Berdon, W. (2001) Estimated risks of radiation-induced fatal cancer from pediatric CT. *American Journal of Roentgenology*, **176** (2), 289–296.
2. Artmann, H., Grau, H., Adelmann, M. and Schleiffer, R. (1985) Reversible and non-reversible enlargement of cerebrospinal fluid spaces in anorexia nervosa. *Neuroradiology*, **27** (4), 304–312.
3. Dolan, R.J., Mitchell, J. and Wakeling, A. (1988) Structural brain changes in patients with anorexia nervosa. *Psychological Medicine*, **18** (2), 349–353.
4. Kornreich, L., Shapira, A., Horev, G. *et al.* (1991) CT and MR evaluation of the brain in patients with anorexia nervosa. *American Journal of Neuroradiology*, **12** (6), 1213–1216.
5. Krieg, J.C., Pirke, K.M., Lauer, C. and Backmund, H. (1988) Endocrine, metabolic, and cranial computed tomographic findings in anorexia nervosa. *Biological Psychiatry*, **23** (4), 377–387.
6. Palazidou, E., Robinson, P. and Lishman, W.A. (1990) Neuroradiological and neuropsychological assessment in anorexia nervosa. *Psychological Medicine*, **20** (3), 521–527.
7. Kohlmeyer, K., Lehmkuhl, G. and Poutska, F. (1983) Computed tomography of anorexia nervosa. *AJNR. American Journal of Neuroradiology*, **4** (3), 437–438.
8. Kiriike, N., Nishiwaki, S., Nagata, T. *et al.* (1990) Ventricular enlargement in normal weight bulimia. *Acta Psychiatrica Scandinavica*, **82** (3), 264–266.
9. Krieg, J.C., Lauer, C. and Pirke, K.M. (1989) Structural brain abnormalities in patients with bulimia nervosa. *Psychiatry Research*, **27** (1), 39–48.
10. Laessle, R.G., Krieg, J.C., Fichter, M.M. and Pirke, K.M. (1989) Cerebral atrophy and vigilance performance in patients with anorexia nervosa and bulimia nervosa. *Neuropsychobiology*, **21** (4), 187–191.
11. Golden, N.H., Ashtari, M., Kohn, M.R. *et al.* (1996) Reversibility of cerebral ventricular enlargement in anorexia nervosa, demonstrated by quantitative magnetic resonance imaging. *Journal of Pediatrics*, **128** (2), 296–301.

12. Katzman, D.K., Lambe, E.K., Mikulis, D.J. *et al.* (1996) Cerebral gray matter and white matter volume deficits in adolescent girls with anorexia nervosa. *Journal of Pediatrics*, **129** (6), 794–803.

13. Kingston, K., Szmukler, G., Andrewes, D. *et al.* (1996) Neuropsychological and structural brain changes in anorexia nervosa before and after refeeding. *Psychological Medicine*, **26** (1), 15–28.

14. Swayze, V.W., Andersen, A., Arndt, S. *et al.* (1996) Reversibility of brain tissue loss in anorexia nervosa assessed with a computerized Talairach 3-D proportional grid. *Psychological Medicine*, **26** (2), 381–390.

15. Katzman, D.K., Zipursky, R.B., Lambe, E.K. and Mikulis, D.J. (1997) A longitudinal magnetic resonance imaging study of brain changes in adolescents with anorexia nervosa. *Archives of Pediatrics and Adolescent Medicine*, **151** (8), 793–797.

16. Lambe, E.K., Katzman, D.K., Mikulis, D.J. *et al.* (1997) Cerebral gray matter volume deficits after weight recovery from anorexia nervosa. *Archives of General Psychiatry*, **54** (6), 537–542.

17. Hoffman, G.W., Ellinwood, E.H. Jr, Rockwell, W.J. *et al.* (1989) Cerebral atrophy in bulimia. *Biological Psychiatry*, **25** (7), 894–902.

18. Husain, M.M., Black, K.J., Doraiswamy, P.M. *et al.* (1992) Subcortical brain anatomy in anorexia and bulimia. *Biological Psychiatry*, **31** (7), 735–738.

19. Doraiswamy, P.M., Krishnan, K.R., Boyko, O.B. *et al.* (1991) Pituitary abnormalities in eating disorders: further evidence from MRI studies. *Progress In Neuro-Psychopharmacology And Biological Psychiatry*, **15** (3), 351–356.

20. Giordano, G.D., Renzetti, P., Parodi, R.C. *et al.* (2001) Volume measurement with magnetic resonance imaging of hippocampus-amygdala formation in patients with anorexia nervosa. *Journal of Endocrinological Investigation*, **24** (7), 510–514.

21. Agzarian, M.J., Chryssidis, S., Davies, R.P. and Pozza, C.H. (2006) Use of routine computed tomography brain scanning of psychiatry patients. *Australasian Radiology*, **50** (1), 27–28.

22. Frampton, I. (2004) Research in paediatric neuropsychology – past, present and future. *Pediatric Rehabilitation*, **7** (1), 31–36.

23. Kuruoglu, A.C., Kapucu, O., Atasever, T. *et al.* (1998) Technetium-99m-HMPAO brain SPECT in anorexia nervosa. *European Journal of Nuclear Medicine*, **39** (2), 304–306.

24. Naruo, T., Nakabeppu, Y., Sagiyama, K. *et al.* (2000) Characteristic regional cerebral blood flow patterns in anorexia nervosa patients with binge/purge behavior. *The American Journal of Psychiatry*, **157** (9), 1520–1522.

25. Rastam, M., Bjure, J., Vestergren, E. *et al.* (2001) Regional cerebral blood flow in weight-restored anorexia nervosa: a preliminary study. *Developmental Medicine and Child Neurology*, **43** (4), 239–242.

26. Takano, A., Shiga, T., Kitagawa, N. *et al.* (2001) Abnormal neuronal network in anorexia nervosa studied with I-123-IMP SPECT. *Psychiatry Research*, **107** (1), 45–50.

27. Key, A., Christie, D., O'Brien, A. *et al.* (2006) Assessment of neurobiology in adults with anorexia nervosa. *European Eating Disorders Review*, **14**, 308–314.

28. Nozoe, S., Naruo, T., Yonekura, R. *et al.* (1995) Comparison of regional cerebral blood flow in patients with eating disorders. *Brain Research Bulletin*, **36** (3), 251–255.

29. Beato-Fernandez, L., Rodriguez-Cano, T., Garcia-Vilches, I. *et al.* (2009) Changes in regional cerebral blood flow after body image exposure in eating disorders. *Psychiatry Research*, **171** (2), 129–137.

30. Yonezawa, H., Otagaki, Y., Miyake, Y. *et al.* (2008) No differences are seen in the regional cerebral blood flow in the restricting type of anorexia nervosa compared with the binge eating/purging type. *Psychiatry and Clinical Neuroscience*, **62** (1), 26–33.

31. Gordon, I., Lask, B., Bryant-Waugh, R. *et al.* (1997) Childhood-onset anorexia nervosa: towards identifying a biological substrate. *The International Journal of Eating Disorders*, **22** (2), 159–165.

32. Chowdhury, U., Gordon, I., Lask, B. *et al.* (2003) Early-onset anorexia nervosa: is there evidence of limbic system imbalance? *The International Journal of Eating Disorders*, **33** (4), 388–396.

33. Frampton, I., Watkins, B., Gordon, I. and Lask, B. (2011) Do abnormalities in regional cerebral blood flow in anorexia nervosa resolve after weight restoration? *European Eating Disorders Review*, **19** (1), 55–58.

34. Ellison, Z., Foong, J., Howard, R. *et al.* (1998) Functional anatomy of calorie fear in anorexia nervosa. *Lancet*, **352** (9135), 1192.

35. Uher, R., Brammer, M.J., Murphy, T. *et al.* (2003) Recovery and chronicity in anorexia nervosa: brain activity associated with differential outcomes. *Biological Psychiatry*, **54** (9), 934–942.

36. Uher, R., Murphy, T., Brammer, M.J. *et al.* (2004) Medial prefrontal cortex activity associated with symptom provocation in eating disorders. *The American Journal of Psychiatry*, **161** (7), 1238–1246.

37. Santel, S., Baving, L., Krauel, K. *et al.* (2006) Hunger and satiety in anorexia nervosa: fMRI during cognitive processing of food pictures. *Brain Research*, **1114** (1), 138–148.

38. Wagner, A., Ruf, M., Braus, D.F. and Schmidt, M.H. (2003) Neuronal activity changes and body image distortion in anorexia nervosa. *Neuroreport*, **14** (17), 2193–2197.

39. Sachdev, P., Mondraty, N., Wen, W. and Gulliford, K. (2008) Brains of anorexia nervosa patients process self-images differently from non-self-images: an fMRI study. *Neuropsychologia*, **46** (8), 2161–2168.

40. Wagner, A., Aizenstein, H., Venkatraman, V.K. *et al.* (2007) Altered reward processing in women recovered from anorexia nervosa. *The American Journal of Psychiatry*, **164** (12), 1842–1849.

41. Wagner, A., Aizenstein, H., Mazurkewicz, L. *et al.* (2008) Altered insula response to taste stimuli in individuals recovered from restricting-type anorexia nervosa. *Neuropsychopharmacology*, **33** (3), 513–523.

42. Redgrave, G.W., Bakker, A., Bello, N.T. *et al.* (2008) Differential brain activation in anorexia nervosa to fat and thin words during a Stroop task. *Neuroreport*, **19** (12), 1181–1185.

43. Zastrow, A., Kaiser, S., Stippich, C. *et al.* (2009) Neural correlates of impaired cognitive-behavioral flexibility in anorexia nervosa. *The American Journal of Psychiatry*, **166** (5), 608–616.

44. Marsh, R., Maia, T.V. and Peterson, B.S. (2009) Functional disturbances within frontostriatal circuits across multiple childhood psychopathologies. *The American Journal of Psychiatry*, **166** (6), 664–674.

45. Frank, G.K., Wagner, A., Achenbach, S. *et al.* (2006) Altered brain activity in women recovered from bulimic-type eating disorders after a glucose challenge: a pilot study. *The International Journal of Eating Disorders*, **39** (1), 76–79.

46. Wagner, A., Aizenstein, H., Venkatraman, V.K. *et al.* (2010) Altered striatal response to reward in bulimia nervosa after recovery. *The International Journal of Eating Disorders*, **43** (4), 289–294.

47. Krieg, J.C., Holthoff, V., Schreiber, W. *et al.* (1991) Glucose metabolism in the caudate nuclei of patients with eating disorders, measured by PET. *European Archives of Psychiatry and Clinical Neuroscience*, **240** (6), 331–333.

48. Delvenne, V., Lotstra, F., Goldman, S. *et al.* (1995) Brain hypometabolism of glucose in anorexia nervosa: a PET scan study. *Biological Psychiatry*, **37** (3), 161–169.

49. Delvenne, V., Goldman, S., De Maertelaer, V. *et al.* (1996) Brain hypometabolism of glucose in anorexia nervosa: normalization after weight gain. *Biological Psychiatry*, **40** (8), 761–768.

50. Delvenne, V., Goldman, S., Biver, F. *et al.* (1997) Brain hypometabolism of glucose in low-weight depressed patients and in anorectic patients: a consequence of starvation? *Journal of Affective Disorders*, **44** (1), 69–77.

51. Wu, J.C., Hagman, J., Buchsbaum, M.S. *et al.* (1990) Greater left cerebral hemispheric metabolism in bulimia assessed by positron emission tomography. *The American Journal of Psychiatry*, **147** (3), 309–312.

52. Andreason, P.J., Altemus, M., Zametkin, A.J. *et al.* (1992) Regional cerebral glucose metabolism in bulimia nervosa. *The American Journal of Psychiatry*, **149** (11), 1506–1513.

53. Delvenne, V., Goldman, S., Simon, Y. *et al.* (1997) Brain hypometabolism of glucose in bulimia nervosa. *The International Journal of Eating Disorders*, **21** (4), 313–320.

54. Frank, G.K., Kaye, W.H., Meltzer, C.C. *et al.* (2002) Reduced 5-HT2A receptor binding after recovery from anorexia nervosa. *Biological Psychiatry*, **52** (9), 896–906.

55. Bailer, U.F., Price, J.C., Meltzer, C.C. *et al.* (2004) Altered 5-HT(2A) receptor binding after recovery from bulimia-type anorexia nervosa: relationships to harm avoidance and drive for thinness. *Neuropsychopharmacology*, **29** (6), 1143–1155.

56. Kaye, W.H., Fudge, J.L. and Paulus, M. (2009) New insights into symptoms and neurocircuit function of anorexia nervosa. *Nature Reviews. Neuroscience*, **10** (8), 573–584.

57. Kaye, W.H., Frank, G.K., Meltzer, C.C. *et al.* (2001) Altered serotonin 2A receptor activity in women who have recovered from bulimia nervosa. *The American Journal of Psychiatry*, **158** (7), 1152–1155.

58. Bailer, U.F., Frank, G.K., Henry, S.E. *et al.* (2005) Altered brain serotonin 5-HT1A receptor binding after recovery from anorexia nervosa measured by positron emission tomography and [carbonyl11C]WAY-100635. *Archives of General Psychiatry*, **62** (9), 1032–1041.

59. Tiihonen, J., Keski-Rahkonen, A., Lopponen, M. *et al.* (2004) Brain serotonin 1A receptor binding in bulimia nervosa. *Biological Psychiatry*, **55** (8), 871–873.

60. Frank, G.K., Bailer, U.F., Henry, S.E. *et al.* (2005) Increased dopamine D2/D3 receptor binding after recovery from anorexia nervosa measured by positron emission tomography and [11C]raclopride. *Biological Psychiatry*, **58** (11), 908–912.

61. Caria, A., Veit, R., Sitaram, R. *et al.* (2007) Regulation of anterior insular cortex activity using real-time fMRI. *Neuroimage*, **35** (3), 1238–1246.

62. Bissada, H., Tasca, G.A., Barber, A.M. and Bradwejn, J. (2008) Olanzapine in the treatment of low body weight and obsessive thinking in women with anorexia nervosa: a randomized, double-blind, placebo-controlled trial. *The American Journal of Psychiatry*, **165** (10), 1281–1288.

63. Heinz, E.R., Martinez, J. and Haenggeli, A. (1977) Reversibility of cerebral atrophy in anorexia nervosa and Cushing's syndrome. *Journal of Computer Assisted Tomography*, **1** (4), 415–418.

64. Sieg, K.G., Hidler, M.S., Graham, M.A. *et al.* (1997) Hyperintense subcortical brain alterations in anorexia nervosa. *The International Journal of Eating Disorders*, **21** (4), 391–394.

65. McCormick, L.M., Keel, P.K., Brumm, M.C. *et al.* (2008) Implications of starvation-induced change in right dorsal anterior cingulate volume in anorexia nervosa. *The International Journal of Eating Disorders*, **41** (7), 602–610.

66. Castro-Fornieles, J., Bargallo, N., Lazaro, L. *et al.* (2009) A cross-sectional and follow-up voxel-based morphometric MRI study in adolescent anorexia nervosa. *Journal of Psychiatric Research*, **43** (3), 331–340.

67. Herholz, K., Krieg, J.C., Emrich, H.M. *et al.* (1987) Regional cerebral glucose metabolism in anorexia nervosa measured by positron emission tomography. *Biological Psychiatry*, **22** (1), 43–51.

68. Hagman, J.O., Buchsbaum, M.S., Wu, J.C. *et al.* (1990) Comparison of regional brain metabolism in bulimia nervosa and affective disorder assessed with positron emission tomography. *Journal of Affective Disorders*, **19** (3), 153–162.
69. Delvenne, V., Goldman, S., De Maertelaer, V. and Lotstra, F. (1999) Brain glucose metabolism in eating disorders assessed by positron emission tomography. *The International Journal of Eating Disorders*, **25** (1), 29–37.
70. Gordon, C.M., Dougherty, D.D., Fischman, A.J. *et al.* (2001) Neural substrates of anorexia nervosa: a behavioral challenge study with positron emission tomography. *Journal of Pediatric*, **139** (1), 51–57.
71. Bailer, U.F., Frank, G.K., Henry, S.E. *et al.* (2007) Serotonin transporter binding after recovery from eating disorders. *Psychopharmacology (Berlin)*, **195** (3), 315–324.
72. Bailer, U.F., Frank, G.K., Henry, S.E. *et al.* (2007) Exaggerated 5-HT1A but normal 5-HT2A receptor activity in individuals ill with anorexia nervosa. *Biological Psychiatry*, **61** (9), 1090–1099.
73. Frank, G.K., Bailer, U.F., Meltzer, C.C. *et al.* (2007) Regional cerebral blood flow after recovery from anorexia or bulimia nervosa. *The International Journal of Eating Disorders*, **40** (6), 488–492.
74. Galusca, B., Costes, N., Zito, N.G. *et al.* (2008) Organic background of restrictive-type anorexia nervosa suggested by increased serotonin 1A receptor binding in right frontotemporal cortex of both lean and recovered patients: [18F]MPPF PET scan study. *Biological Psychiatry*, **64** (11), 1009–1013.
75. Naruo T., Nakabeppu Y., Deguchi D. *et al.* (2001) Decreases in blood perfusion of the anterior cingulate gyri in anorexia nervosa restricters assessed by SPECT image analysis. *BMC Psychiatry*, **1**, 2.
76. Tauscher, J., Pirker, W., Willeit, M. *et al.* (2001) [123I] beta-CIT and single photon emission computed tomography reveal reduced brain serotonin transporter availability in bulimia nervosa. *Biological Psychiatry*, **49** (4), 326–332.
77. Audenaert, K., Van Laere, K., Dumont F. *et al.* (2003) Decreased 5-HT2a receptor binding in patients with anorexia nervosa. *European Journal of Nuclear Medicine*, **44** (2), 163–169.
78. Uher, R., Murphy, T., Friederich, H.C. *et al.* (2005) Functional neuroanatomy of body shape perception in healthy and eating-disordered women. *Biological Psychiatry*, **58** (12), 990–997.
79. Uher, R., Treasure, J. and Heining, M. (2006) Cerebral processing of food-related stimuli: effects of fasting and gender. *Behavioural Brain Research*, **169** (1), 111–119.
80. Mohr, H.M., Zimmermann, J., Roder, C. *et al.* (2010) Separating two components of body image in anorexia nervosa using fMRI. *Psychological Medicine*, **40**, 1519–1529.
81. Roser, W., Bubl, R. and Buergin, D. (1999) Metabolic changes in the brain of patients with anorexia and bulimia nervosa as detected by proton magnetic resonance spectroscopy. *The International Journal of Eating Disorders*, **26** (2), 119–136.
82. Schlemmer, H.P., Mockel, R., Marcus, A. *et al.* (1998) Proton magnetic resonance spectroscopy in acute, juvenile anorexia nervosa. *Psychiatry Research*, **82** (3), 171–179.

4 Neuropsychology

Joanna E. Steinglass and Deborah R. Glasofer

Columbia Center for Eating Disorders, Columbia University Medical Center/New York State Psychiatric Institute, New York, USA

4.1 Introduction

Clinical neuropsychology examines the relationship between brain pathology and behaviour, using standardised measurement instruments [1]. Neuropsychologists are commonly engaged in identifying learning deficits as well as cognitive and perceptual styles. The clinical tools of neuropsychologists have been incorporated into the field of cognitive neuroscience, which aims to elucidate the neural systems underlying behaviours. In early research, the field of neuropsychology was primarily concerned with describing aspects of intellectual functioning. More recently, research has integrated neuropsychological assessments with advances in neuroscience (i.e. neuroimaging) to develop more precise measures of neurobehavioural processes. Whereas earlier work characterised neuropsychological functioning according to domains of performance (attention, memory, etc.), current work seeks to define cognition as it relates to neural mechanisms. Efforts to improve the understanding of eating disorders through the use of neuropsychological testing began in the late twentieth century.

Given the complexity of eating-disorder behaviour and cognition, and the problems that arise in treatment, much attention has been given to understanding cognitive processing in individuals with eating disorders. Cognitive deficits have long been noted, though results have not been entirely consistent [2]. The available data in anorexia nervosa (AN) indicate that some aspects of cognitive functioning, like attention, may be impaired at low weight but tend to improve with weight restoration [3, 4]. Other cognitive deficits, such as visuospatial processing and components of executive functioning, may persist after weight normalisation [5, 6]. In bulimia nervosa (BN), the existing data suggest that the illness is not associated with impairment in basic cognitive processes (e.g. intellectual functioning, memory), though there are mixed results in a few domains, as described below. The most consistent findings to date are neuropsychological correlates of impulsivity, with patients with BN demonstrating impaired decision-making abilities [7–10]. The importance of these deficits in understanding mechanisms of illness has yet to be established. Hypotheses include the notion that

Eating Disorders and the Brain. Edited by Bryan Lask and Ian Frampton.
© 2011 John Wiley & Sons, Ltd. Published 2011 by John Wiley & Sons, Ltd.

areas of cognitive weakness may originate in early childhood and thus may serve as
a risk factor for the development of the disorder [2], and that these areas of relative
weakness contribute to the perpetuation of the eating disorder [6, 11, 12].

This chapter will review the major findings in the neuropsychology of eating disorders, organised by neuropsychological domain. However, no neuropsychological
function is truly independent. Inferences about deficits in a given area are made based
on performance on tasks that may be assessing multiple domains simultaneously. For
example, performance on all measures depends on the individual's ability to attend
to the task, and many also require some memory function. Thus, several tasks can be
understood as assessing multiple functions simultaneously – the Trail Making Task,
for example, measures motor speed, attention and set-shifting. While separation into
clear domains is somewhat artificial, it is nevertheless useful. Similarly, this chapter
will discuss findings for the two primary eating disorders separately, by diagnosis.
However, many of the studies reviewed include both AN and BN groups. Changes to
the diagnostic criteria for AN and BN occurred with the creation of the Diagnostic and
Statistical Manual IV (DSM-IV) [13] in 1994. Consequently, older studies reviewed
here may have made different distinctions between eating disorders, complicating our
ability to make comparisons between diagnostic groups. Nevertheless, consideration of
neuropsychology by diagnosis is worthwhile, given the differences in clinical features
between different eating disorders.

4.2   Intellectual functioning

General intelligence refers to an overall ability to reason and think. Level of intelligence will impact the measurement of cognitive functioning by domain, but intelligence can be intact even with deficits within specific cognitive domains. Tests of
general intellectual functioning (e.g. Wechsler Adult Intelligence Scale) generate an
intelligence quotient (IQ) and assess a range of abilities associated with academic
achievement. Intellectual functioning is separated into verbal and nonverbal abilities.
Verbal IQ measures the ability to think in words and to apply language skills and
verbal information to solve problems. Performance intellect is characterised by the
ability to manipulate and organise visual images with relative speed.

Early on in the neuropsychological evaluation of patients with eating disorders,
it was noted that such patients were 'high achievers' and studies reported they had
above-average intellectual functioning [2, 14]. However, this assertion has since been
refuted, with data indicating that intellectual functioning among individuals with eating
disorders is comparable to the general population [15].

The early literature on cognitive deficits in eating disorders comes from batteries
of tasks that aimed to characterise cognitive functioning. These batteries were scored
by compiling tasks and then creating domain scores. Studies reported the presence
of deficits, but areas of impairment were not consistent across individuals or across
studies [16–18].

Anorexia nervosa

Standard tests of intelligence have been normal among individuals with AN [19, 20].
Gillberg *et al.* [20] reported full-scale IQ ranging from 100 to 106 in a community

sample. In clinical samples, some small studies have reported higher ranges [21, 22] and others have reported significantly lower IQ scores in acutely ill patients [23]. In verbal IQ in particular, no impairment has been demonstrated [15, 24]. Longitudinal studies that have investigated change with treatment have found that any impairments in acutely ill patients with AN improve with weight gain [4, 5]. One study has examined long-term follow-up, and at 10 years after the onset of illness, a group of weight-restored individuals demonstrated fairly normal neuropsychological performance, with a possible deficit in the Object Assembly subscale of the Wechsler Adult Intelligence Scale [25]. In sum, general intellectual functioning is normal in AN. Subtle cognitive deficits appear inconsistently, but with sufficient regularity to warrant further, more targeted research. More recent investigations of neuropsychological functioning have moved away from clinically-oriented batteries and have used cognitive tasks to probe specific hypotheses [26].

Bulimia nervosa

Though few studies have evaluated the intellectual functioning of individuals with BN [14, 15, 17], existing data uniformly suggest that this patient population is of at least average intelligence. A mean full-scale IQ ranging from 102 [15] to 109 [17] has been reported in this group, with one study of highly educated adolescents with BN observing an above-average IQ of 114 in its sample [14]. Individuals with BN do not tend to have any significant discrepancy between verbal and performance abilities, nor has any specific pattern of strengths and weaknesses within these domains been revealed [14, 15, 17]. Finally, individuals with BN do not significantly differ in intellectual functioning as compared to healthy controls or weight-restored individuals with AN [15, 17].

Summary

Some small – or uncontrolled – studies suggested the possibility that individuals with eating disorders may have superior intellectual functioning, but these findings have not been supported by available data. While underweight, some individuals with AN may manifest cognitive impairment, but overall, IQ appears intact among individuals with AN and BN.

4.3   Attention

Attention is highly interrelated with functioning in other domains such as concentration, tracking and memory. Gross attentional deficits are characterised by distractibility or impairment in focused tasks, despite an individual's intention [1]. Efforts to study and measure attention have produced different approaches to understanding the various elements of attention. For example, Mirsky *et al.* [27] identified four factors (focusing, sustaining, shifting and encoding). Others have operationalised the study of attention in different ways, and included the measurement of three subcategories: psychomotor speed, sustained attention and selective attention. Psychomotor speed simply refers to the time an individual requires to complete a task that involves integration of sensory information and motor output, essentially reaction time. Vigilance or sustained attention is commonly measured via accurate responses to a signal (i.e. hit rate) and responses to something that was not a signal (i.e. false alarm) in tasks such as the Continuous Performance Task. Selective attention differs somewhat in that the main measure is the ability to pay attention to an interfering stimulus. For example, in the classic Stroop task [28], individuals are asked to name the colour of ink a word is printed in and ignore the natural (or 'prepotent') tendency to read the word. The task is challenging because the words are colour words ('red', 'green' and 'blue') and lexical processing occurs automatically. Correct responding requires actively overriding this automatic response. In the modified ' Emotional Stroop', colour words are replaced with disorder-relevant words. In eating-disorder populations, food- or body-image-related words have commonly been studied. Scores are determined as the difference between interference on neutral stimuli and interference on salient stimuli. Some have also utilised emotionally salient cues that are not specific to eating disorders (e.g. angry faces). Deficits in attention are measured either by slow reaction time or by increased errors (i.e. impulsivity and poor response-inhibition).

Anorexia nervosa

In a simple reaction-time test, Green *et al.* [29] found that patients with AN were slower than controls in their small study. Others have reported similar deficits [4, 17]. Assessments of focus or vigilance in groups of individuals with AN have had mixed findings. Many studies report decreased vigilance and increased error rates using the Continuous Performance Task [30–32]. One small study reported errors of commission on the same task, suggesting impulsive responding in a group of inpatients with AN [33]. Others found no impairment in vigilance [17, 29, 34]. In the studies that included weight-restored individuals with AN, attention deficits reversed with weight gain [3, 4]. Interestingly, individuals with AN may not be impaired in a classic Stroop task [35]. In numerous modifications of the Stroop using emotionally salient stimuli, individuals with AN were slowed in relation to food and body-image words [36–39], food pictures [40] and other emotional stimuli [40, 41], confirming an attentional bias for disorder-relevant stimuli.

Bulimia nervosa

Individuals with BN perform significantly slower on psychomotor-speed tasks than healthy participants, but with no differences in number of errors [10, 17, 42, 43], and comparably to those with AN [4, 17, 42]. Of note, the data suggest that individuals with BN are not in a clinically impaired range [10].

Sustained-attention assessments in patients with BN have yielded mixed results. Several studies in which individuals with BN performed worse than those without an eating disorder suggest the presence of a vigilance deficit in this diagnostic group [30, 31, 44]. However, Jones and colleagues [17] also used the Continuous Performance Task and did not detect any significant differences in performance between patients with BN and healthy controls. One study reported that performance improved with treatment [4], but its findings may be limited given the lack of a control group and possible practice effects.

Though there are exceptions [45, 46], several investigators have reported no significant differences on classic Stroop performance between those with BN and their healthy counterparts (e.g. [47, 48]). However, a meta-analytic review of studies administering the classic Stroop calculated a moderate effect size for between-group comparisons: patients with BN showed significantly poorer Stroop performance than normal controls [49]. This provides some evidence that patients with BN manifest a deficit in attention and response-inhibition [49].

Findings from studies using the Emotional Stroop indicate that patients with BN do take longer (i.e. display an attentional bias) to name the colours of disorder-salient words than healthy counterparts [45–47, 50, 51]. Meta-analytic results from these studies have also yielded moderate effect sizes [49]. Patients with BN showed similar results in a Stroop using pictures of angry faces [52]. By this measure, individuals with BN have demonstrated general social and angry-threat attentional biases (i.e. significantly longer response times) relative to normal controls, a finding that suggests this may relate to emotion-regulation problems noted in this group [41].

Summary

Psychomotor speed appears to be impaired among acutely ill patients with AN and BN, but the clinical significance of this is unclear. While selective attention may be impaired in underweight individuals with AN, this does seem to improve with weight restoration and is not a clear deficit among individuals with BN. Interestingly, the groups may differ in selective attention. Both groups show impairments when disorder-relevant or emotional stimuli are presented, but patients with BN appear to have a more notable impairment in the classic Stroop. The Stroop has also been interpreted as a measure of impulsivity, suggesting that this finding may relate to the clinical phenomenon of a relationship between BN and impulsivity.

4.4 Memory

Memory is a core cognitive function, commonly impaired in brain disorders. It can be functionally divided into short-term memory and long-term memory. Memory can also be subdivided as explicit memory (for facts and events) and implicit (procedural) memory, which have both been reasonably well characterised with respect to underlying brain structures. Much of memory function is mediated by the hippocampus and related structures, with procedural memory involving primarily basal ganglia structures [53]. Among the best-validated assessments of memory function is the Wechsler Memory Scale [54], which assesses recall and recognition of visual and verbal material. Other commonly used assessments include verbal learning tests such as the California Verbal Learning Test [55] and nonverbal tests such as Digit Span, a subscale of the Wechsler Adult Intelligence Scale that assesses memory for a sequence of numbers. Implicit learning, as mediated by the basal ganglia, has not been studied in eating disorders [11]. Functioning on memory tasks is dependent on other neuropsychological domains, such as attention.

Anorexia nervosa

Some studies of underweight patients with AN have reported impairment in short-term and long-term verbal memory [5, 34, 56]. In one often-cited study, Green et al. [29]

reported that cognitive deficits, including free recall, did not improve after 12 weeks of treatment. In this study, however, patients remained significantly underweight at the final testing time (BMI ~ 16.5 kg m^2). While this small study may suggest that memory impairments are not the result of acute starvation, it does not address the relationship between memory and the underweight state. In the Jones [17] cross-sectional study, there were no memory deficits in the weight-restored group. The few, small studies evaluating patients prospectively have had mixed results. One found continued deficits in memory, in the setting of improvement in attention [5]; others have found normalisation, or at least significant improvement, with weight restoration [4, 57]. Other studies of patients with AN have not demonstrated short- or long-term memory impairments [4, 58]. Similarly conflicting findings have been reported regarding visual memory tasks [59]; these findings are discussed in more detail in the section on Visuospatial processing.

Bulimia nervosa

Memory appears to be unaffected in BN. Patients with BN perform similarly to normal controls on assessments of short- and long-term memory, including immediate-list free recall and 24-hour-list and story free recall [4, 17, 43]. In addition, Lauer and colleagues [4] noted nonverbal memory to be intact during the acute phase of illness, with individuals with BN performing adequately on memory tasks such as reciting a series of digits and pointing to a series of blocks in the same pattern/order as the assessor prior to receiving treatment for their eating disorder.

Summary

Declarative memory seems to be intact overall in individuals with eating disorders. There may be impairments while acutely malnourished among individuals with BN or underweight individuals with AN. However, to the extent that these deficits are present, they do not play a significant role in clinical presentation and have not yet contributed to the mechanisms of illness. Some areas of memory, such as implicit memory, are understudied.

4.5   Visuospatial processing

Visuospatial processing refers to the perception and understanding of spatial relationships. This has emerged empirically as an area of interest, as neuropsychological batteries and assessments of intellectual functioning have suggested the possibility of circumscribed visuospatial deficits in individuals with eating disorders. Furthermore, assessments of executive functioning and higher-order processing have hinted at visuospatial processing as a domain of interest.

However, the relationship between maladaptive eating behaviours and spatial relations is not inherently clear. Neuropsychological batteries have yielded information about visuospatial processing via the Block Design section of performance IQ testing and nonverbal memory tasks (e.g. Benton Visual Retention Test). More complex functioning is measured using tasks that require processing, memory and manipulation of visual material. In the Rey–Osterrieth Complex Figures Test, participants are asked to copy, and then remember and recreate, a complex geometric figure. Other complex tasks evaluate the ability to identify details within a complex figure (e.g. Matching Familiar Figures, Embedded Figures). For example, the Embedded Figures Test [60] measures the time taken to identify and trace a series of simple shapes embedded in complex designs. A shorter response time indicates a bias towards detail and strong 'local processing' [61]. The findings from these tasks have suggested that individuals with eating disorders may be emphasising detail over larger context, or have deficits in 'central coherence'. Central coherence is a perceptual-cognitive 'style' that relates to the ability to integrate detailed information and perceive the overall context. Clinically, patients with eating disorders appear to be overly focused on details (e.g. caloric content of foods, body image, exercise rituals) [62]. Weak central coherence is a cognitive tendency to process information in parts (i.e. a bias towards detail).

Anorexia nervosa

Reviews of neuropsychology in AN have commonly concluded that the salient findings are suggestive of visuospatial deficits [63, 64]. For example, when evaluating overall IQ, there are no consistent impairments. However, pooling individual deficits, they can be understood as falling in the domain of visuospatial functioning [17]. The visuospatial deficits that emerge with reasonable consistency in neuropsychological studies of underweight individuals with AN [23], may persist after weight restoration [24].

Importantly, it has been repeatedly demonstrated that individuals with AN do not have a perceptual deficit. There were initial hypotheses that individuals perceived themselves as 'fat' because they had an abnormality in the ability to perceive their own size. However, it has been repeatedly demonstrated that perception of neutral objects is normal and that while patients do overestimate body size, so do healthy controls [65].

Several studies have suggested abnormalities in tasks that require complex visual memory or visuospatial manipulation. One early study [66] demonstrated that individuals with binge–purge subtype made significantly more errors on the Matching Familiar Figures Task than those with AN restricting subtype and healthy controls. However, another study found no differences between patients and healthy controls on the Matching Familiar Figures Task [67], except in a calculated 'efficiency' score, in which patients exceeded healthy controls. One study of 18 individuals with AN demonstrated poor performance on the Rey–Osterrieth Complex Figures Test [68], with both copying and recall difficulties, suggesting nonverbal memory deficits and organisational strategy problems. Patients with AN generated problem-solving strategies that overly emphasised details, a pattern noted to be similar to that of individuals with obsessive–compulsive disorder.

These findings are consistent with clinical observations that individuals with AN are detail-oriented, and perhaps make cognitive errors for this reason. One group has suggested the presence of weak central coherence in acutely ill individuals with AN, based on a meta-analysis that suggested poor global processing in patients with eating disorders [62]. In a group of individuals who had recovered from an eating disorder, those with a history of AN did not differ significantly from controls on measures of central coherence [62].

Bulimia nervosa

No consistent picture has emerged with regards to visuospatial abilities in individuals with BN. Unlike AN, individuals with BN do not perform significantly differently from healthy controls on Block Design [17, 69]. Studies administering the Rey–Osterrieth Complex Figure Test [70] have yielded mixed results. Murphy and colleagues [64] found that individuals with BN did not differ from healthy individuals in their ability to accurately copy the stimulus [64], but another team of investigators did detect a significant difference in copying ability [61]. Findings on recall accuracy are similarly inconsistent, with some reports suggesting no impairment in individuals with BN as compared to normal controls [17, 64] and others observing poorer performance in the eating-disorder group [61].

Existing data do not clearly suggest weak central coherence in BN. Some studies administering the Embedded Figures Task found individuals with BN took longer to complete the task than healthy controls [17, 71]; others found the opposite, suggesting that individuals with BN were superior in local processing [61]. One study of the Matching Familiar Figures Test found that individuals with BN performed comparably to healthy controls [67].

Summary

Deficits in the visuospatial domain have long been noted in AN and this domain consistently stands out from general intellectual functioning as an area of weakness. Studies targeting visuospatial processing have continued to find deficits that cumulatively suggest the presence of some abnormality, but findings have not been entirely consistent. No clear deficits emerge among patients with BN. Interest in these phenomena is persistent and may be clinically relevant, but the findings remain preliminary. This line of study continues to yield hypotheses about potential mechanisms of illness.

4.6   Executive functioning

The term 'executive functioning' subsumes all higher-order processes involved in integrating information (sensory, emotional and otherwise) and creating goal-directed responses (behavioural and cognitive). These are functions that rely heavily on the frontal lobe. In clinical neuropsychological test batteries, this includes tests of planning, strategy or problem-solving [72]. Research studies have emphasised areas of complex processing that appear to have clinical relevance. In an effort to understand the rigid and 'stuck' nature of AN, the compulsive nature of eating-disorder behaviour, and the preoccupations associated with these disorders, research has focused on areas such as cognitive flexibility, impulsivity and decision-making.

Cognitive flexibility

'Cognitive flexibility' refers to the ability to shift between mental sets either behaviourally or cognitively. This is often assessed in set-shifting tasks, where an individual is asked to change responses based on changing cues, and measured on the number of errors made, or the increase in time to completion. A relatively simple example of this is the Trail Making Task, in which an individual is first asked to connect a sequence of letters (Trails A) and then to switch between letters and numbers (Trails B). The extra amount of time required to complete the second part of the task is thought to quantify the cost of trying to switch between two different rules (sequential letters and sequential numbers). More complex tasks include the Wisconsin Card Sort, in which participants are required to match an index card with a category based on an unknown matching rule. The matching rule changes periodically, without warning to the participant.

Anorexia nervosa

Studies addressing aspects of cognitive flexibility in AN have reported provocative findings. Set-shifting seems particularly relevant to the clinical features of AN, where patients are stuck in maladaptive behaviours, unable to change even when external pressures are clearly altered. Findings from the Trail Making Task have been mixed, with some showing no difference from controls [35] and others finding that patients with AN take more time for Trails B [73]. Individuals with AN make significantly more perseverative errors on this task, indicating difficulty in switching to the new matching rules, and achieve a significantly lower number of categories of classification, further indicating difficulty with identifying the rules [35, 37, 73, 74]. Other set-shifting tasks have yielded similar findings [42, 75] and one meta-analysis has pooled data from all studies with a set-shifting task and confirmed the presence of set-shifting deficits in AN [76].

One group has extended these findings by comparing acutely ill patients with those who have recovered from AN, as well as with healthy siblings of patients with AN. In one study, both acutely ill and recovered patients showed significantly poorer performance on two set-shifting tasks compared to controls [6]. In another study, the healthy sisters of patients with AN showed a deficit in set-shifting compared with unrelated controls [77], suggesting these deficits may have a genetic basis. More recently, this group conducted a study across groups of ill, recovered, related and unrelated participants and found that the healthy siblings did not differ from healthy controls [73]. Another group investigated long-term recovery from AN and found that in a community sample of recovered patients 10 years after the onset of illness, there was no impairment in performance on the Wisconsin Card Sort, compared with healthy controls [25].

Bulimia nervosa

Mental flexibility has been less emphasised in patients with BN as cognitive rigidity is not as prominent in the typical clinical presentation of this disorder [76]. Overall, recent studies have consistently observed those with BN to perform significantly worse than healthy controls on a variety of measures of mental flexibility (including the Wisconsin Card Sort and Trails B) [42, 43, 73]. Consistent with findings in AN family studies, healthy sisters of patients with BN have also been reported to have set-shifting deficits, again suggesting possible heritability [73]. Set-shifting difficulties (cognitive and perceptual) have been associated with more severe variants of BN and additional general psychopathology [73].

Impulsivity and decision-making

A hallmark of behavioural disorders is the presence of behaviours with maladaptive consequences. One attempt to capture this behaviour neuropsychologically relies on conceptualisation of response pattern as a marker of impulsivity. Various assessments, called Go/No-Go tasks, measure an individual's capacity to respond to one cue and to inhibit responding to another. Difficulty with response inhibition can be considered reflective of increased impulsivity. Alternatively, when provided with response options of differing values or saliencies, impulsive choices can be conceptualised as those in which a participant demonstrates a tendency to respond based upon short-term (rather than longer-term) stimulus values. The Iowa Gambling Task [78, 79] attempts to probe 'decision-making' ability via evaluation of short-term and longer-term advantages (i.e. probabilities). Individuals are asked to select cards from any of four decks, with two card decks identified as 'riskier' (i.e. yielding higher potential rewards or losses). Higher numbers of card picks from the 'safer' decks, however, will result in a long-term net win. As with most neuropsychological assessments, multiple domains are involved in completion of the task as the differences between the decks are not explicitly explained, requiring the individual to learn the contingencies over time. This paradigm is intriguing in eating disorders, where patients with AN might be expected to be 'risk-averse' and patients with BN might be expected to be 'impulsive'.

Anorexia nervosa

In behavioural impulsivity Go/No-Go tasks, individuals with AN do not universally manifest impairments [80, 81]. Two studies of the Iowa Gambling Task in patients with AN found that the patients performed poorly and were more likely to choose the disadvantageous cards [82, 83]. In an analysis of decision-making strategy, the authors reported that patients persisted in disadvantageous choices, and did not switch their strategy. Rather than suggesting risk-averse behaviour, these results suggest that while individuals with AN do behave less impulsively, they manifest implicit learning difficulties that result in disadvantageous responding. Some have linked this finding to the set-shifting deficits noted in other paradigms, described above.

Bulimia nervosa

The behavioural symptoms of BN (i.e. binge eating, purging, laxative abuse) suggest impulsivity and maladaptive decision-making [8]. The neuropsychological findings are consistent with this. Mobbs and colleagues [7] administered a Go/No-Go task with affectively relevant stimuli and reported that individuals with BN tended to have greater inhibition problems and poorer discrimination ability than controls when stimuli were food- and body-related [7]. Individuals with BN had significantly faster reaction time to non-neutral stimuli than neutral stimuli, and quicker response time overall compared to healthy controls. Patients with BN also performed poorly on the Iowa Gambling Task and did not demonstrate improvement across trials in learning to avoid risky (i.e. disadvantageous) card picks when compared with healthy controls [8] and those with subthreshold bulimic symptoms [9]. In a modified Iowa Gambling Task, where the rules of gains and losses are explicit and stable during the entire task, allowing individuals to calculate the risk associated with each alternative from the start and to apply strategies for maximum profit [10, 84] (called the Game of Dice Task), patients with BN have been observed to choose disadvantageous alternatives more frequently than healthy controls, resulting in a significantly lower (and sometimes negative) balance across trials [10]. Thus, independent of learning, individuals with BN may make 'riskier' decisions with less regard for explicit short-term consequences.

Summary

Executive functioning studies yield provocative findings in eating disorders. There are compelling data to suggest a set-shifting deficit among individuals with AN. Impulsivity consistently emerges as a concern for individuals with BN, both cognitively and behaviourally. These deficits may be linked to clinical phenomena, though the data supporting this link are preliminary.

4.7   Conclusion

This review of neuropsychology in eating disorders serves to highlight how much remains unknown about cognitive functioning in AN and BN. Findings are often contradictory, most studies are small, and methodologies differ between studies. Considering the overall functioning level of many individuals with an eating disorder (e.g. ability to graduate school, have a job, etc.), the cognitive impairments that underlie eating disorders are likely subtle. And yet, based on the repeated – albeit inconsistent – findings of *some* deficits, underlying impairment seems likely.

In attempting to synthesise across these studies, a picture emerges. AN is characterised by a range of impairments in attention or memory that are present at low weight and differ by individual, but resolve with weight restoration [4, 5, 63]. Impairments in visuospatial processing, on the other hand, appear to be less idiosyncratic and persist after weight normalisation, suggesting a more trait-like phenomenon. Areas of executive functioning with potential clinical relevance may be impaired as well. Set-shifting deficits appear to be present among affected individuals [76], consistent with the cognitive rigidity noted clinically. However, set-shifting deficits are a common finding across psychiatric illnesses, and may not suggest impairment specific to eating disorders. Weak central coherence or insufficient 'global processing' is emerging as a potential area of interest in AN, but results have been mixed. BN appears similar to AN in some respects, with intact intellectual functioning and an attentional bias towards symptom-relevant cues. In BN, however, neuropsychological findings support impulsivity and risky decision-making. These findings are consistent with the clinical presentation of the disorder.

Cognitive functioning in more recently codified eating disorders, such as binge-eating disorder (BED), a provisional diagnosis introduced into the nomenclature in DSM-IV, has not been well-studied. To date, there has been only one investigation assessing executive functioning (via the Iowa Gambling Task and Delay Discounting measure) in individuals with BED, obese controls and normal-weight controls [85]. While the BED and obese groups had significantly worse scores on both tasks than normal-weight controls, they did not differ from each other. When education level was considered in the analyses, those with higher education performed better on both measures and diagnostic-group differences were no longer significant [85]. Further study in these groups is warranted as we improve our understanding of the cognitive mechanisms underlying overeating and weight gain.

Continued efforts to characterise neuropsychological functioning in eating disorders are warranted. Further study is needed to clarify the extent to which these abnormalities represent a preexisting trait that increases the risk of developing illness [2] versus a state-dependent symptom associated with acute illness (e.g. low weight in AN) that resolves with effective treatment [4, 5, 63]. Long-term prospective studies are necessary to clarify the relationship between cognitive deficits and the development of an eating disorder. Cognitive studies have the potential to characterise biobehavioural markers that may discriminate between eating disorders, and to provide information about treatments and prognoses.

Where neuropsychology once relied on brain injury to determine the neural systems of behaviour, advances in neuroimaging now allow for study of the activity that subserves cognitive processes in healthy individuals. By determining the neural systems that mediate specific tasks, inferences can be made about the neurobiology of cognition. These translationally-based tasks can then be applied to specific psychiatric illnesses and used to help determine neural systems that underlie eating disorders. Future work in the understanding of eating disorders will be enhanced by translationally-based cognitive probes that can continue to generate testable models of the neural mechanisms of eating disorders.

References

1. Lezak, M.D., Howieson, D.B. and Loring, D.W. (2004) *Neuropsychological Assessment*, 4th edn, New York, Oxford University Press.
2. Lena, S.M., Fiocco, A.J. and Leyenaar, J.K. (2004) The role of cognitive deficits in the development of eating disorders. *Neuropsychology Review*, **14**, 99–113.
3. Mikos, A.E., McDowell, B.D., Moser, D.J. *et al*. (2008) Stability of neuropsychological performance in anorexia nervosa. *Annals of Clinical Psychiatry*, **20**, 9–13.
4. Lauer, C.J., Gorzewski, B., Gerlinghoff, M. *et al*. (1999) Neuropsychological assessments before and after treatment in patients with anorexia nervosa and bulimia nervosa. *Journal of Psychiatric Research*, **33**, 129–138.
5. Kingston, K., Szmukler, G., Andrewes, D. *et al*. (1996) Neuropsychological and structural brain changes in anorexia nervosa before and after refeeding. *Psychological Medicine*, **26**, 15–28.
6. Tchanturia, K., Morris, R.G., Anderluh, M.B. *et al*. (2004) Set shifting in anorexia nervosa: an examination before and after weight gain, in full recovery and relationship to childhood and adult OCPD traits. *Journal of Psychiatric Research*, **38**, 545–552.
7. Mobbs, O., Van der Linden, M., d'Acremont, M. and Perroud, A. (2008) Cognitive deficits and biases for food and body in bulimia: investigation using an affective shifting task. *Eating behaviors*, **9**, 455–461.
8. Liao, P.C., Uher, R., Lawrence, N. *et al*. (2009) An examination of decision making in bulimia nervosa. *Journal of Clinical and Experimental Neuropsychology*, **31**, 455–461.
9. Boeka, A.G. and Lokken, K.L. (2006) The Iowa Gambling Task as a measure of decision making in women with bulimia nervosa. *Journal of the International Neuropsychological Society*, **12**, 741–745.
10. Brand, M., Franke-Sievert, C., Jacoby, G.E. *et al*. (2007) Neuropsychological correlates of decision making in patients with bulimia nervosa. *Neuropsychology*, **21**, 742–750.

11. Steinglass, J. and Walsh, B.T. (2006) Habit learning and anorexia nervosa: a cognitive neuroscience hypothesis. *The International Journal of Eating Disorders*, **39**, 267–275.

12. Fowler, L., Blackwell, A., Jaffa, A. *et al.* (2006) Profile of neurocognitive impairments associated with female in-patients with anorexia nervosa. *Psychological Medicine*, **36**, 517–527.

13. American Psychiatric Association (1994) *Diagnostic and Statistical Manual of Mental Disorders*, 4th edn, APA, Washington, DC.

14. Blanz, B.J., Detzner, U., Lay, B. *et al.* (1997) The intellectual functioning of adolescents with anorexia nervosa and bulimia nervosa. *European Child and Adolescent Psychiatry*, **6**, 129–135.

15. Ranseen, J.D. and Humphries, L.L. (1992) The intellectual functioning of eating disorder patients. *Journal of the American Academy of Child and Adolescent Psychiatry*, **31**, 844–846.

16. de Hamsher, K.S., Halmi, K.A. and Benton, A.L. (1981) Prediction of outcome in anorexia nervosa from neuropsychological status. *Psychiatry Research*, **4**, 79–88.

17. Jones, B.P., Duncan, C.C., Brouwers, P. and Mirsky, A.F. (1991) Cognition in eating disorders. *Journal of Clinical and Experimental Neuropsychology*, **13**, 711–728.

18. Bayless, J.D., Kanz, J.E., Moser, D.J. *et al.* (2002) Neuropsychological characteristics of patients in a hospital-based eating disorder program. *Annals of Clinical Psychiatry*, **14**, 203–207.

19. Dura, J.R. and Bornstein, R.A. (1989) Differences between IQ and school achievement in anorexia nervosa. *Journal of Clinical Psychology*, **45**, 433–435.

20. Gillberg, I.C., Gillberg, C., Rastam, M. and Johansson, M. (1996) The cognitive profile of anorexia nervosa: a comparative study including a community-based sample. *Comprehensive Psychiatry*, **37**, 23–30.

21. Maxwell, J.K., Tucker, D.M. and Townes, B.D. (1984) Asymmetric cognitive function in anorexia nervosa. *The International Journal of Neuroscience*, **24**, 37–44.

22. Gordon, D.P., Halmi, K.A. and Ippolito, P.M. (1984) A comparison of the psychological evaluation of adolescents with anorexia nervosa and of adolescents with conduct disorders. *Journal of Adolescent*, **7**, 245–266.

23. Mathias, J.L. and Kent, P.S. (1998) Neuropsychological consequences of extreme weight loss and dietary restriction in patients with anorexia nervosa. *Journal of Clinical and Experimental Neuropsychology*, **20**, 548–564.

24. Braun, C.M. and Chouinard, M.J. (1992) Is anorexia nervosa a neuropsychological disease? *Neuropsychology Review*, **3**, 171–212.

25. Gillberg, I.C., Rastam, M., Wentz, E. and Gillberg, C. (2007) Cognitive and executive functions in anorexia nervosa ten years after onset of eating disorder. *Journal of Clinical and Experimental Neuropsychology*, **29**, 170–178.

26. Tchanturia, K., Campbell, I., Morris, R. and Treasure, J. (2005) Neuropsychological studies in anorexia nervosa. *International Journal of Eating Disorders*, **37**, S72–S76.

27. Mirsky, A.F., Anthony, B.J., Duncan, C.C. *et al.* (1991) Analysis of the elements of attention: a neuropsychological approach. *Neuropsychology Review*, **2**, 109–145.

28. Stroop, J. (1935) Studies of interference in serial verbal reactions. *Journal of Experimental Psychology*, **18**, 643–662.

29. Green, M.W., Elliman, N.A., Wakeling, A. and Rogers, P.J. (1996) Cognitive functioning, weight change and therapy in anorexia nervosa. *Journal of Psychiatric Research*, **30**, 401–410.

30. Laessle, R.G., Krieg, J.C., Fichter, M.M. and Pirke, K.M. (1989) Cerebral atrophy and vigilance performance in patients with anorexia nervosa and bulimia nervosa. *Neuropsychobiology*, **21**, 187–191.

31. Laessle, R.G., Fischer, M., Fichter, M.M. *et al.* (1992) Cortisol levels and vigilance in eating disorder patients. *Psychoneuroendocrinology*, **17**, 475–484.
32. Seed, J.A., Dixon, R.A., McCluskey, S.E. and Young, A.H. (2000) Basal activity of the hypothalamic–pituitary–adrenal axis and cognitive function in anorexia nervosa. *European Archives of Psychiatry and Clinical Neuroscience*, **250**, 11–15.
33. Butler, G.K. and Montgomery, A.M. (2005) Subjective self-control and behavioural impulsivity coexist in anorexia nervosa. *Eating Behaviors*, **6**, 221–227.
34. Witt, E.D., Ryan, C. and Hsu, L.K. (1985) Learning deficits in adolescents with anorexia nervosa. *The Journal of Nervous and Mental Disease*, **173**, 182–184.
35. Steinglass, J.E., Walsh, B.T. and Stern, Y. (2006) Set shifting deficit in anorexia nervosa. *Journal of the International Neuropsychological Society*, **12**, 431–435.
36. Sackville, T., Schotte, D.E., Touyz, S.W. *et al.* (1998) Conscious and preconscious processing of food, body weight and shape, and emotion-related words in women with anorexia nervosa. *The International Journal of Eating Disorders*, **23**, 77–82.
37. Fassino, S., Piero, A., Daga, G.A. *et al.* (2002) Attentional biases and frontal functioning in anorexia nervosa. *International Journal of Eating Disorders*, **31**, 274–283.
38. Channon, S., Hemsley, D. and de Silva, P. (1988) Selective processing of food words in anorexia nervosa. *British Journal of Clinical Psychology*, **27** (Pt 3), 259–260.
39. Johansson, L., Ghaderi, A. and Andersson, G. (2005) Stroop interference for food- and body-related words: a meta-analysis. *Eating behaviors*, **6**, 271–281.
40. Stormark, K.M. and Torkildsen, O. (2004) Selective processing of linguistic and pictorial food stimuli in females with anorexia and bulimia nervosa. *Eating behaviors*, **5**, 27–33.
41. Harrison, A., Sullivan, S., Tchanturia, K. and Treasure, J. (2010) Emotional functioning in eating disorders: attentional bias, emotion recognition and emotion regulation. *Psychological Medicine*, **40**, 1–11.
42. Tchanturia, K., Anderluh, M.B., Morris, R.G. *et al.* (2004) Cognitive flexibility in anorexia nervosa and bulimia nervosa. *Journal of the International Neuropsychological Society*, **10**, 513–520.
43. Ferraro, F.R., Wonderlich, S. and Jocic, Z. (1997) Performance variability as a new theoretical mechanism regarding eating disorders and cognitive processing. *Journal of Clinical Psychology*, **53**, 117–121.
44. Laessle, R.G., Bossert, S., Hank, G. *et al.* (1990) Cognitive performance in patients with bulimia nervosa: relationship to intermittent starvation. *Biological Psychiatry*, **27**, 549–551.
45. Lovell, D.M., Williams, J.M. and Hill, A.B. (1997) Selective processing of shape-related words in women with eating disorders, and those who have recovered. *British Journal of Clinical Psychology*, **36** (Pt 3), 421–432.
46. Jones-Chesters, M.H., Monsell, S. and Cooper, P.J. (1998) The disorder-salient Stroop effect as a measure of psychopathology in eating disorders. *The International Journal of Eating Disorders*, **24**, 65–82.
47. Cooper, M.J., Anastasiades, P. and Fairburn, C.G. (1992) Selective processing of eating-, shape-, and weight-related words in persons with bulimia nervosa. *Journal of abnormal psychology*, **101**, 352–355.
48. Black, C.M., Wilson, G.T., Labouvie, E. and Heffernan, K. (1997) Selective processing of eating disorder relevant stimuli: does the Stroop Test provide an objective measure of bulimia nervosa? *The International Journal of Eating Disorders*, **22**, 329–333.
49. Dobson, K.S. and Dozois, D.J. (2004) Attentional biases in eating disorders: a meta-analytic review of Stroop performance. *Clinical Psychology Review*, **23**, 1001–1022.
50. Cooper, M. and Todd, G. (1997) Selective processing of three types of stimuli in eating disorders. *British Journal of Clinical Psychology*, **36** (Pt 2), 279–281.

51. Cooper, M.J. and Fairburn, C.G. (1994) Changes in selective information processing with three psychological treatments for bulimia nervosa. *British Journal of Clinical Psychology*, **33** (Pt 3), 353–356.
52. Ashwin, C., Wheelwright, S. and Baron-Cohen, S. (2006) Attention bias to faces in Asperger Syndrome: a pictorial emotion Stroop study. *Psychological Medicine*, **36**, 835–843.
53. Squire, L.R. and Zola, S.M. (1996) Structure and function of declarative and nondeclarative memory systems. *Proceedings of the National Academy of Sciences of the United States of America*, **93**, 13515–13522.
54. Wechsler, D. (1945) A standardized memory scale of clinical use. *Psychology*, **19**, 87–95.
55. Delis, D.C., Kramer, J.H., Kaplan, E. and Ober, B.A. (1987) *California Verbal Learning Test: Adult Version*, The Psychological Corporation, San Antonio, TX.
56. Fox, C.F. (1981) Neuropsychological correlations of anorexia nervosa. *International Journal of Psychiatry in Medicine*, **11**, 285–290.
57. Moser, D.J., Benjamin, M.L., Bayless, J.D. *et al.* (2003) Neuropsychological functioning pretreatment and posttreatment in an inpatient eating disorders program. *The International Journal of Eating Disorders*, **33**, 64–70.
58. Bradley, S.J., Taylor, M.J., Rovet, J.F. *et al.* (1997) Assessment of brain function in adolescent anorexia nervosa before and after weight gain. *Journal of Clinical and Experimental Neuropsychology*, **19**, 20–33.
59. Duchesne, M., Mattos, P., Fontenelle, L.F. *et al.* (2004) Neuropsychology of eating disorders: a systematic review of the literature. *Revista Brasileira de Psiquiatria*, **26**, 107–117.
60. Witkin, H., Oltman, P., Raskin, E. and Karp, S. (1971) *A Manual for the Embedded Figures Test*, Consulting Psychologists Press, Palo Alto, CA.
61. Lopez, C.A., Tchanturia, K., Stahl, D. and Treasure, J. (2008a) Central coherence in women with bulimia nervosa. *The International Journal of Eating Disorders*, **41**, 340–347.
62. Lopez, C., Tchanturia, K., Stahl, D. and Treasure, J. (2008b) Central coherence in eating disorders: a systematic review. *Psychological Medicine*, **38**, 1393–1404.
63. Szmukler, G.I., Andrewes, D., Kingston, K. *et al.* (1992) Neuropsychological impairment in anorexia nervosa: before and after refeeding. *Journal of Clinical and Experimental Neuropsychology*, **14**, 347–352.
64. Murphy, R., Nutzinger, D.O., Paul, T. and Leplow, B. (2004) Conditional-associative learning in eating disorders: a comparison with OCD. *Journal of Clinical and Experimental Neuropsychology*, **26**, 190–199.
65. Cash, T.F. and Deagle, E.A. III (1997) The nature and extent of body-image disturbances in anorexia nervosa and bulimia nervosa: a meta-analysis. *The International Journal of Eating Disorders*, **22**, 107–125.
66. Toner, B.B., Garfinkel, P.E. and Garner, D.M. (1987) Cognitive style of patients with bulimic and diet-restricting anorexia nervosa. *The American Journal of Psychiatry*, **144**, 510–512.
67. Southgate, L., Tchanturia, K. and Treasure, J. (2008) Information processing bias in anorexia nervosa. *Psychiatry Research*, **160**, 221–227.
68. Sherman, B.J., Savage, C.R., Eddy, K.T. *et al.* (2006) Strategic memory in adults with anorexia nervosa: are there similarities to obsessive compulsive spectrum disorders? *The International Journal of Eating Disorders*, **39**, 468–476.
69. Galderisi, S., Mucci, A., Monteleone, P. *et al.* (2003) Neurocognitive functioning in subjects with eating disorders: the influence of neuroactive steroids. *Biological Psychiatry*, **53**, 921–927.
70. Osterrieth, P. (1944) The test of copying a complex figure: a contribution to the study of perception and memory. *Archives de Psychologie*, **30**, 206–356.

71. McLaughlin, E., Karp, S. and Herzog, D.B. (1985) Sense of ineffectiveness in women with eating disorders: a clinical study of anorexia nervosa and bulimia. *The International Journal of Eating Disorders*, **4**, 511–523.

72. Yudofsky, S.C. and Hales, R.E. (eds) (2000) *The American Psychiatric Publishing Textbook of Neuropsychiatry and Clinical Neurosciences*, 4th edn, American Psychiatric Publishing, Inc, Washington, DC.

73. Roberts, M.E., Tchanturia, K. and Treasure J.L. (2010) Exploring the neurocognitive signature of poor set-shifting in anorexia and bulimia nervosa. *Journal of Psychiatric Research*, **44**, 964–970.

74. Nakazato, M., Tchanturia, K., Schmidt, U. *et al.* (2009) Brain-derived neurotrophic factor (BDNF) and set-shifting in currently ill and recovered anorexia nervosa (AN) patients. *Psychological Medicine*, **39**, 1029–1035.

75. Tchanturia, K., Serpell, L., Troop, N. and Treasure, J. (2001) Perceptual illusions in eating disorders: rigid and fluctuating styles. *Journal of Behavior Therapy and Experimental Psychiatry*, **32**, 107–115.

76. Roberts, M.E., Tchanturia, K., Stahl, D. *et al.* (2007) A systematic review and meta-analysis of set-shifting ability in eating disorders. *Psychological Medicine*, **37**, 1075–1084.

77. Holliday, J., Tchanturia, K., Landau, S. *et al.* (2005) Is impaired set-shifting an endophenotype of anorexia nervosa? *The American Journal of Psychiatry*, **162**, 2269–2275.

78. Bechara, A., Damasio, H., Tranel, D. and Damasio, A.R. (1997) Deciding advantageously before knowing the advantageous strategy. *Science*, **275**, 1293–1295.

79. Bechara, A., Damasio, A.R., Damasio, H. and Anderson, S.W. (1994) Insensitivity to future consequences following damage to prefrontal cortex. *Cognition*, **50**, 7–15.

80. Claes, L., Nederkoorn, C., Vandereycken, W. *et al.* (2006) Impulsiveness and lack of inhibitory control in eating disorders. *Eating Behaviors*, **7**, 196–203.

81. Rosval, L., Steiger, H., Bruce, K. *et al.* (2006) Impulsivity in women with eating disorders: problem of response inhibition, planning, or attention? *The International Journal of Eating Disorders*, **39**, 590–593.

82. Tchanturia, K., Liao, T., Uher, R. *et al.* (2004) A neuropsychological examination of the ventromedial prefrontal cortex using the Iowa Gambling Task in anorexia nervosa (AN). *Eating Disorders Research Society, Amsterdam, Netherlands*, **56**.

83. Cavedini, P., Bassi, T., Ubbiali, A. *et al.* (2004) Neuropsychological investigation of decision-making in anorexia nervosa. *Psychiatry Research*, **127**, 259–266.

84. Brand, M., Fujiwara, E., Borsutzky, S. *et al.* (2005) Decision-making deficits of Korsakoff patients in a new gambling task with explicit rules: associations with executive functions. *Neuropsychology*, **19**, 267–277.

85. Davis, C., Patte, K., Curtis, C. and Reid, C. (2010) Immediate pleasures and future consequences. A neuropsychological study of binge eating and obesity. *Appetite*, **54**, 208–213.

5 Neurochemistry: the fabric of life and the fabric of eating disorders

Kenneth Nunn

Molecular Neuropsychiatry Service, Department of Psychological Medicine, The Children's Hospital at Westmead, Westmead, Australia

5.1 Introduction

This chapter has five aims, five propositions, five implications of these propositions and five recommendations for future research.

5.2 Five aims

1. **To justify diverting precious time to a subject which may appear to be of limited relevance**

   Why should someone trained in social science or psychotherapy devote precious time to understanding a subject full of obscure chemical, molecular and enzymatic interactions which take a lifetime to master? A primary aim of this chapter is to convey both the importance and value of this aspect of eating disorders.

2. **To describe a neurochemistry approach to eating disorders and explore how this perspective might complement existing understandings**

   There are extensive reviews of biochemical and neurochemical studies in eating disorders which are difficult to read, hard to interpret, lacking a broader research context and unlinked to current understanding of the neurochemistry. They read like fishing and hunting expeditions for the 'eye of newt and wing of bat' which will, through appropriate scientific hubbling and bubbling, produce the answer to whatever human problem is under consideration. The chemical of the day, or neurotransmitter in fashion (cholecystokinin, substance P, galanin, serotonin, leptin, noradrenalin, opioids, oxytocin, orexigenic peptides), may be presented as the verge of a breakthrough. The researchers involved may often have a clear rationale but their papers do not commonly indicate this. This chapter has a more limited goal in that it seeks to provide a neurochemical perspective on a clinical problem.

Eating Disorders and the Brain. Edited by Bryan Lask and Ian Frampton.
© 2011 John Wiley & Sons, Ltd. Published 2011 by John Wiley & Sons, Ltd.

3. **To place eating disorders within a neurochemical context**

   This chapter aims to give some idea, for the neurochemically disinclined, of how the eating disorder field looks from a neurochemistry perspective, without losing sight of existing perspectives that have proved to be of value.

4. **To consider the possible impact of a neurochemistry perspective on the treatment of eating disorders**

   How would our practice change and our research agenda be affected if this perspective had a greater impact? How would environmental influences be conceptualised if food were counted as one of them? How would food be reconsidered if it were seen as the provision of the molecules of experience and mind? How might we understand the whole enterprise of treatment if food were no longer primarily symbolic, metaphor-fraught and meaning-bearing, but actually the very basis of these functions?

5. **To suggest some directions for future research**

   There is much activity, research and clinical effort which needs to be garnered and targeted strategically if there is to be a shift in *causal understanding* towards defeating the devastating impact of eating disorders. Including a neurochemistry perspective will be one essential component in that strategy.

5.3 Five propositions relating neurochemistry to the field of eating disorders

1. **Our bodies and the universe are a single fabric**

   Believed by physicists to be about 13.7 billion years old, the universe is so large that it challenges our ability to believe and to conceive. It is estimated that the universe consists of around 100 billion galaxies [1]! In this chapter we will be looking at a world within ourselves that will also challenge our ability to believe and conceive. This is the universe within our selves: the universe of the brain. It too has 100 billion galaxies of activity, and each is called a 'neuron'.

   Life appears to have emerged on earth about 3.5 billion years ago. It is built from a small number of chemical elements abundant in the atmosphere at that time, such as nitrogen, and from those needed to make life sustainable in water: oxygen and hydrogen. Water is incredibly versatile in providing an environment for dynamic chemical interaction but at the same time keeping the mix as stable as possible. Without water, irreversible bodily changes occur in a little over three days.

   Ninety-nine percent of the mass of the human body is made up of six elements: oxygen, carbon, hydrogen, nitrogen, calcium and phosphorus [2]. The remaining one percent includes potassium, sodium, chlorine, sulfur, magnesium, iron, iodine, zinc, copper and chromium. Each has a unique character with an immediate functional association:

   Oxygen is needed to liberate energy, such as the light of a candle or the wood in a warm fire. The site for oxygen activity is usually thought to be the lungs. But every cell has its own set of 'lungs' for respiration: the mitochondria. The human brain is packed full of mitochondria. Neurons are heavy users of oxygen and without oxygen humans only last about 3−5 minutes before permanent brain damage occurs.

Carbon makes up only 0.09% of the earth's crust but is the element most essential for life. It has the capacity to form relationships with other substances, as well as long chains of itself. Carbon is the 'great networker' of the elements. The whole of life on earth is carbon-based and the only known forms of self-replicating chemistry – DNA and RNA – are carbon-based.

Hydrogen produces weak bond between chains of amino acids and nucleic acids in the long chains of proteins and in molecules of RNA and DNA. Proteins are the chemical workhorses in the body. They are everywhere and involved in everything. Each protein folds uniquely to operate optimally based on these hydrogen bonds. In states of dehydration and starvation these hydrogen bonds experience changes and these changes affect the efficiency of the proteins formed.

Nitrogen, which dominates the air we breathe, forms a significant part of our DNA and is used in the storage of such living matter as sperms, ova and embryos.

Calcium is mostly found in the bone – 90% of the body's calcium – but it has a vital role in neuronal activity too. It acts as a 'go signal' for much of the complicated machinery of the neurons. It signals the release of neurochemical signals from the ends of neurons, and almost every signal involves calcium. In fact, if too much calcium is released, neurons suffer from 'burn out' or excitotoxicity, which in turn may lead to brain cell loss. It should also be noted that the calcium mobilisation associated with bone loss in anorexia nervosa (AN) can have an excitatory effect on the brain.

Phosphorus is the energy currency that trades in phosphate groups, combining energy production (oxygen) with the energy money market (metabolism). When refeeding occurs in patients with eating disorders, food has to be processed and existing phosphorus may become rapidly depleted. Many of the usual foods containing phosphorus (dairy products, meat, eggs) are high on the 'to avoid' list of those with restrictive eating disorders. Phosphorus must be supplemented to avoid the nerves supplying the heart from misfiring and causing fatal arrhythmias.

Magnesium counteracts calcium by stabilising overexcited neurons. It interacts with those neurons containing information (DNA and RNA) and energy (ATP and other enzymes that use phosphate groups). More than 300 enzymes require magnesium ions for their catalytic action.

Potassium is chemically very similar to sodium and acts to move water around the body compartments as required. It is used to keep fluids in balance inside the cells, particularly the brain cells.

Sodium is water-attracting, chloride-stabilising and a 'dancing partner' with potassium in the human body. It is used to keep fluids in balance, especially in the space outside the brain cells.

Chloride is a salt-former that associates with metals (like potassium, sodium and calcium). It is used in the body, along with sodium and potassium, to support fluid balance and electrical activity. Nowhere is this more relevant than in the brain. Chloride content is not only depleted by food restriction, but also by vomiting, as hydrochloric acid is lost from the stomach along with food.

Sulfur forms strong bonds with almost any protein or nucleic acid chain, which are held permanently in their vital shape by two sulfur atoms 'holding hands'.

Iron is the great carrier of oxygen, with electrons to give and take in abundance. It is used in haemoglobin in the blood and myoglobin in the muscles. It is also part of the electron-transport chain, required in every cell to extract the final energy from our food.

Iodine has the biggest atom of all the elements in the human body and as a result can easily give and take electrons, acting as an electron go-between. It is used in the body to regulate metabolism through its role in the thyroid gland. If iodine is lacking in the diet, thyroid activity slows, and with it the entire metabolism of the body.

Zinc, *Copper* and *Chromium* are subtle cameo players in the metabolism of life. They are associated with hundreds of metabolic pathways, especially those involving RNA, DNA and neuronal transmission.

All of these minerals are threatened by restrictive diets unless specifically supplemented.

2. **The fabric of our daily lives is woven from the food in our environment**

   Although only 2% of total body weight, human brains take up 20% of the body's energy supplies [3]. This energy is obtained from those parts of the environment we eat and hence enables construction of our experience. Brain cells need high-energy foods because each cell relates to up to 100 000 others. In the context of severe food restriction, there is a fall in core body temperature, blood pressure and respiratory and heart rates. Major enzyme systems can no longer operate efficiently and immune function, blood clotting and muscle function, including heart muscle, may all be impaired.

3. **DNA is the golden thread tying it all together**

   We have moved from the material of the universe to biochemistry. The golden thread tying together the whole fabric of life is DNA. DNA holds the key to the very nature of living matter [4]. It stores the hereditary information that is passed from one generation to another – the genetic instructions for our bodies (see below). The components of DNA that carry this genetic information are called genes, and other components regulate its use.

4. **Genes are the spinning wheels, shuttles, bibs and bobs for the fabric of life**

   The genes, of which there are 20 000, are chemical memories of information on how to build the proteins that make our bodies work. Their entirety is known as the genome, the set of genetic instructions in the nucleus of every cell [5]. They are written in an ancient language that only has three letters in each word (codon) and only four letters altogether (A – adenine; G – guanine; T – thymine; C – cytosine). The genes regulate the activity of the neurotransmitters.

5. **Neurotransmitters are the words of a chemical conversation**

   Internal communication is dependent upon a system containing a sender (pre-synaptic neurone), a receiver (post-synaptic neuron), a place to meet (synapse) and carriers for the messages: the neurotransmitters. The neurotransmitters need to be highly specialised to ensure accuracy and precision in the context of one trillion synapses [6]! The main neurotransmitters are summarised below, with key references for each, but fuller details can be found in [7].

   Glutamate is a universal accelerator of neuronal activity [8]. It maintains cognitive arousal, enables long-term memory and provides the 'go' signal (calcium release) for activating neurons. It may give rise to a sense of overstimulation, as may be experienced after some Chinese meals that use monosodium glutamate as flavouring.

GABA (gamma amino butyric acid), a chemical sibling of glutamate, which inhibits neuronal activity by acting as the universal brake in the central nervous system [9]. Antiepileptic, anti-anxiety and anti-chronic-pain drugs often increase GABA, which provides the 'no go' to inhibit neurons.

Encephalin is one of the key neurotransmitter substances in the body's own morphine system [10]. The experience of being injured, for example whilst playing a sport, but only becoming aware of this later, is due to the release of encephalins. Similarly, the enhanced sense of well-being after particularly vigorous exertion arises from release of encephalins.

Dopamine has many functions [11] but those of particular relevance to eating disorders relate to movement and motivation. The movement centres (basal ganglia) are fuelled by dopamine. Excessive dopamine activity gives rise to agitation and motor restlessness (often misinterpreted and managed by clinicians as a deliberate attempt to lose weight). Reduced dopamine activity leads to anergia and Parkinsonian symptoms. Dopamine also serves the motivational centre in the brain – the nucleus accumbens – which both produces and uses dopamine. When dopamine is released, it acts as a reward, increases motivation and enables reinforcement. Dopamine increases in response to praise and results in the person feeling good. Cocaine, amphetamines and nicotine stimulate dopamine release and increase dopamine levels in the synapses.

Serotonin is fundamental to many functions [12]. It induces and maintains sleep [13] through the sleep centres of the brainstem (the Raphe nuclei). It also regulates moods such as depression, aggression and irritability, and is involved in checking for errors and omissions. The building block for serotonin is carbohydrate, and when there is carbohydrate depletion, as occurs in AN, there is serotonin depletion, with consequent lowering of mood, irritability and, in some, excessive checking (obsessive–compulsive disorder). This depletion explains why selective serotonin reuptake inhibitors do not work in states of malnutrition: there is no serotonin for them to act upon.

Acetylcholine also has many functions [13]. It fuels the parasympathetic nervous system, responsible for 'rest and digest', and is particularly active in meditation. It assists the calming system (the insula and the parasympathetic nervous system) in its balancing of the alarm system (amygdala and sympathetic nervous system). In states of depletion, the calming system becomes unstable and may become over- or underactive. With overactivity of acetylcholine, the heart and respiration slow down and blood pressure and temperature fall, as in AN. Finally, acetylcholine is also relevant to the retrieval of visual memory, often impaired in AN.

Nitric oxide, once proclaimed 'molecule of the year' [14], is involved in many physiological processes, one of the most important of which is vasodilatation. The process of thinking about a specific body part causes vasodilatation in that part and at the site of its cortical representation. The consequent increase in cerebral perfusion has treatment implications for AN (see Chapter 8), in which there is such preoccupation with specific parts of the body.

Noradrenalin is central to alertness, threat-detection, fear, fight and flight [15]. The alarm system (amygdala and sympathetic nervous system) is powered by noradrenalin. Thus, anxiety and panic are fuelled and sustained by noradrenalin. Noradrenalin also plays a major role in regulating cerebral blood flow [16] and facilitating neuroplasticity [17]. Excessive noradrenaline activity may be a key factor in the pathogenesis of AN [18]. Chapter 8 outlines in depth a noradrenergic dysregulation hypothesis for the pathogenesis and maintenance of AN.

5.4 Five implications of these propositions

1. Understanding the construction of the bodily experience means having some appreciation for the 20 or so natural elements central to the process.
2. The adequacy of nutrition will have an impact on the capacity to construct accurately that bodily experience.
3. Eating disorders, with their nutritional depletion and imbalance, represent a major threat to that accurate construction.
4. Adequate nutrition is part of the therapeutic modification of that inaccurate construction.
5. What makes each individual unique, whether in a starved or a well-fed state, is mediated by DNA, and by its expression through the genes.

5.5 Five directions for future research

1. Chemists, especially medical biochemists and molecular geneticists, should be recruited to the research endeavour.
2. Psychonutrition should be developed as a critical part of the profile of theoretical understanding and practical management of eating disorders.
3. The impact of disturbed neurochemistry on eating-disorder psychopathology should be examined directly and precisely, for example by correlating variations in elements, such as sodium, potassium and phosphate, with the clinical phenomena and the course of the illness.
4. The current sporadic 'fishing expeditions' for key molecules in eating disorders should be abandoned in favour of a broad theoretical and hypothesis-driven framework.
5. The genetic regulation of sense of bodily self, and the impact of sense of bodily self on genetic regulation, should be given a higher profile.

5.6 Conclusion

Our bodies and our universe are a single fabric. This fabric of our daily lives is woven from the food in our environment. The golden thread running through and tying together the whole fabric of life is DNA. This is a thread inscribed with writing so small, so miniscule and yet so vital that each word (gene) is a fragment of our genesis and of the story that will unfold in the life we are to live. The genes are both the weaver and the woven: the recurring motifs across the vast fabric of life in the 'mind' of the weaver and in each individual living tapestry. The neurotransmitters are the narratives recorded as they happen, yet fulfiled as they are written along the golden thread: commands announced, conversations communicated, instruction given on which words are to be spoken, when and where. Amidst the infinitely subtle variations in the tight and loose weaves, the density and colouring of thread, emerges the muddle that is eating disorder.

Acknowledgement

I am deeply grateful for the many insights of and countless discussions with Dr Ruth Urwin, Principal Scientist in the Molecular Neuropsychiatry Service at the Children's Hospital Westmead in Sydney, Australia.

References

1. Christian, D. (2008) *Big History: The Big Bang, Life on Earth and the Rise of Humanity*, The Great Courses, The Teaching Company, Chantilly, VA.
2. Swertka, A. (1998) *A Guide to the Elements*, Oxford University Press, Oxford.
3. Nunn, K., Hanstock, T. and Lask, B. (2008) *Who's Who of the Brain*, Jessica Langley Press, London and New York.
4. Collins, F. (2010) *The Language of Life*, Profile Books, London.
5. Watson, J. (2004) *DNA: The Secret of life*, Arrow Books.
6. Blier, P. (2001) Crosstalk between the norepinephrine and serotonin systems and its role in the antidepressant response. *Journal of Psychiatry and Neuroscience*, **26** (Suppl.), S3–S10.
7. Siegel, G., Albers, R., Brady, S. and Price, M.D. (2005) *Basic Neurochemistry: Molecular, Cellular and Medical Aspects*, Lippincott, Williams & Wilkins, Philadelphia, PA.
8. Nakazato, M., Hashimoto, K., Schmidt, U. *et al.* (2010) Serum glutamine, set-shifting ability and anorexia nervosa. *Annals of General Psychiatry*, **9**, 29–37.
9. Ganguly, K., Schinder, A.F., Wong, S.T. and Poo, M. (2001) GABA itself promotes the developmental switch of neuronal GABAergic responses from exitation to inhibition. *Cell*, **105** (4), 521–532.
10. Cabyoglu, M.T., Ergene, N. and Tan, U. (2006) The mechanisms of acupuncture and clinical applications. *International Journal of Neuroscience*, **116** (2), 115–125.
11. Björklund, A. and Dunnet, S.B. (2007) Dopamine neuron systems in the brain: an update. *Trends in Neurosciences*, **30** (5), 194–202.
12. Kaye, W.H., Frank, G.K., Bailer, U.F. *et al.* (2005) Serotonin alterations in anorexia nervosa and bulimia nervosa: new insights from imaging studies. *Physiological Behavior*, **85** (1), 73–81.
13. Jones, B.E. (2005) From waking to sleeping: neuronal and chemical substrates. *Trends in Pharmacological Sciences*, **26** (11), 578–586.
14. Culotta, E. and Koshland, D.E. (1992) No news is good news. *Science*, **258** (5090), 1862–1865.
15. Bremner, J.D., Krystal, J.H., Southwick, S.M. and Charney, D.S. (1996) Noradrenergic mechanisms in stress and anxiety: II. Clinical studies. *Synapse*, **23**, 39–51.
16. Nathanson, J.A. and Glaser, G.H. (1979) Identification of *B*-arenergic-sensitive adenylate cyclase in intracranial blood vessels. *Nature*, **278**, 567–569.
17. Gu, Q. (2002) Neuromodulatory transmitter systems in the cortex and their role in cortical plasticity. *Neuroscience*, **111** (4), 815–835.
18. Urwin, R.E. and Nunn, K.P. (2005) Epistatic interaction between the monoamine oxidase A and serotonin transporter genes in anorexia nervosa. *European Journal of Human Genetics*, **13** (3), 370–375.

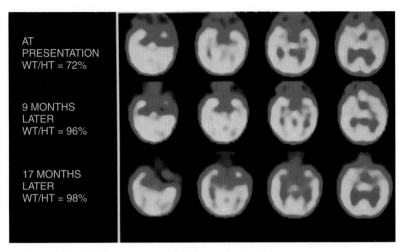

Plate 1 SPECT image of regional cerebral blood flow in a patient with AN, at initial presentation and then following weight restoration. (See Page 91)

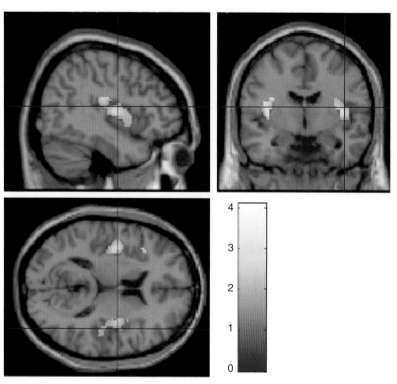

Plate 2   Composite fMRI image comparing brain activation in response to a mental rotation task in a group of patients with AN versus matched control participants. (See Page 93)

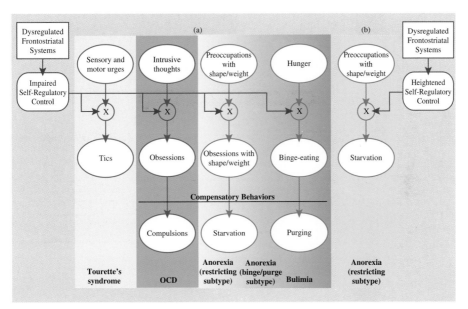

Plate 3 The role of dysregulated frontostriatal systems in Tourette's syndrome, OCD, AN and BN. The top row of panel (a) represents urges, thoughts and drives that are present in both healthy and patient populations. An impaired capacity for self-regulatory control interacts with these normal urges, thoughts and drives to produce ego-dystonic symptoms or behaviours (middle row) Attempts to relieve the anxiety associated with these symptoms or to compensate for these behaviours produce further behavioural abnormalities (bottom row). BN and AN restricting subtype are on opposite ends of a continuum. AN binge-purge subtype is positioned within the middle of this continnum, since it shares features with both BN and AN restricting subtype. Panel (b) illustrates an alternative conceptualisation of AN restricting subtype: preoccupation with body shape and weight interact with heightened, rather than impaired, self-regulatory control, producing starvation directly [9] Reproduced from Marsh, R., Maia, T.V., and Peterson, B.S. (2009). Functional Disturbances Within Frontostriatal Circuits Across Multiple Childhood Psychopathologies. *American Journal of Psychiatry*, **166**, 664–674; with permission from APA. (See Page 154)

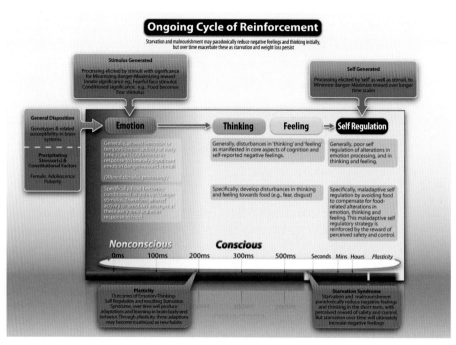

Plate 4   The Integrative Neuroscience Model of Anorexia Nervosa (INTEGRATE-AN) [11]. (See Page 159)

6 Body-image disturbance

Maria Øverås

Regional Eating Disorders Service, Oslo University Hospital, Oslo, Norway

6.1 Introduction

Body-image disturbance is a core symptom of all eating disorders. Studies have found that a disturbed body image often precedes and predicts the development of eating disorders [1, 2]. Also, body-image disturbance at discharge from treatment is associated with higher rates of relapse [3]. In consequence, understanding how disturbed body image develops and persists is of crucial importance for successful prevention and treatment.

There can be no doubt that cultural, social and psychological factors influence body image. The body is a central aspect of all cultures. It is our 'shop window to the world'. It conveys who we are, what we stand for and where we belong. In Western societies the current body ideal for women is extremely thin, and hence unrealistic and unhealthy for most people. The result is a society where it is quite common to be unhappy with one's body weight or shape. In other words, cultural, social and psychological factors must clearly be taken into account when trying to understand the body-image disturbance of patients with eating disorders.

However, body-image disturbance seen in patients with eating disorders is both qualitatively and quantitatively different from the worry or dissatisfaction seen in the general population. Why do some people develop this extreme form of body-image disturbance, while most do not? Could individual differences in brain functioning render some people more vulnerable than others to developing the body-image disturbances seen in eating disorders?

This chapter starts with a review of the definition of body image, followed by a section exploring how body image is normally constructed in the brain, and a description of the specific body-image disturbance of patients with eating disorders. There is then an exploration of some of the theories and empirical findings that might help us understand the brain's involvement in body-image disturbance, and finally, a summary of knowledge to date and consideration of some possible directions for future research.

Eating Disorders and the Brain. Edited by Bryan Lask and Ian Frampton.
© 2011 John Wiley & Sons, Ltd. Published 2011 by John Wiley & Sons, Ltd.

6.2   What is body image?

Bruch is often credited as the first to describe body image as a central feature in eating disorders [4]. In 1997 she stated: 'the expression "body image" is so widely used in the psychiatric evaluation of patients that it is surprising to note how vague the concept is' [5]. This statement is still valid, reflecting how difficult it is to capture the complexity of the concept in one simple definition. A useful working definition is given by Slade [4], suggesting that body image relates to: '. . . the picture we have in our minds of the size, shape and form of our bodies; and to our feelings concerning these characteristics and our constituent body parts' (p. 20).

This definition is simple, but reflects the general agreement that body image is a multidimensional construct. Furthermore, it takes into account the different elements of body-image disturbance. Body image is often divided into two main elements: perceptual and attitudinal [6]. The perceptual aspect concerns how we *experience* our body (e.g. size and shape), while the attitudinal aspect concerns how we *evaluate* our body (e.g. the thought 'I am fat' followed by feelings of disgust or shame). Obviously, these elements are closely connected and interact in complex ways. Although artificial, this division is heuristically useful and maybe even necessary for us to explore the construct scientifically.

6.3   How is body image constructed in the brain?

We can access and decode knowledge of our own body without effort. We can name different body parts, locate them, and tell if they are warm or cold, in pain or just fine. We are never confused about whether or not another object is part of our body, nor do we misinterpret someone else's hand as our own [7]. We know whether we feel fat or thin, and how happy we are about different parts of our body. Much research has been conducted into how this experience of our body is constructed and represented in the brain. Despite all these efforts, it has not been possible to identify a single location in the brain that contains the 'body image', indicating that several structures are involved in this process [8, 9]. Body image is experienced through somatotopic representations, known as sensory homunculi (homunculus = little human). These homunculi emanate from the somatosensory cortex, located in the parietal lobes and the insula (see also Chapter 8).

The somatosensory cortex

The somatosensory cortex may broadly be divided into three main components:

1. Primary (sensory and perceptual), located in the superior aspect of the anterior parietal cortex, immediately posterior to the central sulcus, and which deals with perception of the somatosensory experience (e.g. touch, temperature, posture);
2. Secondary (or interpretative), located in the inferior aspect of the anterior parietal lobe. Even though specific cells in the brain receive sensory information about size, shape, texture and temperature, we do not perceive the world in such a fragmented way. Quite effortlessly, the information is integrated and decoded as something meaningful, like a cup, a lighter or someone else's hand [10]. This interpretation of somatosensory information occurs in the secondary somatosensory cortex, the

region responsible for combining information about the body, including somatosensory and visual data, into a coherent sense of the body [11, 12]. In this region of the brain the ventral visual pathway [13] sends visual data to left-hemisphere temporal-lobe regions hosting neural networks that contain semantic details about visual information [14]. It appears that the temporoparietal junction has a specific function in distinguishing between mental imagery of one's own body and other neutral objects [12].

3. Tertiary (or integrative), located in the insula, which integrates and provides meaning to the experience. The final element of this integrated network is the insula cortex, located within the Sylvian fissure. It has been suggested that this cortex has a specialised function in the integration of emotion and bodily perception [15] and in producing an integrated internal 'map' of the body in the brain [16, 17] (see also Chapter 8).

These levels of homuncular activity blend into each other.

Each homunculus provides 'representational space' for each part of the body. However, certain parts are represented in greater detail than others. In the sensory homunculus, the face, hands and genitals have greater representation because of their larger amount of sensory innervation. Other body parts, for example the trunk, limbs and internal organs, have less representation given their smaller amount of sensory innervation (see also Chapter 8).

Different parts of the primary somatosensory cortex receive information from different parts of the body. If one traces where input from each body part is located in the parietal cortex, the resulting map will look like an odd little human (see Figure 6.1). The representation in the brain does not correspond with the size of the body part itself, but rather with the density of sensory nerve endings. For example, sensitivity in the hands, mouth and genitals is vital for survival and reproduction, and therefore these parts contain high sensory nerve density. On the other hand, the elbows and knees do not need as much sensitivity to serve their function, and are therefore represented with fewer neurons [10]. Information about the left side of the body is represented on the right side of the brain, and vice versa [7, 10].

It is important to note at this point that activation in the parietal cortex does not only depend on sensory input, but also requires that attention is directed towards the stimuli [11]. Indeed, an attentional model of body image suggests that sensory input is not continuously integrated into a coherent image of the body in the brain, but rather that diverse information about the body is integrated only when attention is directed towards it [8]. Studies of parietal lesions and their effects have led to speculation about lateralisation of such attentional functions. It has been proposed that the left parietal lobe is involved in attention towards motor activity, while the right parietal lobe is more specialised for spatial attention [9], a hypothesis supported by the clinical observation that only patients with right-sided stroke typically experience visual-neglect phenomena.

Taken together, these findings suggest that there is not yet a clear consensus on the processes involved in construction of body image and how the different structures work together. Furthermore, a broader perspective on body image as involving not only perception of body shape and size, but also body ownership, agency, thoughts, feelings and identity, suggests that structurally the whole brain is involved at some level.

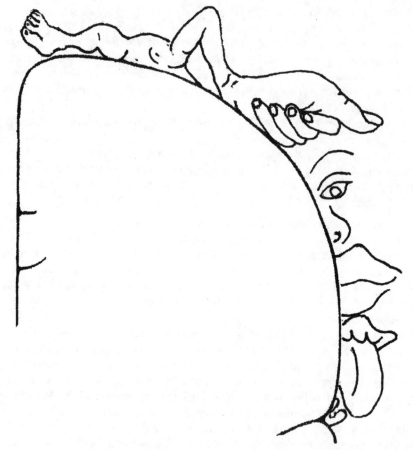

Figure 6.1 The sensory homunculus. Source: http://spinacare.wordpress.com/category/pain-and-the-brain/.

Online and offline representations of the body

The previous section reviewed some of the brain areas thought to be involved in the construction of body image. Another way of approaching this question is to describe the construction of body image from a theoretical perspective. A theoretical model proposed by Carruthers [18] suggests that there are two levels of bodily representation in the brain: online and offline. He suggests that online representation results from the direct monitoring of how the body is here-and-now, based on current incoming sensory information about, for example, touch and posture (i.e. perception). This online representation of the body is dynamic: it changes as the input from the body changes.

Offline representations of the body on the other hand, are stored representations of *what the body normally is like* (i.e. memory). Carruthers suggests that the offline representation is based mainly on earlier online representations. However, the offline model does not seem to change at the same rate at which new online information enters. This is illustrated for example by the fact that people tend to retain an image of their self as relatively young when growing older, sometimes resulting in surprise when they catch a glimpse of themselves in a mirror.

Another example is the phenomenon of phantom limbs, where a person feels that their arm or leg is still there long after the limb has been amputated [19]. Further, there are examples of phantom limbs in patients who are born without one or more limbs, and hence have never experienced any online representations of the missing limb [20]. This implies that the offline representation of the body consists of some innate aspects (e.g. number of limbs, left vs right limbs) that are relatively stable throughout life, in addition to more dynamic aspects formed and changed by online information (e.g. changing length of body) [15, 21].

6.4   Body-image disturbance in eating disorders

As identified earlier, it is common to distinguish between attitudinal and perceptual aspects of body image. In eating disorders the attitudinal aspects include a strong sense of dissatisfaction with one's weight and shape, and the feeling that weight and shape define one's value as a person. The perceptual aspect, on the other hand, involves a distorted experience of the size of one's body. This distortion is most prominent for patients with anorexia nervosa (AN), who often report seeing themselves as fat, even when they are so thin that they are in severe danger of physical collapse [1].

Research into the attitudinal aspects has tended to focus mostly on the influence of cultural and psychological factors, with the role of thin-ideals in Western societies being central to the development of negative attitudes towards body shape and size. However, some twin studies have indicated that there is also a genetic contribution to the development of body attitudes in women, independent of body mass index (BMI) (e.g. [22, 23]). Research into the perceptual component of body image has been more influenced by a neuroscience perspective, with exploration of how a normal body image is constructed and represented in the brain and how changes in the brain could result in a distorted experience of one's body. In the remainder of this chapter, I will focus on the research on neuroscience and body-size perception in eating disorders. A fuller description and discussion of the attitudinal component of body image can be found in [8].

One of the most challenging phenomena in the field of eating disorders is that of distorted body image, particularly in the presence of overwhelming evidence against the false image. Patients know what their weight is, and how it compares to the general population. They know that they are fitting into the smallest sizes available for clothes. They know that their parents and friends are extremely worried about their low weight. When talking to patients with AN, confronting them with the evidence of their extreme underweight status, it is obvious that they are able to grasp the logic of what they are told but remain hesitant to accept that they are in fact very thin. The responses differ. Some argue that there is something wrong with the weighing equipment. Others say that their parents and friends are overreacting. Yet others say that their body is different from everyone else's. A common response, however, can be summarised with this statement from one patient:

I understand what you are saying, and agree to the logic, but I still FEEL fat, and that feeling is so strong that it MUST be true.

It is important to note at this point that there is great variability in how patients with AN experience their body, and that not all experience body-image distortions. Interviews of women with AN about their body image have indicated that some patients do not have a distorted experience of their body at all; others feel that they are fat, but know that they are not; while others again both feel that they are fat and believe they really are so [24].

Several studies have confirmed the clinical observations that patients with AN over-estimate the size of their body more than healthy controls [25]. However, the findings are conflicting, and some studies have shown that the estimation of own-body size can be affected by both contextual and psychological variables, such as mood, how much was eaten at the last meal and how the question was asked [26–28]. This has led some researchers to question the meaningfulness of this research, as it suggests that body-size estimation is not a static construct and that the results might depend on the timing or setting of the experiment. However, a review of several studies of body-size estimation confirms the finding that patients with AN generally overesti-mate their body size more than healthy controls [25], indicating that even though the experience of body size is dynamic, it involves some degree of stability. The finding that patients with AN only overestimate the size of their own body, not the sizes of other bodies or neutral objects, has led to the conclusion that the overestimation does not reflect a general problem with size estimation [25].

It should be mentioned that most of the research on body-image disturbance has focused on patients with AN. The remainder of this chapter will therefore focus on AN, unless stated otherwise.

6.5 The neuroscience of body-image distortion in anorexia nervosa

In the light of these findings, how can we understand the body-image disturbance in AN? I will begin by looking at how the theory of online and offline representations applies to body-image disturbance in AN. Then I will describe some syndromes fol-lowing lesions in the brain that result in a disturbed body image and discuss their relevance for the understanding of body-image disturbance in AN. Finally, I will dis-cuss some of the findings from studies using neuroimaging techniques to explore body image in eating disorders, and briefly discuss the possible influence of the neuropsy-chological functioning of patients with AN on body image.

Online and offline representations

As discussed above, Carruthers [18] suggests that body image contains information from both online and offline representations. In other words, a person uses both the memory of how the body 'normally is' (offline representation) and perception of the body 'here-and-now' (online representation) to construct their body image. This could explain the finding that the body image of patients with AN seems to have some stability (offline), and at the same time to fluctuate depending on context (online).

However, this distinction does not explain how interactions between online and offline body representations are played out over time. Tsakiris [29] suggests a 'test-for-fit' model that accounts for the interaction between online and offline information.

In line with Carruthers' theory, Tsakiris suggests that there is a preexisting stored (offline) model of the body in the brain. Further, he suggests that current (online) information about the body is integrated and compared to the existing model.

This model was originally developed to explain the concept of body ownership in the context of 'out-of-body' experiences. However, it could be hypothesised that similar mechanisms might be involved in the process of amending offline representations based on new online information. Tsakiris suggests that this process involves a network in the brain, including the right temporoparietal junction, the secondary somatosensory cortex, the posterior parietal and ventral premotor cortices and the right posterior insula [29, 30].

Based on this model, it might be expected that someone who loses large amounts of weight will adapt their body image accordingly, as the new online information is received. However, this does not seem to be the case with AN. On the contrary, many of these patients seem to have a persistent experience of being fat even when they are in fact extremely underweight. This could imply a problem in the transaction between online and offline information.

An alternative approach is based on Kosslyn's [31] general theory of mental imagery. In this theory she distinguishes between prototypes and exemplars. The prototype is described as a less precise representation including only the properties that are general across different examples (e.g. birds in general), while the exemplar is a specific representation of an object and how it looks at one particular time (e.g. an eagle you just saw). This division has some parallels to Carruthers' model, with the prototype corresponding to the offline representation and the exemplar corresponding to the online representation.

Research has suggested that prototypes and exemplars are represented differently in the brain, with the prototypes stored more efficiently in the left cerebral hemisphere and the exemplars in the right hemisphere [32, 33]. Smeets and Kosslyn [34] have hypothesised that the experience of being fat in patients with eating disorders is a prototype and therefore will be more efficiently stored in the left hemisphere. This was indeed what they found in a divided-visual-field experiment. More specifically, patients with AN were found to process a picture of themselves as fat faster when it was presented to the left hemisphere (via right visual field) than to the right hemisphere (via left visual field) [34].

Several other studies have indicated that the right hemisphere is central to the processing of bodies (e.g. [35, 36]). However, these findings need not be contradictory, as there might be different areas involved in different aspects of body processing, with the processing of prototypes of own-body represented in the left hemisphere and other processes represented in the right hemisphere. More research is needed to reach any conclusion about lateralisation of body-image processes.

Body-image distortions due to brain lesions

An important source of knowledge about how the body image is constructed, and sometimes disrupted, comes from studies of patients with brain lesions. Several striking syndromes involving the body have been found as the result of damage in particular areas of the brain. This section considers some of these syndromes and the possible parallels to the body-image disturbance found in AN.

Damage in the right parietal lobe sometimes results in *neglect syndrome* [37], whereby patients deny the existence of a part of their own body. For example, there have been cases of patients neglecting to recognise the left side of the body as their own. There are indications that these patients can see their body accurately but overlook its existence, with striking results such as failing to wash or dress one side of their body. When confronted with a neglected body part, these patients do not acknowledge it as a part of themselves, but tend to confabulate and offer alternative explanations. For example, one patient who woke up and saw his neglected foot in the bed insisted that someone must have left a fake leg in his bed as a joke [10].

Another syndrome, *anosognosia for hemiplegia*, can arise from lesions in the right insula cortex [38]. In this condition patients are unaware of being paralysed on one side of the body. If asked to do something that normally would include the use of both arms, such as lifting a tray with glasses of water, they will often attempt to do so, with unfortunate results such as dropping the tray. When asked why this happened these patients often come up with an explanation other than their being paralysed, for example that they did not use both arms because they have pains in one shoulder [39].

These examples have some striking parallels to the body-image disturbance of patients with AN. Like those with unilateral neglect or anosognosia for hemiplegia, patients with AN are surrounded with evidence that they fail to accept. Patients know their weight and how it compares to the normal population, they know the size of the clothes they are wearing, and they observe the reaction of people they love and trust. All this is pointing to the fact that they are not fat, but rather dangerously underweight. However, as in the cases of unilateral neglect and anosognosia for hemiplegia, patients with AN resist accepting what one might normally see as the most logical explanation. Instead they tend to come up with an alternative explanation that can account for what they *feel* is right (see section on 'Body-image disturbance in eating disorders').

Could this *feeling* of what the body is really like be accounted for by the stored offline representation of what the body is normally like? Carruthers [18] argues that this is the case. He suggests that patients with anosognosia for hemiplegia or unilateral neglect are less able to adapt their offline representation to the current online information. Could this also be true for patients with AN?

Another possible explanation could be that these patients are unable to construct an accurate online representation of their body in the first place [16, 17]. This might explain why many patients with AN insist that they are fat, even though they obviously are not. However, it does not explain why some patients with eating disorders also report *seeing* themselves as fat when they look in the mirror. Could the feeling of how the body is also affect how patients with eating disorders see themselves?

Carruthers [18] argues that the experience of visual input can indeed be affected by offline representations of the body. He gives several examples of this. First, he points to studies using the *rubber hand illusion paradigm*. In this paradigm, participants watch a rubber hand being stroked at the same time as their own unseen hand. Several studies have demonstrated that participants in this condition will attribute the rubber hand as part of their own body [40, 41]. Some studies using this paradigm have also found that some participants who experience the rubber hand as their own report seeing the rubber hand as more similar to their actual hand (e.g. in shape and colour) than it really is (e.g. [40]). Carruthers' explanation for this is that when one starts to *feel* like the rubber hand is one's own, the visual experience changes so that it fits better with the offline representation of what one's hand normally looks like [18].

In a second example, Carruthers points to the cases of patients with anosognosia for hemiplegia. Remember how these patients often offer an explanation for why they did not use both arms when asked to lift a tray with glasses: in some cases these patients would actually claim to have used both arms, and even report that they saw their paralysed arm move [42].

In both these examples, the feeling of how the body is seems to affect the visual experience. In the same way, one could hypothesise that the feeling of being fat is so strong in some patients with AN that this biases their visual perceptual processing to the extent that they start to see themselves as fat when looking in the mirror.

fMRI studies of body image in eating disorders

A few studies have been conducted using functional magnetic resonance imaging (fMRI) to explore body image in patients with eating disorders. Uher *et al.* [36] found that patients with AN or bulimia nervosa (BN), when compared to healthy controls, had reduced activity in several brain areas when exposed to drawings of bodies in different sizes. More specifically, the areas with reduced activation included the occipitotemporal and parietal regions, with the reduced activation being more pronounced for the patients with AN than those with BN. Uher *et al.* suggest that these findings indicate dysfunction in circuits involved in body-image processing [34].

In a study exploring brain activation during exposure to images of self and others, Sachdev *et al.* [43] found that patients with AN and healthy controls had similar activation for nonself-images. However, when exposed to self-images, the controls showed considerably greater activation in attentional systems and the insula than did the patients with AN. These findings suggest that those with AN process images of others similarly to controls, but when it comes to processing of self-image there is a discrepancy between the two groups. Sachdev *et al.* suggest that this discrepant processing might underlie the distortion of body image in AN.

Some of these findings were replicated by Vocks *et al.* [44]. More specifically, they found that both patients with AN and patients with BN had reduced activity in areas of the brain involved in attentional processing when exposed to pictures of themselves compared to nonself pictures. This reduced activation was not found in healthy controls. The authors suggest that the reduced activation in areas associated with attentional processes could reflect patients' engagement in body-avoidance behaviour during exposure to pictures of themselves. This is in line with clinical observations that some patients do avoid exposure to their own appearance because of the high level of anxiety such exposure elicits.

The lack of activation in the insula found by Sachdev *et al.* [43] is interesting theoretically, as this area has been indicated as a central brain structure in eating disorders [16]. Further, as the insula is anatomically placed as a centre for communication between several areas assumed to be involved in the construction of body image, it makes sense that problems in this area could affect the ability to construct and maintain an accurate body image [17].

Clearly, more research is needed on this area to help us make sense of these findings. However, it is noteworthy that two of the recent neuroimaging studies [44, 34] found similar patterns for patients with AN and those with BN, possibly indicating that the brain processes underlying body-image disturbance in these two conditions are more similar than we might have anticipated.

Body-image distortion and neuropsychology

Research has not yet focused on the association between neuropsychological functioning and body-image disturbance in AN (or any other eating disorder). However, it seems plausible that the way people organise information in general will not only affect how they experience the outside world, but also how they experience their own body.

Findings from research on the neuropsychological profile in patients with AN (see Chapter 4) have been relatively consistent. For example, several studies have found that patients with AN tend to have a detailed, focused processing style (often called weak central coherence) compared to healthy controls. Another relatively stable finding has been that many patients with AN perform poorer on tasks requiring set-shifting (mental flexibility). Finally, several studies indicate that patients with AN are poorer at visuospatial memory than healthy controls.

How could these findings contribute to our understanding of body-image disturbance in AN? One could hypothesise that a person who tends to get caught up in details in general would also apply this processing style when attending to her own body. Jansen et al. [45] found that patients with AN who were exposed to pictures of themselves looked more at the body parts with which they were unhappy, compared to a group of healthy controls. In other words, patients with AN not only focus on details when evaluating their own body, but also seem to have an attentional bias towards negatively charged detail. This could affect both the direct perception of the body (online representation) and how the body is remembered (offline representation). Poor flexibility, on the other hand, could affect the ability to adapt mental schemas (offline representation) based on new information (online representation). Finally, poor visuospatial memory could affect the ability to form a correct visual representation of the body in the brain (offline representation). More research is needed to explore the relationship between neuropsychological functioning and aspects of body-image disturbance such as body-size estimation error in eating disorders.

6.6   Conclusion

Neuroscience research to date has failed to locate a specific area in the brain associated with the body-image disturbance characteristically seen in eating disorders. This could indicate that body-image disturbance is the result of a neural network problem, rather than damage in one specific structure. If a network problem is involved, we must assume that this contributes to the development of body-image disturbances in interaction with psychological and sociocultural variables. For example, a network problem could affect how the individual responds to the thin-body ideals conveyed by society. Furthermore, a network problem in the brain could be intensified by aspects of the eating disorder such as extreme low weight or preoccupation with weight and shape over extended periods of time. Longitudinal and prospective studies will be needed to clarify whether such neural factors are a cause or consequence of eating disorders, or both.

In order to understand more about the neural basis for body-image disturbance, we need first to find out more about how a mental image of the body is constructed in normal development, both online (what is my body image today?) and offline (what is my memory of my body?). Such a complex representation of the body will necessarily encompass visual, tactile, vestibular, somatosensory and visceral perceptual information, matched against stored template memories. Perhaps the next step could be for researchers in the field to work together to develop a more coherent conceptual model of body-image representation and its disturbance, which can be tested empirically.

References

1. Garner, D.M. (2002) Body image and anorexia nervosa, in *Body Image: A Handbook of Theory, Research, and Clinical Practice* (eds T.F. Cash and T Pruzinsky), The Guilford Press, New York, pp. 295–303.
2. Killen, J.D., Taylor, C.B., Hayward, C. *et al.* (1996) Weight concerns influence the development of eating disorders: a 4-year prospective study. *Journal of Consulting and Clinical Psychology*, **64**, 936–940.
3. Farrell, C., Shafran, R. and Fairburn, C.G. (2003) Body size estimation: testing a new mirror-based assessment method. *International Journal of Eating Disorders*, **34**, 162–171.
4. Slade, P.D. (1988) Body image in anorexia nervosa. *British Journal of Psychiatry*, **153**, 20–22.
5. Bruch, H. (1997) Body image and self-awareness, in *Food and Culture: A Reader* (eds C. Counihan and P. Van Esterik), Routledge, New York, pp. 211–225.
6. Bell, L. and Rushforth, J. (2008) Body image and body image disturbances, in *Overcoming Body Image Disturbance: A Programme for People with Eating Disorders* (eds L. Bell and J. Rushforth), Routledge, New York.
7. Ames, F.R. (2002) The neurological basis of body image, in *Disorders of Body Image* (eds D.J. Castle and K.A. Philips), Wrightson Biomedical Publishing, Petersfield.
8. Cash, T.F. and Pruzinsky, T. (2002) *Body Image: A Handbook of Theory, Research, and Clinical Practice*, The Guilford Press, New York.
9. Trimble, M. (2007) Body image and the parietal lobes. *CNS Spectrums*, **12**, 540–544.
10. Bear, M.F., Connors, B.W. and Paradiso, M.A. (2001) *Neuroscience: Exploring the Brain*, Lippincott Williams & Wilkins, Baltimore.
11. Brodal, P. (2001) *Sentralnervesystemet*, Universitetsforlaget, Oslo.
12. Blanke, O., Mohr, C., Michel, C.M. *et al.* (2005) Linding out-of-body experience and self processing to mental own-body imagery at the temporal junction. *The Journal of Neuroscience*, **25**, 550–557.
13. Grill-Spector, K. (2003) The neural basis of object perception. *Current Opinion in Neurobiology*, **13**, 1–8.
14. Tranel, D., Damasio, H. and Damasio, A.R. (1998) The neural basis of lexical retrieval, in *Fundamentals of Neural Network Modeling: Neuropsychology and Cognitive Neuroscience* (eds R.W. Parks, D.S. Levine and D.L. Lond), The MIT Press, Cambridge, pp. 271–296.
15. Berlucchi, G. and Aglioti, S.M. (2010) The body in the brain revisited. *Experimental Brain Research*, **1**, 25–35.
16. Nunn, K., Frampton, I., Gordon, I. and Lask, B. (2008) The fault is not in her parents but in her insula: a neurobiological hypothesis of anorexia nervosa. *European Eating Disorders Review*, **16**, 355–360.

17. Nunn, K., Frampton, I., Fuglset, T. *et al.* (2011) Anorexia nervosa in the insula. *Medical Hypotheses*, **76**, 353–357.
18. Carruthers, G. (2008) Types of body representation and the sense of embodiment. *Consciousness and Cognition*, **17**, 1302–1316.
19. Ramachandran, V.S. and Hirstein, W. (1998) The perception of phantom limbs. *Brain*, **9**, 1603–1630.
20. Scatena, P. (1990) Phantom representations of congenitally absent limbs. *Perceptual and Motor Skills*, **70**, 1227–1232.
21. Tsarkiris, M. and Fotopoulou, A. (2008) Is my body the sum of online and offline body-representations? *Consciousness and Cognition*, **17**, 1317–1320.
22. Keski-Rahkonen, A., Bulik, C.M., Neale, B.M. *et al.* (2005) Body dissatisfaction and drive for thinness in young adult twins. *International Journal of Eating Disorders*, **37**, 188–199.
23. Spanos, A., Burt, S.A. and Klump, K.L. (2010) Do weight and shape concerns exhibit genetic effects? Investigating discrepant findings. *International Journal of Eating Disorders*, **43**, 29–34.
24. Espeset, E.M., Nordbø, R.H., Gulliksen K.S. *et al.* (2011) The concept of body image disturbance in anorexia nervosa: an empirical inquiry utilizing patients' subjective experiences. *Eating Disorders*, **19** (2), 175–193.
25. Farrell, C., Lee, M. and Shafran, R. (2005) Assessment of body size estimation: a review. *European Eating Disorders Review*, **13**, 75–88.
26. Garner, D.M. and Moncrieff, C. (1988) Body image distortion in anorexics as a non-sensory phenomenon: a signal detection approach. *Journal of Clinical Psychology*, **44**, 101–107.
27. Taylor, M.J. and Cooper, P. (1992) An experimental study of the effect of mood on body size perception. *Behaviour Research and Therapy*, **30**, 53–58.
28. Thompson, J.K., Coovert, D.L., Pasman, L.N. and Robb, J. (1993) Body image and food consumption: three laboratory studies of perceived calorie content. *International Journal of Eating Disorders*, **14**, 445–457.
29. Tsakiris, M. (2010) My body in the brain: a neurocognitive model of body-ownership. *Neuropsychologia*, **48**, 703–712.
30. Tsakiris, M., Costantini, M. and Haggard, P. (2008) The role of the right temporo-parietal junction in maintaining a coherent sense of one's body. *Neuropsychologia*, **46**, 3014–3018.
31. Kosslyn, S.M. (1994) *Image and Brain: The Resolution of the Imagery Debate*, MIT Press, Cambridge, MA.
32. Laeng, B., Zarrinpar, A. and Kosslyn, S.M. (2003) Do separate processes identify objects as exemplars versus members of basic-level categories? Evidence from hemispheric specialization. *Brain and Cognition*, **53**, 15–27.
33. Kosslyn, S.M. (1987) Seeing and imagining in the cerebral hemispheres: a computational approach. *Psychological Review*, **94**, 148–175.
34. Smeets, M.A.M. and Kosslyn, S.M. (2001) Hemispheric differences in body image in anorexia nervosa. *International Journal of Eating Disorders*, **29**, 409–416.
35. Frassinetti, F., Maini, M., Romualdi, S. *et al.* (2008) Is it mine? Hemispheric asymmetries in corporeal self-recognition. *Journal of Cognitive Neuroscience*, **20**, 1507–1516.
36. Uher, R., Murphy, H.C., Freiderich, T. *et al.* (2005) Functional neuroanatomy of body shape perception in healthy and eating-disordered women. *Biological Psychiatry*, **58** (12), 990–997.
37. Pinto, L.R. (1990) Unilateral neglect syndrome: clinical and topographic study of 20 subjects. *Arquivos de Neuro-Psiquiatria*, **48**, 188–194.
38. Karnath, H.O., Baier, B. and Nägele, T. (2005) Awareness of the functioning of one's own limbs mediated by the insular cortex? *The Journal of Neuroscience*, **25**, 7134–7138.
39. Ramachandran, V.S. (1995) Anosognosia in parietal lobe syndrome. *Consciousness and Cognition*, **4**, 22–51.

40. Botvinick, M. and Cohen, J. (1998) Rubber hand 'feel' touch that eyes see. *Nature*, **391**, 756.
41. Costantini, M. and Haggard, P. (2007) The rubber hand illusion: sensitivity and reference frame for body ownership. *Counsciousness and Cognition*, **16**, 229–240.
42. Ramachandran, V.S. and Blakeslee, S. (2005) *Phantoms in the Brain: Human Nature and the Architecture of the Mind*, Harper Perennial, London.
43. Sachdev, P., Mondraty, N., Wen, W. and Gulliford, K. (2008) Brains of anorexia nervosa patients process self-images differently from non-self-images: an fMRI study. *Neuropsychologia*, **46**, 2161–2168.
44. Vocks, S., Busch, M., Grönemeyer, D. *et al.* (2010) Neural correlates of viewing photographs of one's own body and another woman's body in anorexia nervosa and bulimia nervosa: an fMRI study. *Journal of Psychiatry and Neuroscience*, **35**, 163–176.
45. Jansen, A., Nederkoorn, C. and Mulkens, S. (2005) Selective visual attention for ugly and beautiful body parts in eating disorders. *Behaviour Research and Therapy*, **43**, 183–196.

7 Conceptual models

Mark Rose[1] and Ian Frampton[2]

[1] *Huntercombe Group, UK*
[2] *College of Life and Environmental Sciences, University of Exeter, UK*

7.1 Introduction

Back to basics: what is a conceptual model?

Before describing a number of conceptual models on the neuroscience of eating disorders, it is worth considering the nature and origins of conceptual models. If we consider science in general, the ultimate goal is to describe phenomena that exist in nature and organise them in order to increase our understanding. Research about causality, predictions of associations and consequences allow us to make rules and exert control over these phenomena. In the field of nuclear physics, Nils Bohr revolutionised how physicists described and understood atomic particles by introducing a model to represent an atom.

A conceptual model is a map of concepts and their relationships. It describes the key elements of a system, their characteristics and the associations between them. The aim of a conceptual model is to simplify and describe a theory and to identify interrelationships between and among its component concepts; to capture and describe the workings of natural phenomena.

It is worth noting that the terms 'theory' and 'model' are often used interchangeably but are quite distinct. The Concise Oxford English Dictionary [1] defines a theory as 'a supposition or system of ideas explaining something, especially one based on general principles independent of the particular thing to be explained' (p. 1266). A model is simply a representation to help us understand and make predictions about the related phenomena described by a theory.

Walker [2] suggested that the purpose of science is to accurately predict events in nature. Any prediction based on a model must be independently validated by empirical methods such as observations or measurements. The correspondence between the model and its predictions is an indication of its validity. It is fair to say that conceptual models are not 'fixed'. As empirical methods of validation become more sophisticated, a model may become outdated and thus need revision.

What a conceptual model must include

There are several general principles that make a good conceptual model. These have been summarised by Fawcett [3]: comprehensiveness of content, logical congruence, conceptual clarity and level of abstraction.

Comprehensiveness of content refers to the depth and breadth of a model. Depth can be specified in terms of the adequacy of descriptions of constructs, and explanation of interrelationships between them. Breadth on the other hand refers to the scope of the model and its applicability across various fields or clinical contexts. Logical congruence refers to the logic of the internal structure of the model and the extent to which the components of the model fit together in a coherent way. Conceptual clarity refers to the identification and explicit description of the concepts and the relationships between them. Level of abstraction refers to the representation of concepts that range from concrete to abstract. In contrast to concrete concepts, abstract concepts are not directly measurable.

With any theory or model within the field of mental health, one must also consider its clinical utility. This refers to the applicability and relevance of the model to the real world of practice. Does the model address clinical issues; that is, does it account for the clinical presentation of a disorder and what are the practical implications for clinical treatment?

7.2   Conceptual models in anorexia nervosa

Seven neuroscience-based conceptual models that endeavour to explain the pathogenesis and maintenance of eating disorders have been selected. These appear in chronological order and cover a wide range of perspectives, from genes to thoughts and behaviours. An overview of each model is given and the evidence base offered by the original authors is summarised, before a brief commentary is offered about the model's *key characteristics*, *evidence base*, *clinical applicability* and *testability*.

Model 1: a neurodevelopmental model for anorexia nervosa (Connan, Campbell, Katzman, Lightman and Treasure, 2003) [4]

Overview

This model (Figure 7.1) focuses on pre- and perinatal factors and childhood stages of development. The authors propose there is an interaction between genes, early life experience and biopsychosocial environment at puberty which may make an individual susceptible to developing anorexia nervosa (AN) via alteration of appetite and emotion-regulation systems. At the heart of this model is the proposed poor regulation of the stress response due to modification of the hypothalamic–pituitary–adrenal (HPA) axis. This consequently leaves an individual with chronic stress and maladaptive coping strategies.

The model suggests that several factors in early life may interact and contribute to the development of AN. The authors propose that genetic factors may confer risk of developing AN. Perinatal factors such as high levels of anxiety during pregnancy may contribute to overcontrolling and overprotective parenting styles. Neonatal development may be affected by anxious, insecure or dismissive attachment styles.

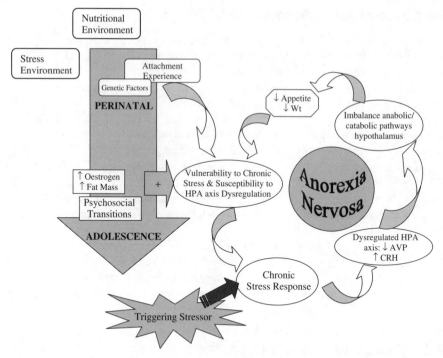

Figure 7.1 Early attachment experiences interact with genetic factors to modulate personality features, childhood psychosocial development and HPA axis development. In individuals at risk of AN, these factors result in impaired coping and a tendency to submissive responses. By the time of adolescence, there is increased vulnerability to chronic stress and susceptibility of the HPA axis to dysregulation. These vulnerabilities are exacerbated by the biological and psychosocial changes associated with puberty, especially in females. Exposure to a significant stressor at this critical time triggers a dysregulated HPA axis response, which is characterised by a failure to upregulate AVP activity and persistently elevated CRH activity. This results in disruption of the balance between anabolic and catabolic pathways of the hypothalamus, causing loss of appetite and weight. Once initiated, underlying susceptibility factors and the impact of starvation upon psychological and biological systems maintain the vicious cycle of AN [5] Reproduced from *Journal of Mental Health*, **14**, 553–566, with permission from Informa Health Care.

Early functional alteration of the HPA axis and serotonergic system may impact on appetite regulation in later life. Childhood risk factors may be due to interaction between genes, early life experience and biopsychosocial environment. For example, poor social skills and lack of parental attachment may result in dismissive- or avoidant-type behaviours and impairments in theory of mind and/or metacognitions in later life. This may lead to overdependence on cognitive systems; that is, rigidity. An impaired ability to manage stressful events may contribute to susceptibility of developing AN. When entering adolescence, individuals may have compromised self-management processes, interpersonal skills, stress response and appetite systems.

Additional factors in adolescence may add further risk of developing AN. It is a time of psychosocial, cultural and biological transition. Cognitively, this time requires great flexibility. This may be challenging for rigid individuals and could further affect the dysregulation of biopsychosocial systems. Biologically, sex differences occur at puberty. Oestrogen may affect mood, stress and appetite and account for the sexual dimorphism of AN. Peripubertal genetic factors acting on biological systems (such as leptin and fat stores) may be more important as a risk factor than environment (media and dieting) for AN. Neurologically, a failure of synaptogenesis, pruning and myelination could lead to emotional and neuropsychological impairments. All of these risk factors come together at puberty to make it a vulnerable period.

Early modification of the HPA stress-response system due to both the genetic context in which environmental factors operate and the interaction between pre- and post-natal factors leads to HPA dysfunction. It is not HPA dysfunction itself, rather the nature by which it has occurred, that is specific to AN. Serotonergic dysfunction has been shown in AN and is associated with key clinical features. It is suggested that serotonergic overactivity is a trait-related phenomenon.

According to social-ranking theory, individuals in a low social hierarchy cannot usually win conflicts, thus resolution of conflict is either by submissive responses or escape. If there is no escape then submission is the only option. Trauma or other life difficulty, low self-esteem, lack of mastery and helplessness, combined with placation and perfectionism of AN, may result in a submissive response from which chronic stress results. Chronic social stress may lead to alteration of the HPA and serotonergic systems.

Evidence base

Evidence from several perspectives has been used to support this model, ranging from genetics to social-ranking theory.

Evidence for the role of *genetics* in the model is drawn from studies showing an increased risk of eating disorders in relatives of patients and a genetic liability to subthreshold forms of eating disorder. The authors stress that although genetic factors are believed to confer 58–88% risk of developing AN, there is unlikely to be a single responsible gene, since linkage studies using broad diagnostic criteria have found no evidence of linkage in the entire genome. However, in family studies of those with restricting AN, there is evidence of linkage to chromosome 1p34. The eating disorder traits of drive for thinness and obsessionality have been linked to chromosomes 1, 2 and 13, and self-induced vomiting linked to chromosome 10.

Evidence for the role of *perinatal factors* is drawn from studies showing obstetric difficulties in 25% of mothers of a child with AN compared to 7.5% in controls and a 2–36-fold increase in prematurity and birth trauma in AN.

Evidence for the role of *early life experience and the HPA axis* is drawn from animal studies in which rats deprived of maternal care show hyperactivity of the HPA axis mediated by frontal and hippocampal regions. The authors also draw on evidence that hyperactivity of the HPA leads to increased cortisol-releasing hormone (CRH) production and hence to hypercortisolaemia. The increased levels of cortisol in turn lead to hippocampal atrophy, which is associated with impaired learning and memory.

The contribution of *early life experience and appetite regulation* is supported by studies showing that by adolescence, maternally deprived rats weigh less than normal rats and that reduced nutrition during lactation is associated with reduced appetite in later life. Poor nutrition during pregnancy is associated with the so-called 'thrifty phenotype', which increases risk of obesity and type 2 diabetes in later life.

The contribution of *childhood development* (in the domains of affect, cognition and interpersonal style) is supported by studies implicating minimal parental involvement and affection, lack of close friends and poor recall of attachment-related memories.

Evidence for *impaired interpersonal skills* includes theory of mind, self-reflective function, metacognition, alexithymia and impaired emotional regulation. Unresolved trauma, helplessness and lack of mastery prior to onset and avoidant coping response to a triggering event have all been documented.

Evidence for the importance of *adolescent transition and maturation* includes studies of metabolic changes such as increased fat stores associated with leptin and the role of oestrogen on endocrine function. Evidence of altered serotonergic function has also been found and is associated with common features of AN, obsessive–compulsive symptomatology and enhanced satiety.

Research evidence for the contribution of *submissive response and chronic stress* is drawn from studies identifying an increase in significant severe life events before onset, low self-esteem, lack of mastery and helplessness. Animal models such as 'thin-sow syndrome' (by which sows at the lower end of social ranking develop anorexia, infertility, overactivity and weight loss) and low-ranking animals developing reduced aggressiveness, altered psychomotor activity and reduced sexual, reproductive and appetitive behaviours all support the importance of chronic stress. Chronic social stress also results in elevated arginine vasopressin (AVP), an adrenocorticotrophic hormone, and increased numbers of AVP receptors, which sensitises the HPA axis. In the final step of the chain, effective cortisol feedback is lost, resulting in a catabolic spiral of loss of appetite and weight loss.

Commentary

- **Characteristics:** The strength of this model is that it encompasses a very broad range of developmental factors, from genetic and perinatal to endocrine changes associated with adolescence.
- **Evidence base:** A vast amount of research evidence is drawn on to support the model.
- **Clinical applicability:** The authors suggest that many of the risk factors in the model are irreversible (i.e. perinatal factors or genetic loading). However, psychotherapy could target some risk factors. For instance, attachment style (insecure, anxious and dismissive) could be targeted with cognitive behavioural theory (CBT) and attachment interventions; submissive response behaviour may have implications during therapy sessions, such that the therapist should avoid power differentials, and work towards enhancing self-esteem and self-efficacy. In terms of psychopharmacological treatments, CRH antagonists have been shown to work in animal studies. The model predicts that they may help with stimulating appetite and reducing anxiety in AN.
- **Testability:** The main weakness of this model is that no recommendations are made about how to test it.

Model 2: building a model of the aetiology of eating disorders by translating experimental neuroscience into clinical practice (Southgate, Tchanturia and Treasure, 2005) [5]

Overview

This model (Figure 7.2) focuses on factors that may be involved in the development and maintenance of eating disorders, such as disruption in brain development, emotion processing and complex inhibitory and reflective processing. There are three components to the model: (i) underlying vulnerability to an eating disorder; (ii) precipitating features in adolescent brain development, including maturational changes in collaborative brain function and the social information processing network (SIPN); and (iii) factors which shape the reaction to the illness, including personality traits and information-processing style, emotional responsivity, attachment style and cultural context.

The first component of the model is based on Connan *et al.* [4] and covers the same underlying vulnerability factors as the earlier model. The second component incorporates the concept of *collaborative brain function*: during adolescence, two major processes occur in the brain. First, synaptic pruning strips down connections to maximise circuitry and second, myelination speeds up neural transmission for increased signal speed. These two processes support the collaboration of widely distributed circuitry, a move from localised to distributed functioning. By improving the connections between the prefrontal cortex and subcortical regions (i.e. basal ganglia and thalamus), the subcortical regions are modulated by the executive areas to enable collaborative brain function. In terms of brain functioning, inhibitory and reflective processes become more efficient.

In parallel with these processes, adolescent development of the *SIPN* occurs in affect and detection 'nodes' that undergo synaptic pruning and myelination, modulated by gonadal hormones during adolescence. Maturation of the cognitive node occurs after maturation of the affective node, thus resulting in a 'mismatch'. As described by Nelson *et al.* [6], 'thus in individuals who have powerful emotional responses to social stimuli, the ability to regulate, contextualise, plan or inhibit newly emergent and motivated behaviour in a context-appropriate manner is far from mature'. This mismatch is hypothesised to result in the onset of behavioural difficulties in some individuals.

In the third component of the model, maladaptive coping mechanisms interact with personality traits involved in determination of eating disorder phenotype in order to maintain the illness.

Evidence base

Evidence for *dysfunction in collaborative brain function* is drawn from a range of neuroimaging studies showing several regions of abnormal functioning operating in parallel, supporting the hypothesis of dysfunction in a network of regions rather than in one region in isolation.

Evidence for *disturbance in the SIPN* and *affect regulation* is drawn from studies showing that patients with eating disorders have difficulty in emotion recognition and abnormal activation of the appetite-motivational system in response to pleasant stimuli.

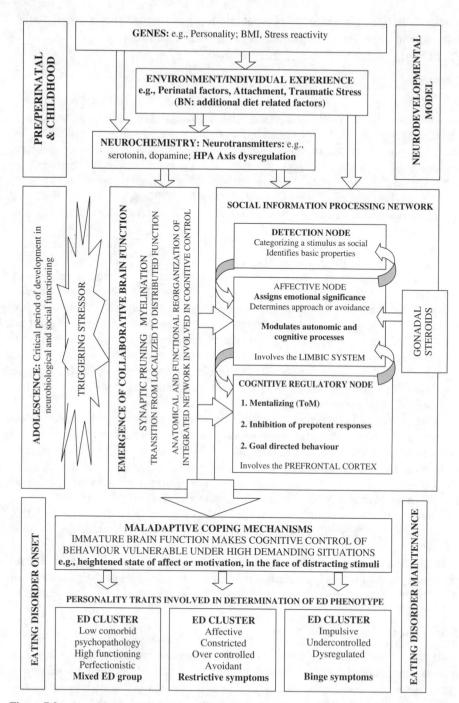

Figure 7.2   A working model of eating-disorder development and maintenance [4] Reproduced from *Physiology and Behaviour*, **79**, 13–24 with permission from Elsevier.

Evidence for *cognitive dysfunction* is drawn from a wide range of neuropsychological studies of inhibition, set-shifting, goal-directed behaviour, central coherence and theory of mind.

Evidence for the involvement of *personality traits* and *impaired coping mechanisms* is drawn from a wide range of sources.

Commentary

- **Characteristics:** The strength of this model is that it builds on the authors' previous work and again covers a very diverse range of factors in early development, adolescence and illness maintenance.
- **Evidence base:** A large amount of research evidence is drawn on to support the model.
- **Clinical applicability:** The model predicts a range of therapeutic implications. For example, it suggests that therapy must address the cognitive and affective nodes of SIPN and maximise emotional intelligence. In the case of AN, this suggests a focus on accepting and reflecting on emotions rather than using displacement or avoidance. In the case of bulimia nervosa (BN), it suggests a focus on moderating emotional responses. The model predicts that patients with eating disorders may have difficulty learning new responses as they have an insensitivity of reward pathways, and thus change may take time. The model suggests that therapy should address information-processing style by working with strengths in focused goal-planning and attention to detail, and weaknesses in broader functioning and flexibility of thinking. Finally, the authors suggest that specific personality traits should be targeted in treatment, but do not specify which.
- **Testability:** The main weakness of this model is that no recommendations are made about how to test it.

Model 3: habit learning and anorexia nervosa: a cognitive neuroscience hypothesis (Steinglass and Walsh, 2006) [7]

Overview

This model is based on the cognitive and neurobiological literature of habitual behaviours in obsessive–compulsive disorder (OCD) and how such knowledge may contribute to our understanding of AN. Given the similarity between many of the clinical features of OCD and AN (repetitive and stereotyped behaviours and preoccupation with specific thoughts and ideas), the high degree of comorbidity between these two disorders, case reports of AN and OCD developing after an infection (autoimmune AN), and evidence of serotonin dysfunction in both disorders, the authors argue that it is plausible that both of these conditions 'share a similar neurobiologic foundation'.

The authors begin by drawing an analogy between implicit learning and stimulus-response learning. Implicit learning refers to learning processes that occur outside of consciousness and are distinct from conscious or declarative learning. Stimulus-response learning is based on the behaviourist principles of classical and operant condition: the pairing of a stimulus and behaviour toward a reward. Even though these models were originally developed using animal models, it has been shown that such mechanisms can govern human behaviour. Humans show both implicit and explicit elements in their learning, as demonstrated by probabilistic classification tasks. Subjects learn to associate particular stimuli with a response but cannot report the rules they are using to make such choices. Once stimulus-response learning has occurred, it results in habitual behaviours that are performed in response to the stimulus without conscious awareness. Similarly, implicit learning leads to a response set without conscious knowledge of the association.

When most individuals lock a door they have implicitly learnt that the door is now locked. In OCD, this implicit learning has failed, thus to reduce doubt associated with the thought 'What if I haven't locked the door?', the solution is to repeatedly lock the door to compensate for the failed implicit learning. This model of implicit-learning failure can also be applied to AN. When most individuals eat cake, they have implicitly learnt that the cake alone will not immediately make them fat (but rather interacts over a longer period of time with other lifestyle factors such as activity levels). In AN, this implicit learning has failed, thus in order to answer the question 'Will this cake make me fat?', the answer is to resist eating cakes to compensate for the failed implicit learning. Implicit-learning dysfunction in AN may contribute to the explicit, routine and repetitive behaviours observed, further reinforced by set-shifting difficulties, which may make it difficult for a patient to change or stop established routines.

The model is therefore functionally defined in terms of an implicit-learning deficit, and how this subsequently interacts with neuropsychological dysfunction in set-shifting, leading to compensatory repetitive behaviours. Structures hypothesised to be implicated in these processes include the prefrontal cortical regions (anterior cingulate cortex (ACC) and orbitofrontal cortex), basal ganglia and thalamus.

Evidence base

Evidence for *implicit-learning deficits* is drawn from studies showing different patterns of brain activation between control participants and patients with OCD on implicit-learning tasks that correlate with regional cerebral blood flow in frontostriatal areas, regions implicated in implicit learning. By contrast, there is currently no direct evidence for implicit-learning deficits in AN, although studies using the Iowa Gambling Task, which draws on nondeclarative aspects of decision-making (similar to implicit learning), have shown that patients with AN perform poorly relative to controls.

Evidence for *set-shifting deficits* is drawn from a wide range of neuropsychological studies in AN.

Evidence for *structural and functional involvement of specific brain regions* in the case of OCD is drawn from a range of studies implicating altered activation of orbitofrontal cortex in response to symptom provocation and anterior cingulate and caudate nucleus at rest, with a suggestion that different brain regions may be associated with specific symptom profiles (caudate nucleus with washing symptoms and putamen/globus pallidus with checking symptoms). In the case of AN, evidence is drawn from studies showing structural differences in thalamus and midbrain regions in patients with AN and BN compared with controls, and positron emission tomography (PET) studies revealing a higher metabolic rate in the thalamus, caudate and brainstem in patients at rest compared to controls, normalised with weight gain. Several functional imaging studies are reported which indicate activation of the amygdala fear network in patients with eating disorders in response to food-related anxiety.

Commentary

- **Characteristics:** The strength of this model is that it draws on the existing literature in OCD and applies it to eating disorders. The model encompasses underlying neurobiological characteristics, neuropsychological processes and functional elements.
- **Evidence base:** The evidence base for abnormalities at the neurobiological, neuropsychological and functional levels is well made in the case of OCD; the authors acknowledge that the evidence in the case of eating disorders is less well established.
- **Clinical applicability:** This model suggests that modified CBT focused on behavioural repetition rather than cognitive restructuring may be beneficial for those with implicit-learning difficulty. Also, the authors suggest that understanding more about the cognitive and biological aspects of eating disorders may guide the development of new pharmacological treatments.
- **Testability:** The model is testable through further clarification of cognitive dysfunction and exploration of implicit learning through tasks that assess motor and cognitive skills. Such exploration could guide neuroimaging studies to substantiate and localise the neural mechanisms.

Model 4: the fault is not in her parents but in her insula: a neurobiological hypothesis of anorexia nervosa (Nunn, Frampton, Gordon and Lask, 2008) [8]

Overview

The authors propose a dysfunction within a single brain region that can account for the aetiology and maintenance of AN (Figure 7.3). Research has identified abnormal functioning in several cortical structures in AN (frontal, somatosensory and parietal cortices) as well as in subcortical structures (amygdala, hippocampus, hypothalamus and the striatum). Rather than predicting damage to each of these regions, the authors argue it is more likely that there is damage or dysfunction within a part of the brain that connects between them: the insular cortex or insula. This dysfunction means that the insula is unable to perform its functions to integrate information from cognitive, affective and physiological systems. These functions include:

- Regulation of the autonomic nervous system;
- Regulation of appetite and eating;
- Monitoring of the body state;
- Perception and integration of disgust;
- Reception, perception and integration of taste;
- Monitoring and evaluation of digestive-system status;
- Integration of thoughts and feelings;

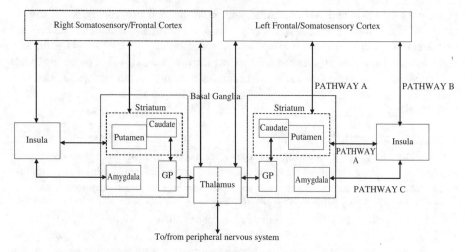

Figure 7.3 Schematic bilateral coronal section illustrating functional insular networks that regulate direct cortical–subcortical pathways: (the proposed pathways are labelled on one side only for visual simplicity) pathway A – insula via striatum to frontal cortex, pathway B – insula to somatosensory cortex, pathway C – insula to amygdala. GP, globus pallidus [8] Reproduced *European Eating Disorders Review*, **16**, 355–360, with permission.

- Investment of emotion in language;
- Regulation of the experience of pain.

The model therefore predicts that the clinical phenomena of AN can be explained by a rate-limiting dysfunction in the insula which reduces its capacity to integrate information from cognitive, affective and physiological systems. This underlying risk factor may interact with precipitating risk factors such as sociocultural pressures, life events such as puberty and additional psychosocial stressors to precipitate the manifest illness during adolescence.

Evidence base

Evidence for *abnormal functioning of cortical and subcortical structures* is drawn from many sources, together with evidence for *the role of the insula* in the wide range of functions described.

Commentary

- **Characteristics:** This model is empirically based in earlier studies demonstrating functional abnormalities in the temporal-lobe regions that contain the insula. It also has the strength of parsimoniously accounting for a wide range of eating-disorder dysfunctions through impairment of a single connecting structure.
- **Evidence base:** A large amount of research evidence is drawn on to support the model, including studies of the functions of the insula in normal development and special populations (such as people with insula stroke).

- **Clinical applicability:** The model predicts psychopharmacological treatments (either by psychoactive agents that act on specific neurotransmitters or by vasoactive agents to address blood-flow abnormalities), psychological treatments such as mindfulness approaches to enhance self-awareness of cognitive, emotional and physiological states, and cognitive remediation techniques to address neuropsychological processing style.
- **Testability:** The authors suggest that future studies should use brain-imaging technology alongside neurocognitive tests to investigate activity within the fronto–insula–limbic–striatal circuit. Specifically, functional neuroimaging tasks that are known to activate insula cortex should reveal significant differences between patient and matched-control participants, both in the acute stage and (assuming that the underlying risk factor does not remit) following weight-restoration treatment. A failure to demonstrate such between-group differences would disprove the hypothesis.

Model 5: functional disturbances within frontostriatal circuits across multiple childhood pychopathologies (Marsh, Maia and Peterson, 2009) [9]

Overview

The authors suggest that self-regulation encompasses cognitive and inhibitory control: being able to organise thoughts, emotions and behaviours to attain goals (Figure 7.4). Disturbance in this process is a common characteristic of many disorders: in Tourette's syndrome, failure in behavioural self-regulation manifests in uncontrollable tics; OCD is characterised by uncontrollable thoughts (obsessions), which lead to uncontrollable compensatory behaviours (compulsions); and in eating disorders, BN is characterised by binge episodes and impulsive acts while the core feature of AN is extreme dietary restriction and intrusive thoughts about weight and shape.

Evidence has shown that frontostriatal neural circuits are recruited by self-regulatory processes. Broadly speaking, there is a cortico–striato–thalamo–cortical network or loop; this network directs information from the cerebral cortex to the subcortex and then back again to specific regions of the cortex. Structures in this network include the supplementary motor area, frontal eye fields, dorsolateral prefrontal cortex, lateral orbitofrontal cortex and ACC, dorsal striatum, ventromedial striatum and the nucleus accumbens.

In this model, anatomical and functional disturbance in frontostriatal circuits leads to a failure to control thoughts and behaviours, for instance uncontrollable motor tics, or instructive thoughts about contamination, weight or shape. These elicit compensatory or maladaptive thoughts and behaviours to reduce the anxiety associated with the original intrusive thoughts and behaviours. This eventually manifests itself in a variety of ways, such as compulsions, rigid and ritualistic behaviour and purging.

The authors propose that bingeing and preoccupation with weight and shape in BN are a result of diminished regulatory control. Dysfunction of the orbital frontal cortex and ventral striatum may also be implicated as these are linked to reward and motivation. Eating food releases dopamine (DA) in these circuits, and increased DA levels are also associated with food-seeking behaviour in humans and other animals. Bulimic

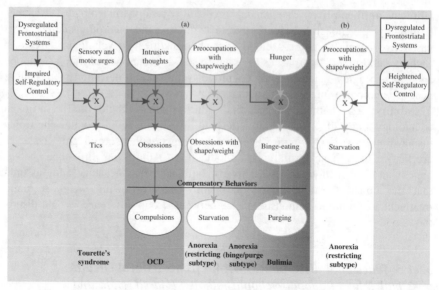

Figure 7.4   The role of dysregulated frontostriatal systems in Tourette's syndrome, OCD, AN and BN. The top row of panel (a) represents urges, thoughts and drives that are present in both healthy and patient populations. An impaired capacity for self-regulatory control interacts with these normal urges, thoughts and drives to produce ego-dystonic symptoms or behaviours (middle row) Attempts to relieve the anxiety associated with these symptoms or to compensate for these behaviours produce further behavioural abnormalities (bottom row). BN and AN restricting subtype are on opposite ends of a continuum. AN binge–purge subtype is positioned within the middle of this continnum, since it shares features with both BN and AN restricting subtype. Panel (b) illustrates an alternative conceptualisation of AN restricting subtype: preoccupation with body shape and weight interact with heightened, rather than impaired, self-regulatory control, producing starvation directly [9] Reproduced from Marsh, R., Maia, T.V., and Peterson, B.S. (2009). Functional Disturbances Within Frontostriatal Circuits Across Multiple Childhood Psychopathologies. *American Journal of Psychiatry*, **166**, 664–674; with permission from APA. (See Plate 3 for colour figure.)

symptoms could be further exacerbated by a failure to control the time delay of reward (to obtain gratification by immediate reward rather than waiting for a later reward). These may all interact with the precipitating risk factor of serotonin dysfunction in the frontal region. Serotonin has been shown to be associated with impulsive behaviour in humans and animals. Furthermore, increased levels of serotonin are associated with feelings of satiety. This view is supported by evidence that patients with BN treated with specific serotonin reuptake inhibitors (SSRIs) tend to decrease their frequency of binges.

There are many parallels between BN and AN. Both illnesses predominantly affect women and age of onset is usually during adolescence. Phenotypically, both disorders show an intense preoccupation with food, weight, shape or calories. There is also a high degree of diagnostic drift between BN and AN, which has led some to suggest that these disorders share a common neural substrate. AN is characterised by restrictive dieting, with an intense fear of fat. The failure of self-regulation in AN lies in the obsessive preoccupation with food and the inability to shift from food-related thoughts. This leads to rigid and ritualistic behaviours that manifest as excessive dietary restriction. Reward pathways may also be altered. Dysfunction in these circuits may explain why there is diminished motivation to eat and lack of avoidance of negative consequences, and why food no longer holds rewarding properties.

Evidence base

Evidence for *the role of specific brain structures* in self-regulation is drawn from studies using experimental manipulation of inhibitory control such as the Stroop task. Brain activity when naming the colours of incongruent stimuli is greater than when naming the colours of congruent stimuli, particularly in the ACC, prefrontal and parietal cortices and striatum, in both adults and children. There appears to be a developmental trajectory to self-regulation, associated with increases in brain volume, grey-matter density and cortical thickness, later maturation of prefrontal cortices and changes in prefrontal white matter. These changes most likely mediate more advanced, higher-order control functions and reflect the myelination of axons.

For BN, evidence for *dysfunctional frontal control systems* is drawn from functional magnetic resonance imaging (fMRI) studies of self-regulation, revealing that relative to controls, patients with BN respond more impulsively, make more errors and do not activate frontostriatal regions including the inferolateral prefrontal cortex and ACC, inferior frontal gyrus, putamen and caudate nucleus.

In AN, there is evidence of *reduced brain volume* in the dorsal anterior cingulate, *decreased blood flow* in the ACC and *alterations in post-synaptic receptors* for serotonin. Given their inhibitory and excitatory roles on other neurons, dysfunction in these receptors may have a knock-on effect on other regions of the brain, giving rise to further functional abnormalities.

Finally, there is evidence that *reward pathways* may also be altered. Studies using a guessing game showed that patients with AN recruit ventral striatum in response to negative and positive feedback, whereas healthy controls only show activation when receiving positive feedback.

Commentary

- **Characteristics:** This model creates links between a range of neurodevelopmental disorders that clinically do seem to be linked – especially eating disorders and OCD. However, this strength begs the question about why individuals go on to develop one disorder rather than another, and also why the characteristic clinical features of the disorders are so different (preoccupation with dirt and contamination in OCD, overvalued ideas about weight and shape in AN).
- **Evidence base:** A large amount of research evidence is drawn together from imaging studies across the disorders, which may help in the design of future studies using common experimental paradigms for participants with different diagnoses.
- **Clinical applicability:** The authors suggest that their model can contribute to the nosological debate about whether mental illness should be characterised as dimensional or categorical. Shared neural substrate and phenotype suggest a dimensional approach; however, where different regions are specific to different disorders, a categorical approach to diagnosis may be more appropriate.

- **Testability:** The main weakness of this model is that no recommendations are made about how to test it.

Model 6: new insights into symptoms and neurocircuit function of anorexia nervosa (Kaye, Fudge and Paulus, 2009) [10]

Overview

This model (Figure 7.5) identifies premorbid traits that make some individuals more susceptible to developing AN, including temperament and personality traits such as perfectionism and harm-avoidance. These may have a genetic basis, since such traits are present before illness onset and persist after recovery.

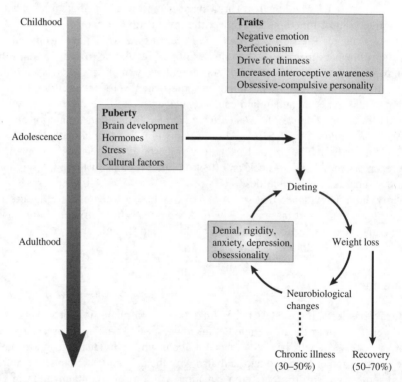

Figure 7.5 The time course and phenomenology of AN. Childhood personality and temperament traits, which contribute to a vulnerability for developing AN, become intensified during adolescence as a consequence of the effects of multiple factors, such as puberty and gonadal steroids, development, stress and culture. Individuals with AN find that dieting reduces, and eating enhances, dysphoric mood. But with chronic dieting and weight loss, there are neurobiological changes which increase denial, rigidity and obsessions, as well as depression and anxiety, so that individuals often enter a downward spiral. Although 50% or more of individuals with AN recover by their early- to mid-20s, a significant proportion of subjects develop a chronic illness or die [10] Reproduced from *Nature Reviews: Neuroscience*, **10**, 573–584, with permission from Nature.

The model suggests that a core characteristic of AN is disturbed appetite and reduced food intake. Appetite is a drive governed by a complex interaction of psychobiological factors, including the reward properties of food, homeostatic needs and flexible approaches to eating. Numerous structures are involved, including taste receptors in the tongue, the medulla and nucleus tractus solaris of the brainstem, the thalamus, anterior insula and gustatory cortex, amygdala, frontal and parietal cortex. As a result, numerous psychological processes are involved, including interoceptive awareness, affective relevance, conflict-monitoring, flexibility, working memory, planning and reward-processing.

The model also predicts how serotonin (5-HT) and dopamine (DA) may confer additional risk and sustain symptoms of AN. Alterations in the 5-HT system may contribute to restricted eating, behavioural inhibition and a bias towards anxiety and error-prediction. Disturbance in the DA system may lead to a maladaptive reward response.

In this model, the anterior insula plays a crucial role in AN (see also section on 'Model 5'). This region is involved in interoceptive awareness, the integration of internal sensations such as muscle tension, stomach acidity and subjective hunger. This structure forms the physiological basis of the sense of self and provides the link between the condition of the body and cognitive and affective states. Core features of AN such as disturbed body image, increased pain threshold and lack of symptom recognition or motivation to change may therefore be due to dysfunction in the anterior insula. Food may evoke an aversive visceral response that might lead to altered processing of its reward qualities and activation of cognitive processes governing harm-avoidance. Signals promoting immediate reward-processing such as reducing hunger may be dampened down, while signals associated with long-term reward such as losing weight may become more valued. The insula has also been shown to be involved in risk-related processing. Dysfunction in the anterior insula could lead to inappropriate appraisal of risk and contribute to harm-avoidance.

Evidence base

Evidence for *genetic risk factors* for AN is drawn from studies showing that behavioural traits such as weight and shape preoccupation and bingeing are heritable. Also, predisposing factors such as perfectionism and harm-avoidance precede the onset of illness, persist after recovery, are present in nonaffected relatives and are independent of weight.

Evidence for the *effect of disturbed appetite and reduced food intake* is drawn from studies showing that starvation leads to reduced 5-HT concentration and subsequent increased numbers of post-synaptic receptors (as the brain adapts to lower levels of the neurotransmitter in attempting to help the neurochemical signals get through). Since eating carbohydrate increases levels of 5-HT, the post-synaptic receptors are overstimulated, leading to dysphoric mood. Dieting, on the other hand, reduces this negative feeling and is therefore reinforced. Studies have also shown that starvation may have effects on the brain and other organs. Brain structural changes include reduced brain size and altered metabolism in all cortical regions. Animal studies have shown that experimental manipulation of endocrine factors can produce physiological and behavioural changes that are very similar to the symptoms of AN, including decreased feeding activity. Neuroimaging studies have consistently shown that there is altered binding potential for post-synaptic 5-HT receptors in currently ill and recovered AN patients, indicating that serotonin alteration is a trait-related feature.

There is also evidence of altered DA-receptor binding in PET studies, with those who have recovered from AN showing an increased binding in the ventral striatum relative to currently ill patients. DA-receptor binding in the putamen has also been shown to be correlated with harm-avoidance in recovered AN patients.

Evidence for *the role of the insula* is drawn from studies showing that administration of sucrose or water to participants recovered from AN results in reduced activity in the insula, ACC and striatum compared to controls. In healthy controls, self-ratings of pleasantness of the sugar taste correlate positively with activity in the insula, the ACC and the ventral and dorsal putamen; no such relationship is observed in patients recovered from AN. Finally, showing food pictures to underweight participants with AN leads to altered activity in the insula and other brain regions compared with healthy controls.

Commentary

- **Characteristics:** This model offers a very comprehensive overview of factors ranging from genetic risk to psychosocial functioning, based on empirical studies conducted by the authors and others. Its strengths lie in the explanatory detail it provides at each level to account for the research evidence, and in the way it creates links between the levels.
- **Evidence base:** A vast amount of research evidence is drawn together in support of the model.
- **Clinical applicability:** The model can account for why there is surprisingly little evidence of a positive effect on symptoms of AN when treating with SSRIs, due to the inhibitory effect of 5-HT receptors and reduced levels of 5-HT due to starvation. The model suggests that atypical antipsychotics which work on the DA system may be more useful in reducing anxiety to aid weight gain. From a psychological perspective, therapies may need to address specific structures and their corresponding functions. An example could be insula-specific interventions such as sensitisation or habituation of interoceptive sensitivity through real-time monitoring of insular cortex activation.
- **Testability:** The main weakness of this model is that no recommendations are made about how to test it.

Model 7: anorexia nervosa: towards an integrative neuroscience model (Hatch, Madden, Kohn, Clarke, Touyz and Williams, 2010) [11]

Overview

This model (Figure 7.6) is based on INTEGRATE, a generic integrative neuroscience framework in which the core motivation for humans is to minimise danger and maximise reward. This principle organises brain–body activity and behaviour over time. Concepts that are traditionally considered as dichotomous (cognition–emotion;

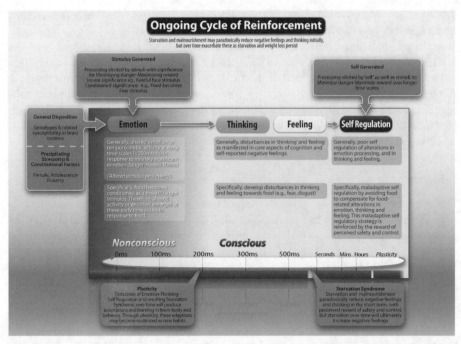

Figure 7.6   The Integrative Neuroscience Model of Anorexia Nervosa (INTEGRATE-AN) [11].   (See Plate 4 for colour figure.)

conscious–nonconscious and cortical–subcortical) are rearranged by this framework along a dynamic time continuum consisting of three phases:

1. **Emotion (<200 ms):** Adaptive action tendencies in response to cues. Rely on evolutionary context and not on subjective experience.
2. **Thinking and feeling (200 ms and beyond):** Distinguished by subjective experiences and conscious awareness of information and emotions (being able to represent or describe them). This allows selective attention and understanding of context, and guides controlled voluntary responses with feedback from higher cortical regions.
3. **Self-regulation (seconds and longer):** Management of thinking and feeling to maximise reward and minimise danger. This phase allows self-awareness, capacity for planned behaviour and linking to stimuli and previous experiences held in long-term memory. Uses feedback and feed-forward brain–body interactions.

Two types of factor can contribute to individual differences in the model: dispositional factors such as genes, age and so on, and adaptive factors such as brain plasticity. This model can be applied to normal functioning as well as dysfunction within mental disorders.

Applying this framework to AN, in the emotional phase (<200 ms) there is a disturbance in early, nonconscious processing of emotional stimuli, with automatic processing towards negative emotionality. In the thinking and feeling phase (200 ms and beyond), there is an increased vulnerability due to abnormal processing of danger cues, which is further exacerbated by cognitive deficits that predispose an individual to a rigid and detail-bound thinking style. Food cues may signal less of a reward than in normal individuals and may trigger the avoidance of food.

In the self-regulation phase, a threshold is reached when avoidance of food becomes more rewarding than eating and so food avoidance compensates for emotional disturbance in the short term. Food is then conditioned as a negative cue that leads to further reward via dietary restraint. This forms a maladaptive cycle of attempted self-regulation that eventually develops into starvation syndrome. This may interact with or exacerbate preexisting levels of other disturbances, such as anxiety, depression, rigidity and detail focus.

Evidence base

Evidence for *abnormalities in emotion processing* is drawn from studies using event-related potentials (ERPs) to measure neural activity within the first 200 ms after the presentation of a stimulus, which show differences in participants with AN relative to controls. Studies using fMRI suggest altered activation in limbic–medial prefrontal networks during perception of emotion or AN-related cues, which may be a trait marker given its stability as a feature of AN. Single-photon emission computed tomography (SPECT) studies have also shown reduced metabolism in the temporal lobe and associated emotional brain systems (thalamus and ventral medial prefrontal cortex). In studies of body arousal, AN-relevant stimuli have been associated with increased heart rate, greater skin conductance and exaggerated eye-blink startle responses. Emotional non-food-related stimuli have also been linked to arousal dysfunction in those with AN.

Evidence for *abnormalities in feeling and thinking* is drawn from studies of alexithymia (difficulty in distinguishing and describing feelings) and social cognition, in which patients with AN exhibit lower levels of emotional awareness, an inability to identify and describe their own emotions and a 'mentalising' impairment in understanding other people's emotional experience. Studies have also found high rates of comorbidity between mood disorders and AN and between AN and OCD. In studies of cognition, consistent deficits have been found in attention, speed of processing, memory, executive functioning, set-shifting and central coherence in patients with AN.

Commentary

- **Characteristics:** This model offers a fresh perspective in linking eating-disorder psychopathology to a generic neuroscience framework – INTEGRATE – and thereby benefits from the evidence base used to develop the latter. It also emerges from the work this group of authors has already contributed to the literature concerning ERPs, neuropsychology and brain functioning in AN.
- **Evidence base:** A broad evidence base is drawn upon to support the model.
- **Clinical applicability:** If, as the model predicts, there is a core disturbance in nonconscious emotional processing which has generalised to food cues then refeeding to reverse this is an obvious treatment strategy. However, understanding more about the nature and extent of these nonconscious processes will inform innovative treatments, including emotion-based psychological therapies and pharmacotherapy.

These approaches may prove to be more successful than cognitive-based treatments that require patients to be consciously aware of their feelings and thoughts.
* **Testability:** The authors suggest that tests of their framework include exploring the brain correlates of altered processing of innately significant emotion cues in AN to answer these questions: Is altered activation a general disturbance in emotional processing or is it specific to food/illness cues? Are alterations in processing emotional cues present from the earliest, automatic phases of neural activity (within 200 ms)? Are alterations in emotional processing state or trait? Is maladaptive self-regulation, reflected in a starvation syndrome in AN, reversible?

7.3 Conclusion

This chapter shows that in the past decade there has been a surge of activity in creating new neuroscience models for eating disorders. To some extent, this activity reflects the state of the neuroscience, with a critical volume of empirical studies published to enable us to begin to model the relationships between constructs.

One of the problems for this endeavour has been the lack of a common framework for developing models, with the result that some have adopted a 'neurocircuitry' approach [10, 12], while others have used novel alternative frameworks such as INTE-GRATE [11]. Such diversity contributes to a rich description of the neuroscience but makes it difficult to test one model directly against another.

In 2010 the US National Institute of Mental Health published its Research Domain Criteria (RDoC) Project (http://www.nimh.nih.gov/research-funding/rdoc.shtml). The project has defined six *classes* or levels of description for neuroscientific constructs (genetic, molecular, cellular, neural circuits, behavioural and self-reports). For the purposes of models developed before the publication of this framework, we can collapse the molecular and cellular classes into a single 'neurotransmitter' class, and include neuropsychological data in the 'behavioural' class.

Review of Table 7.1 suggests that the models have become more comprehensive over time and that some authors have taken testability into account. With the benefit of the RDoC, it should now be possible for future models to be built on a common

Table 7.1 Focus of each model relative to NIMH Research Domain Criteria.

Research Domain Class	Connan (2003)	Southgate (2005)	Steinglass (2006)	Nunn (2008)	March (2009)	Kaye (2009)	Hatch (2010)
Self-reports[a]	X	X	X	X	X	X	X
Behavioural[b]	–	X	X	X	–	X	X
Neural circuits	X	X	X	X	X	X	X
Neurotransmitter[c]	X	–	–	–	X	X	X
Genetic	X	–	–	–	–	X	X
Model test defined	–	–	X	X	–	–	X

[a] Includes cognitive, behavioural and affective functioning.
[b] Includes neuropsychological functioning.
[c] Includes molecular and cellular descriptions.

framework, which should help to foster comparisons between them. Ideally, opposing models should be directly testable (and falsifiable) against each other. In this regard it is encouraging that different authors are positing distinct features at each level (such as different key neurotransmitters or neural circuits), which should help in designing experimental tests to decide between them. It may be that this is a good stage of the neuroscience for researchers to focus their activity on designing tests to falsify existing models (see Nunn et al. [12] and Chapter 8, for example), rather than creating more novel ones. Experimental tests of the predictions arising from the existing models will enhance our understanding of eating-disorder neuroscience more than the creation of new models.

Finally, what are the implications of all these models for clinical practice? Arguably, one of the major reasons why the eating disorders (especially AN) have proven so difficult to treat is that we have lacked a coherent understanding of what causes them. By testing and refining models incorporating the range of classes defined in the RDoC, we should improve our ability to design and target specific treatments.

The authors of all seven models reviewed here say something about how their models may affect clinical practice. Connan et al. suggest that although many of the risk factors in their model are irreversible (such as perinatal factors or genetic risk), psychotherapy could still effectively target-attachment style and submissive-response style, and enhance self-esteem and self-efficacy. Psychopharmacological treatments that stimulate appetite and reduce anxiety in AN could be effective. Southgate et al. suggests that therapy must address the cognitive and affective nodes of their SIPN and maximise emotional intelligence. Steinglass et al. suggest a modified CBT to target implicit-learning difficulty by focusing on behavioural repetition rather than cognitive restructuring. They also hope that understanding more about the neurobiology may guide the development of new drug treatments.

Nunn et al. suggest potential psychopharmacological treatments (using agents that act on specific neurotransmitters or that address blood-flow abnormalities). They also promote psychological treatments such as mindfulness approaches in order to enhance self-awareness of cognitive, emotional and physiological states. They predict that neuropsychological impairments could be addressed through cognitive remediation therapy. Marsh et al. hope that their model can contribute to the diagnostic debate about whether eating disorders should be characterised as dimensional or categorical.

Kaye et al. help us to understand why SSRIs are not effective in the treatment of AN, which opens up possibilities for the development of new drug treatments based on this knowledge. In order for SSRIs to be effective, extracellular 5-HT needs to be present. They also suggest novel treatments such as sensitisation or habituation of interoceptive sensitivity through real-time neurobiofeedback of insular cortex activation. Finally, Hatch et al. predict innovative emotion-based psychological and pharmacological treatments, which according to their model will be more effective than existing cognitive-based approaches.

In Chapter 8 a novel model for AN is proposed, building on the work reviewed above. The development of models and testable hypotheses about the cause and maintenance of eating disorders has arguably reached the stage where we can now directly compare one against another and thereby refine our understanding as well as explore the treatment implications.

References

1. *Concise Oxford English Dictionary*. (1990), Oxford University Press, Oxford.
2. Walker M. (1963) *The Nature of Scientific Thought*, New York, Prentice Hall.
3. Fawcett, J. (1995) *Analysis and Evaluation of Conceptual Models of Nursing*, F. A. Davis Company, Philadelphia, PA.
4. Connan, F., Campbell, I.C., Katzman, D. *et al.* (2003) A neurodevelopmental model for anorexia nervosa. *Physiology and Behaviour*, **79**, 13–24.
5. Southgate, L., Tchanturia, K. and Treasure, J. (2005) Building a model of the aetiology of eating disorders by translating experimental neuroscience into clinical practice. *Journal of Mental Health*, **14**, 553–566.
6. Nelson, E.E., Liebenluft, E., McClure, E.B. and Pine, D.S. (2005) The social re-orientation of adolescence: A neuroscience perspective on the process and its relation to psychopathology. *Psychological Medicine*, **35**, 163–174.
7. Steinglass, J. and Walsh, T. (2006) Habit learning and anorexia nervosa: a cognitive neuroscience hypothesis. *International Journal of Eating Disorders*, **39**, 267–275.
8. Nunn, K.P., Frampton, I., Gordon, I. and Lask, B. (2008) The fault is not in her parents but in her insula – a neurobiological hypothesis of anorexia nervosa. *European Eating Disorders Review*, **16**, 355–360.
9. Marsh, R., Maia, T.V. and Peterson, B.S. (2009) Functional disturbances within frontostriatal circuits across multiple childhood psychopathologies. *American Journal of Psychiatry*, **166**, 664–674.
10. Kaye, W.H., Fudge, J.L. and Paulus, M. (2009) New insights into symptoms and neurocircuit function of anorexia nervosa. *Nature Reviews: Neuroscience*, **10**, 573–584.
11. Hatch, A., Madden, S., Kohn, M. *et al.* (2010) Anorexia nervosa: towards an integrative neuroscience model. *European Eating Disorders Review*, **18**, 156–179.
12. Nunn, K., Frampton, I., Fuglset, T. *et al.* (2011). Anorexia nervosa and the insula. *Medical Hypotheses*, **76** (3), 353–357.

8 Towards a comprehensive, causal and explanatory neuroscience model of anorexia nervosa

Kenneth Nunn[1], Bryan Lask[2, 3, 4] and Ian Frampton[5]

[1]*Molecular Neuropsychiatry Service, Department of Psychological Medicine, The Children's Hospital at Westmead, Westmead, Australia*
[2]*Regional Eating Disorder Service, Oslo University Hospital, Oslo, Norway*
[3]*Ellern Mede Service for Eating Disorders, London, UK*
[4]*Great Ormond Street Hospital for Children, London, UK*
[5]*College of Life and Environmental Sciences, University of Exeter, UK*

8.1 Introduction

It is clear from the previous chapter and the wider literature that to date there has been no comprehensive, causal, explanatory, specific and testable model that accounts for the pathogenesis, phenomenology and maintenance of anorexia nervosa (AN). Any such model would need to integrate genes and environment, psyche and soma, and predisposing, precipitating and perpetuating factors. Furthermore, it should be able to inform both a future research agenda and treatment. We present in this chapter a model that attempts to fulfil all these demands and to provide a credible explanation of AN.

8.2 The model

Given the complexity of AN, any explanatory model is in itself bound to be multi-faceted. Specifically, there will be genetic and environmental components, and each of these in turn will have multiple constituents. The environmental components have been broadly disseminated, discussed and generally agreed in the wider literature [1]. In this section, given the sociocultural context in which AN occurs, we offer an explanation

Eating Disorders and the Brain. Edited by Bryan Lask and Ian Frampton.
© 2011 John Wiley & Sons, Ltd. Published 2011 by John Wiley & Sons, Ltd.

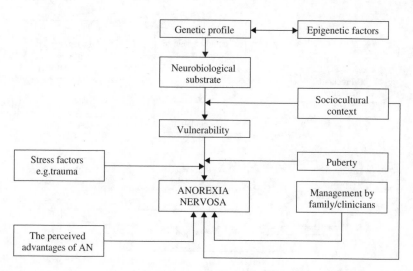

Figure 8.1 Aetiology and maintenance of AN.

of how the genetic component contributes to the pathogenesis, phenomenology and maintenance of AN. In other words, we do not in any way intend to minimise the importance of environmental factors, but rather we will try to show how genetically mediated neurobiological factors are absolutely essential. To achieve this, we extend the notion of environment to include food and the impact upon the developing central nervous system of factors such as ultraviolet radiation and obstetric complications. We argue that without taking into account the genetically determined neurobiological substrate it is not possible to account for the aetiology and phenomenology of AN.

Figure 8.1 illustrates at a macro-level how the genetic and environmental factors interact. A specific genetic profile contributes to the development of a neurobiological substrate that operates within the context of specific sociocultural influences. This combination renders the individual vulnerable to the development of AN. The combination of the onset of puberty and other stress factors, such as trauma, peer-group or other school-related difficulties, family problems, and so on, precipitates the onset of AN. This in turn can be maintained by persisting sociocultural influences and stress factors, the manner in which the illness is managed by the family and clinicians, and the perceived advantages of the illness, such as sense of achievement, enhanced self-esteem, sense of control and well-being.

Figure 8.2 illustrates the genetically mediated pathogenesis of the neurobiological substrate of AN, which we now explore in depth.

This model has numerous important components, with significant interactions amongst them.

Noradrenergic genetic profile

Previous studies of neurotransmitter systems in AN have emphasised serotonergic mechanisms [2]. Though very informative from a descriptive point of view, such studies have not to date provided a comprehensive nor a causative explanation of AN. Furthermore Pinheiro *et al.* [3] have concluded that no assumptions can be made concerning the implication of abnormalities in this mechanism for the vulnerability to AN.

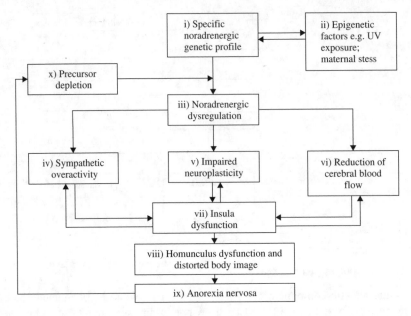

Figure 8.2   A neurobiological model for the pathogenesis of AN.

Our model of AN begins with those aspects of the genome specifically related to noradrenergic function. However, it differs from generic noradrenergic models of anxiety, depression and post-traumatic stress disorder in two ways. First, it implicates noradrenergic function in a very specific manner that goes beyond sympathetic arousal and amygdala overactivity. Second, it also focuses on the differential effects of the noradrenergic system in different states of nutrition. We expand on these points in the section on 'Critical appraisal'.

Urwin *et al.* [4–6] have demonstrated differences in the noradrenergic genetic profiles of those with and without AN. Odds ratios indicate the increased likelihood of specific gene variants contributing to AN, varying from a very modest 1.4 for the long variant (L4) of the monoamine oxidase gene on the X chromosome, to 11 for interactions between the MAO long variant and genes on very different chromosomes (16 and 17) regulating both noradrenergic and serotonergic genes. Other researchers [7, 8] have found hyperfunctioning variants in the genes specifying the COMT enzyme, on chromosome 22. The serotonergic genes had no independent capacity to predict differences between those with and without AN.

Epigenetic factors

These are factors that influence the gene expression, for example ultraviolet light exposure, as expressed by season of birth (SoB) bias or obstetric complications.

Season of birth

Amongst the identified risk factors for AN is a consistent finding of a spring SoB bias. Winje *et al.* [9] have outlined a number of hypotheses to explain this bias. The most relevant to this model is the proposal that exposure to high levels of sunlight radiation during early pregnancy may contribute to abnormal neurodevelopment [10]. The genes most likely to be affected in this or other ways are the so-called homeobox genes, including PHOX 1 and PHOX 2. These genes regulate the development of the brain, the sympathetic nervous system and the noradrenergic system itself [11]. Factors that alter expression of these homeobox genes during early development of the embryo may influence the lifelong stress response.

Obstetric complications

There is substantial evidence that obstetric complications are a risk factor for psychosis [12] and other brain disorders. In contrast, very little work has been done exploring these in eating disorders. Favaro *et al.* [13] have identified high rates in a population birth cohort study of adults aged 18–25 with AN. Neurodevelopmental adversities (particularly during early foetal life) and subsequent obstetric complications may be markers of the interaction between genetic processes in early brain development and epigenetic factors.

Noradrenergic dysregulation

In this model we propose an interaction between a specific noradrenergic genetic profile – see section on 'Noradrenergic genetic profile' – and epigenetic factors – see section on 'Epigenetic factors' – to produce the potential for noradrenergic dys-regulation.

Noradrenalin has multiple functions. In relation to this model, these include:

1. regulating sympathetic arousal and, therefore, the neurochemical underpinnings of anxiety [14];
2. the regulation of cerebral blood flow (CBF) generally, including the middle cerebral artery and its supply to the insula [15];
3. the mediation of cortical neuroplasticity, including cortical representation [16].

In this model there is increased noradrenergic activity in the brain premorbidly. This increased activity is due to one or more of the regulatory enzymes having variants with higher levels of activity than the enzymes in the general population. The variety and activity of the enzyme is specified by the gene for that enzyme. The more high-activity genes there are for the noradrenergic system ('the genomic dose'), the greater the activity or turnover of the system and the greater the 'fuel' consumed. This leads to increased resting sympathetic 'tone' or activity and consequent increased likelihood of high-arousal and high-sensitivity states, including anxiety. In addition there is reduced CBF and impaired neuroplasticity.

In contrast, once dieting has commenced, with its subsequent nutritional and nora-drenaline precursor depletion, there is reduced noradrenergic activity, with rapid reduction in anxiety. Changes to CBF and neuroplasticity modify slowly over weeks to months. The short-term changes adjust over time to increased (the default position) or decreased activity, depending on the nutritional state of the individual.

Anxiety dysregulation

It can be argued that all psychiatric disorders represent some aspect of affective dys-regulation. However, the focus in this model is on the way in which anxiety plays a major role in AN, both premorbidly (and therefore contributing to pathogenesis) and in subsequent states of nutritional depletion. What distinguishes the anxiety in AN is its tendency to be focused on the body and food. In particular, although much has been written about other neurotransmitter systems, such as the serotonergic and glutaminergic systems, this model quite specifically predicts that noradrenaline has a primary role and that other neurotransmitter systems will play secondary or supportive roles.

As stated above, the model specifies that patients with AN are genetically prone to metabolise noradrenaline more quickly. In the premorbid state, this is reflected by increased sympathetic activity and heightened levels of anxiety. The greater the genomic 'dose' of higher-activity noradrenergic genes and the greater the criticality of the sites, the greater the resting level of anxiety and therefore the greater the sensitivity to change in response to substrate depletion (i.e. dietary restriction).

Once dieting commences, a number of changes occur:

1. **Early stages (days to weeks):** There is a relative depletion of noradrenaline and its precursors, such as tyrosine. The consequent reduced noradrenergic activity leads to a reduction in anxiety and an enhanced sense of well-being. This in turn reinforces the wish to diet.
2. **Medium term (weeks to months):** Gradually the noradrenergic system adjusts to the lack of nutritional precursors of noradrenaline, with subsequent re-emergence of anxiety. As with all reinforcement schedules, intermittent and unpredictable responses are most powerful.
3. **Refeeding:** With the accompanying refeeding there is a repletion of noradrenaline precursors, restoration of premorbid noradrenergic activity and increase in anxiety.
4. **Chronic adjustments (months to years):** In contrast, if refeeding does not occur, or is vigorously resisted, chronic depletion of 'fuel' for the noradrenergic system leads to a failure of the capacity to adjust (the adaptive response) noted above and to the emergence of depression. The loss of anxiety at this stage may reflect a failing, and essentially nonadaptive, sympathetic arousal system.
5. **Persistent in extremis (years to decades):** In the long term, when nutritional depletion is chronic and severe, the noradrenergic system becomes so severely compromised that the capacity for anxiety is lost, and profound depression, apathy and death may supervene.

Middle cerebral artery

Patients with AN have consistently demonstrated hypoperfusion in the medial temporal region ([17], see also Chapter 3). The location of this hypoperfusion implicates the middle cerebral artery, of which a major segment supplies the insula (M2: [18]). Since noradrenergic mechanisms are implicated in the regulation of cerebral vasculature, and in cortical microvasculature in particular [19, 20], reduced flow in the insula segment flow territory could explain the hypoperfusion abnormalities observed on single-photon emission computed tomography (SPECT) [21, 22] and subsequently on functional magnetic resonance imaging (fMRI) [23].

Impaired neuroplasticity

Neuroplasticity is the capacity of the nervous system to modify its organisation. This occurs as a consequence of many events, including the normal development and maturation of the organism, the acquisition of new skills ('learning') in immature and mature organisms, damage to the nervous system and sensory deprivation. Cortical neuroplasticity, a human variable with individual differences just like height and weight, is mediated through noradrenergic, anticholinergic, serotonergic and glutamate receptors (see Chapter 5). Dysregulation in any of these neurotransmitter systems could lead to impairment of cortical neuroplasticity in the tertiary somatosensory cortex, located in the insula. It is therefore possible that those with AN (or at least a significant subgroup of them) have a genetically determined, reduced capacity to respond to the neuroplasticity demands of puberty, the cortical pruning of adolescence and extreme dieting and its consequent noradrenergic substrate depletion (see Figure 8.2). We have focused on noradrenergic mechanisms for conceptual economy, convergent explanations and specificity of prediction for testing.

Insula dysfunction

We have previously hypothesised that AN can be explained by a neural circuit abnormality, at the centre of which is the insula [24] (see Figure 8.3). The rationale for this hypothesis is outlined in Nunn *et al.* [25] and the hypothesis is explored in depth in Chapter 7. The predominant role of the insula is to orchestrate the balance between those parts of the brain that deal with adaptation to the external environment and those responsible for internal stability or homeostasis. It is also a bridge between the right and left sides of the brain (intersecting as it does the anterior and posterior commissures: [26]), between the feeling brain and the thinking brain, and between the expression and reception of speech and emotions [27–29]. The insula might be compared to an Internet server, which has the potential to facilitate communication between millions of people [24]; it facilitates and regulates communication between the

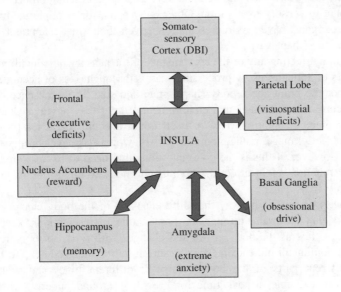

Figure 8.3 The insula's integral role in AN.

billions of brain cells in the various structures to which it is connected. Dysconnection or dysfunction in this network could lead to a wide range of abnormalities, the specific nature of which would be determined by the exact type and location of the insula dysfunction. Figure 8.3 outlines our model of how insula dysfunction accounts for many of the characteristic features of AN.

Homunculus dysfunction and distorted body image

In general terms, therefore, many of the clinical phenomena of AN can be accounted for on the basis of insula dysfunction [24]. However, this leaves the question of the more specific pathogenesis of distorted body image (DBI), a feature that has defied any satisfactory explanation to date. We need therefore to consider specifically body-image representation and how this becomes distorted in AN.

The experience of body image is mediated through somatotopic representation, or body maps, more commonly known as sensory homunculi (homunculus = little human). The modern notion of the sensory homunculus has three components, with a degree of overlap between them:

1. primary (sensory and perceptual), located in the post-central gyrus (the somatosensory cortex) of the anterior parietal lobe, which deals with perception of the somatosensory experience;
2. secondary (or interpretative), located in the inferior post-central gyrus of the anterior parietal lobe, which deals with interpretation of that experience;
3. tertiary (integrative and multisensory), located in the insula, which integrates and provides meaning to that experience.

Each homunculus provides 'representational space' for each part of the body. However, certain parts are represented in greater detail than others. In the sensory homunculus, the face, hands and genitals have greater representation because of their larger amount of sensory innervation. Other body parts, for example the trunk, limbs and internal organs, have less representation, given their smaller amount of sensory innervation (see Chapter 6).

Dysfunction affecting any of the components of the sensory homunculi may lead to impairments of somatosensory processing, with subsequent loss of accurate feedback to the rest of the brain about body shape, state and size. In the absence of accurate feedback, current mood states and environmental input may aggravate the misinterpretation of bodily condition. This in itself could account for at least some of the distortion of body image, pathognomonic of AN, which has never been satisfactorily explained. However, if this is the case, questions that need to be answered are: what form of dysfunction might affect the homunculi and how might this relate to insula dysfunction?

At the heart of this is the way that different parts of the body change over time, and the way that the brain, through the homuncular representations, keeps up with these changes. Just as the body grows and changes with time, so its representations through the homunculi must keep apace, ensuring utility and accuracy. To complicate matters, different parts of the body change at different times and with different velocities. For example, a peak time for growth is around puberty, when there is considerable expansion of the limbs and the trunk, along with the development of secondary sexual characteristics. Thus the space for homuncular representation of these structures must also increase. This representational change occurs through neuroplasticity (see section on 'Impaired neuroplasticity').

However, neuroplasticity is challenged by the fact that there is finite representational space in the brain for which different body parts compete and for which there are changing demands over time. The actual change in brain size is constrained by the skull and thus there is much less change in brain size than in the size of other body parts. Clearly, puberty is the time that imposes the greatest challenge upon the neuroplasticity process. During puberty the body is growing far more rapidly than the brain – indeed this is actually a time of neuronal pruning [30] – thus the amount of brain volume available for representation is static, or even reducing. The body changes that take place during adolescence are not uniform and differ between boys and girls. Most of this growth occurs in the long bones (thighs), hips and trunk, with relatively smaller changes in face, arms and lower legs.

This pubertal growth spurt creates competition between (i) the available representational space for areas requiring expansion because of pubertal change and (ii) other areas such as the face and hands that already have disproportionate representation. Girls change faster and earlier than boys, over a shorter duration, and therefore experience greater demands on neuroplasticity mechanisms. Thus an internal neuroplasticity challenge is set in process, which, in the majority, is satisfactorily resolved. However, should neuroplasticity be impaired, as for example when there is noradrenergic dysregulation, with subsequent major discrepancy between actual body size and body representations (the homunculi), DBI is likely to arise. It is worth noting here that the parts of the body most commonly misrepresented in AN are those that grow fastest in puberty and proportionately have the least sensory representation.

In summary, we are proposing that DBI arises as a result of genetically determined noradrenergic dysregulation. This predisposes some individuals to an impaired response to the neuroplasticity challenge of puberty, with subsequent discrepancy of representational space for the rapidly changing body, giving rise to DBI.

This phenomenon in turn links to insula dysfunction in that the tertiary or integrative homunculus is to be found in the insula itself. It is possible that broader insula activity is compromised by the neuroplasticity challenge, with subsequent impairment of insula function. In any event the failure to withstand this challenge could explain why AN arises in the peripubertal period, why it selectively affects girls more than boys, given the more rapid and extensive growth spurt of the former, and why those parts of the body most commonly 'misrepresented' are the hips, thighs and trunk.

Furthermore, a common finding in AN is that of weak global sensory processing, with greater attention to fine detail [31]. Global processing of body image occurs in the tertiary homuncular representations in the insula [25, 32]. Impairment of insula activity, including homuncular activity, would lead to higher priority being given to the fine-detail processing of body image occurring in the primary and secondary homunculi. This would explain the intense focus on the minutiae of the somatosensory experience, at the expense of the 'big picture' in the insula.

Anorexia nervosa onset

The clinical phenomena of AN are extraordinarily plentiful and diverse (see Chapter 2). Some may be explained by nutritional inadequacy, such as the physical sequelae of weight loss and some of the cognitive impairments, for example poor concentration, memory and motor performance (see Chapter 4). However, such characteristics reverse with refeeding and are therefore most likely to be secondary phenomena.

Other features are far harder to account for on the basis of nutritional inadequacy alone. These include high levels of premorbid anxiety, morbid dread of weight gain, body-image disturbance or distortion, relentless pursuit of thinness, self-disgust (abhorrence of self), anosognosia (unawareness of illness), raised pain threshold, inability to integrate thoughts and feelings, dysregulation of the reward system, obsessive–compulsive behaviour and perfectionism, excessive exercising, cognitive deficits such as poor cognitive flexibility and inhibition, impaired visuospatial memory and weak central coherence (see Chapter 4), and the very localised abnormalities of regional cerebral blood flow (rCBF) (see Chapter 3).

To date there has been no adequate explanation of this miscellany of pathology. If nutritional deficiency were the cause then it would be hard to understand why the vast majority of those who diet do not develop AN nor its accompanying features.

This model, with its basic premise of genetically determined noradrenergic dysregulation, probably mediated by certain epigenetic phenomena, does seem to offer a coherent explanation, however. The high levels of premorbid anxiety and their reduction after dieting can be accounted for by noradrenergic dysregulation. There is however a rebound phenomenon in which the previous high levels of anxiety return as homeostasis of the noradrenergic system takes over. The noradrenergic dysregulation gives a plausible account of impaired rCBF and neuroplasticity, with subsequent dysfunction in the insula.

Most other features can be accounted for by this insula dysfunction, through (i) its intrinsic functions, that is regulation of pain and disgust, interpretation of body image, autonomic regulation and central coherence, and (ii) its extrinsic provision of connectivity, viz. its role as the 'central station of the brain'. The disturbance of body image is explained by the inability of the tertiary somatosensory cortex in the insula to accommodate to the pubertal growth spurt; the high levels of self-disgust may be accounted for by the insula's failure to regulate disgust; and a similar failure of regulation explains the raised pain threshold.

The networking failure and its consequent impaired communication with other key structures surrounding the insula could explain the remaining phenomena. Failure of adequate communication between the insula and the frontal lobes would explain the executive-functioning deficits such as weak cognitive flexibility, inhibition and central coherence. Similarly impaired communication between the insula and the nucleus accumbens accounts for faulty reward regulation, and that between the insula and the parietal lobe for deficits in visuospatial memory. Emotional regulation, and especially that of anxiety, is dependent upon the integrity of the relationship between the insula and the limbic system, most particularly the amygdala for activation of emergency emotions, such as fear and anxiety, and the insula for calming emotions and stabilising emergency responses. Impairment of insula function could account for the failure in integration of thoughts and feelings, the inability to self-soothe and the weakness in central coherence. Failure of the insulo–striatal (basal ganglia) network could explain the excessive motor agitation and consequent drive to exercise, as well as the obsessive–compulsive behaviour. The very localised abnormalities in rCBF are likely a reflection of this impairment in insula activity.

Precursor depletion and other perpetuating factors

Recursive interactions and the consequent perpetuation of AN are integral to this model. A number of factors play a significant part in the maintenance of the illness (see Figures 8.1 and 8.2). Dieting subsequently leads to depletion of noradrenaline precursors and initial reduction of noradrenergic activity, with subsequent consolidation of longer-term changes in noradrenergic dysregulation. This depletion reinforces impairment of insula function with further anxiety, distortion of body image and cerebral artery hypoperfusion, which in turn reinforces insula dysfunction. This sets up a malignant feed-forward system (goal-directed attempts at anticipated relief based on reward reinforcement) as well as a feedback (incorrect assessment of bodily condition) system, from which habitual or 'instinctive' responses by the individual are only likely to worsen the situation. In these circumstances external intervention (i.e. treatment) may be needed to reestablish homeostasis (i.e. appropriate feedback control) and enable meaningful adaptation (readjustment of goals and anticipated outcomes).

8.3   Critical appraisal

As discussed in Chapter 7, there are several principles required for a conceptual model: comprehensiveness of content, logical congruence, conceptual clarity and level of abstraction [33], all of which we have tried to ensure apply to this model. However, though it may satisfy the above principles, for a model to have real value it also needs to fulfil the demands of (i) necessity, (ii) sufficiency, (iii) specificity, (iv) empirical derivation and (v) refutability.

1. **Necessity:** For the model to fulfil the requirement of necessity it must be able to explain those elements of the causal pathway without which the illness cannot emerge and then be maintained. The sine qua non of AN, DBI, is accounted for at three explanatory levels:

   a. the molecular level: noradrenergic dysregulation;
   b. the neuroanatomical and neurocircuitry levels: insula dysfunction;
   c. the cortical representational level: homuncular misrepresentation.

   The necessity to explain symptom and illness maintenance requires persistent negative recursion and this occurs at numerous levels (see Figure 8.2).

2. **Sufficiency:** For the model to fulfil the demands of sufficiency it must be able to account for the full range of phenomena of the illness. This model accounts for all the neurocognitive, emotional and behavioural components of AN.

3. **Specificity:** For the model to fulfil the demand of specificity it must account for those aspects of the condition that differ from other conditions. In AN, no one component alone is specific. For example, DBI can be found in dysmorphobia; weak central coherence occurs in autistic spectrum disorder; intense body-focused anxiety can also be found in dysmorphophobia and in hypochondriasis; and extreme food restriction can be found in food-avoidance emotional disorder and severe depression. However, the specificity of this model for AN is based upon its explanation of age of onset, gender bias and the convergence, persistence and severity of all the features, which do not occur in this combination in any other disorder.

4. **Empirical derivation:** For the model to fulfil the demands of empirical derivation, each major component requires empirical support. In relation to this model, we consider the core components of the cascade (see above). The noradrenergic profile has been demonstrated by Urwin *et al.* [4–6]; the noradrenergic dysregulation, even after refeeding, has been demonstrated by Kaye *et al.* [34]; high levels of body-focused anxiety are very commonly reported [35]; impaired neuroplasticity due to noradrenergic dysregulation has been documented by Gu [36]; regional hypoperfusion has been documented in numerous studies (see Brewerton *et al.* [37] for a review) [37]; insula dysfunction [24, 25] is currently being investigated using fMRI paradigms, with early results showing reduced insular activation compared to controls [23]; and homuncular misrepresentation has been shown to be related to insular dysfunction [38]. The process of neuroplasticity and the differential growth rate of different parts of the body at puberty (especially the secondary sexual characteristics), as well as the differential growth rate between boys and girls, are well-recognised and empirically-supported phenomena [39].

5. **Refutability:** Ultimately a model stands or falls upon its being able to fulfil the demands of refutability. Each component should be open to empirical testing.

The relevant noradrenergic profile could be refuted either by full genomic studies of patients with AN failing to find such a profile in significant numbers or by evidence of a more compelling alternative explanation. In this model, noradrenergic dysregulation is both a cause and a consequence of starvation, or both. To refute this would require demonstration of no dysregulation or dysregulation being exclusively causative or consequential, but not both.

The component of anxiety could be refuted by showing that it is not primarily noradrenergically mediated.

The neuroplasticity component could be refuted by demonstration either of no impairment in AN or that an alternative neurotransmitter system, for example acetylcholine, serotonin or glutamate, is primary to impairment. All of these transmitters have also been implicated in different ways in cortical neuroplasticity and could end up providing a more compelling causal explanation.

The component relating to middle cerebral artery hypoperfusion could be refuted by demonstrating that the hypoperfusion is an epiphenomenon of other cerebral regulators such as nitrous oxide, serotonin, glutamate or a host of others (see Chapter 5).

The insula dysfunction component could be refuted by showing normal insula activation in fMRI studies or by showing that other structures or regions of interest are just as salient, such as the anterior cingulate, the amygdala or the basal ganglia.

The homuncular component could be refuted by one of two studies. The first would involve using standard growth charts [40] to compare rate of change in body size with that of the changing activation patterns within the somatosensory cortices and the insula, using existing normative data and paradigms analogous to the pain research literature [41]. The model would be refuted if there were no discrepancy in AN patients or no relationship in controls between the respective rates of change. The second study, using fMRI, would involve application of gentle sensory stimuli to different parts of the body, including those of specific relevance in AN such as hips, thighs and trunk, to compare activation patterns in the somatosensory cortex and insula between subjects with AN and age-matched controls. The hypothesis would be refuted if there were no significant difference in levels of activation between the two groups.

Finally, the component of recursivity due to dietary depletion could be refuted by showing that the specific noradrenergic profile, combined with dieting, does not necessarily lead to AN; that is, the dieting is an epiphenomenon.

Possible criticisms of the model include:

1. It does not fully explain later onset of AN; that is, those who have passed the peripubertal period. It is possible that other events such as trauma, pregnancy (a body-distorting event), acute weight gain or other stress may contribute.
2. It does not explain the 30% of those with AN who appear to show no regional cerebral hypoperfusion on the earlier SPECT studies [21, 22]. However, this raises the fact that SPECT does not measure absolute levels of perfusion, providing only a strong indication of relative perfusion between the two hemispheres and between different regions in the same hemisphere. As scanning techniques become more sophisticated, with far greater degrees of resolution and with a shift from qualitative to quantitative assessment, it should be possible to assess more accurately regional levels of perfusion and laterality differences. In fact, it is quite possible that all cases of AN have both generalised and regional hypoperfusion, as indicated in an ongoing fMRI study [23].
3. It fails to take into account issues of laterality. This concern is addressed in point 2. It is likely that the apparent lateralisation of hypoperfusion is relative rather than absolute, and that there is bilateral hypoperfusion. In other words, we suggest that the final picture represents a failure of integrity of the bilateral insula system. Developmental effects on laterality and the fact that there is interhemispheric compensation make any quick judgements at this stage premature.

8.4   Clinical implications

Confirmation of the model's validity would open avenues for novel approaches to treatment (see Chapter 10). Examples include:

Medical therapies

1. The reduction in noradrenergic precursors might be remedied by tyrosine supplementation to the refeeding programme or by other precursors. This is currently being tested by a randomised controlled trial in young people [42]. Other possibilities include the use of L-Dopa, which has a known profile of side effects from its long-term use in Parkinson's disease.
2. Excessive post-synaptic noradrenergic activity, as manifested by high levels of anxiety, might be attenuated by the use of noradrenergic antagonists such as beta-blockers and presynaptic autoreceptor agonists (braking mechanisms) such as clonidine. There is some reason to believe these might be especially helpful where trauma is a known recursive contributor.

3. The rate of breakdown of noradrenaline might be reduced by blocking the activities of mono-amine-oxidase or COMT, once repletion is complete.
4. Reuptake might be reduced by using noradrenergic reuptake inhibitors such as reboxetine, mirtazepine or venlafaxine once repletion of precursors has taken place.
5. Compounds which enable cerebral vasodilatation, such as endothelial nitric oxide synthase agonists, might be used to reduce cerebral hypoperfusion.
6. Other more general non-adrenergic anxiolytics that have reduced potential for addiction, such as hydroxyzine, might be considered to address the central experience of anxiety, such as hydroxyzine.

Psychological interventions

1. Individual, group and family psycho-education are likely to take some new and different directions in light of this model.
2. Therapies which address serious, severe and pervasive anxiety, such as cognitive behavioural theory (CBT) and relaxation techniques, could be used to target the central anxiety.

Neuropsychological interventions

1. Cognitive remediation therapy (CRT) – see Chapter 10 – may assist with the common cognitive deficits, such as executive impairments, poor visuospatial memory and weak central coherence – see Chapter 4 – each of which could be attributed to insula dysfunction and its subsequent failure to process relevant information. The task here would be the same as in any remediation programme; that is, to determine what function can be recovered and therefore needs to be 'exercised' and supported with 'scaffolding', and what functions represent permanent deficits which must be 'got around' and for which environmental or human 'prostheses' must be found to substitute for them. Important examples include emotional and social processing.
2. Specifically addressing anosognosia, empathy deficits and social skills would represent a major aspect of neurodevelopmental understanding and intervention. Much could be learned from the interventions of those with autistic-spectrum disorders, especially the social narrative interventions.
3. Visuospatial memory difficulties could be explored within a traumatic brain-injury model of rehabilitation and recovery. This would effectively bring to bear a whole literature of intervention wisdom that has largely remained untapped to date.
4. Neurobiofeedback using real-time feedback of insula activation in the scanner has been shown to be effective [43]. Since significant changes to insula function have been achieved within three 5 minutes trials in the scanner, adapting these paradigms for patients with AN, with their impaired insula functioning, could prove to be helpful.

Physical therapies

1. The role of exercise as part of the solution, rather than part of the problem, needs to be considered once repletion and refeeding have taken place. Exercise's role as

an anxiolytic and antidepressant, as well as a stimulant to basal ganglia function and somatotopic activation, needs further consideration.

2. Mirror therapy might be used to reflexively stimulate mirror neurons and to enable prefrontal evaluation (more 'objective' or 'as if for another') of the self, to counteract distortions created by insula dysfunction.

3. Somatotopic electrodermal stimulation to those body parts that are currently underrepresented, and therefore perceived as fat, may offer opportunity to increase the competitive advantage of those areas that give rise to maximal distress and disgust.

8.5 Conclusion

To our knowledge there has been no causal model that explains the pathogenesis, phenomenology and maintenance of AN. In this chapter we have proposed just such a model. It is rooted in genetically determined noradrenergic dysregulation, which in combination with epigenetic factors, leads to high levels of anxiety, impaired neuroplasticity and regional cerebral hypoperfusion. These, in combination, lead to insular dysfunction, with deficits in information processing and dysfunctional homuncular representation. The consequent body-image distortion and high levels of body-focused anxiety give rise to intense dieting, noradrenergic precursor depletion, initial reduction in anxiety followed by a rebound exacerbation, and a vicious cycle of maintenance.

We do not claim that this model offers the definitive causal explanation for AN but it does seem to offer a coherent account of its pathogenesis, phenomenology and maintenance, at least in a majority of cases. Its value is supported by it seeming to fulfil the criteria of necessity, sufficiency, specificity, empirical derivation and refutability. This latter is of particular significance as the model clearly needs to be empirically tested. We have attempted to show how such studies could be conducted in future research.

Acknowledgements

Ken Nunn is particularly indebted to Ruth Urwin for so many conversations in and around the noradrenergic system. He also wishes to acknowledge the collegiate support and encouragement of Mel Hart, Bridget Wilkins, David Sibbritt and Lauren Williams.

References

1. Treasure, J., Claudino, A. and Zucker, N. (2010) Eating disorders. *Lancet*, **375**, 583–593.

2. Kaye, W., Frank, G., Bailer, U. *et al.* (2005) Serotonin alterations in anorexia nervosa and bulimia nervosa – new insights from imaging studies. *Physiological Behaviour*, **85**, 73–81.

3. Pinheiro, A., Root, T. and Bulik, C. (2009) The genetics of anorexia nervosa: current findings and future perspectives. *International Journal of Child and Adolescent Health*, **2**, 153–164.

4. Urwin, R., Bennets, B., Wilcken, B. *et al.* (2002) Anorexia nervosa (restrictive subtype) is associated with a polymorphism in the novel norepinephrine transporter gene promoter polymorphic region. *Molecular Psychiatry*, **7**, 652–657.

5. Urwin, R., Bennets, B., Wilcken, B. *et al.* (2003) Investigation of epistasis between the serotonin transporter and norepinephrine transporter genes in anorexia nervosa. *Neuropsychopharmacology*, **28**, 1351–1355.

6. Urwin, R. and Nunn, K. (2005) Epistatic interaction between the monoamine oxidase A and serotonin transporter genes in anorexia nervosa. *European Journal of Human Genetics*, **13**, 370–375.

7. Frisch, A., Laufer, N., Danziger, Y. *et al.* (2001) Association of anorexia nervosa with the high activity allele of the COMT gene: a family-based study in Israeli patients. *Molecular Psychiatry*, **6** (2), 243–245.

8. Funke, B., Malhotra, A.K., Finn, C.T. *et al.* (2005) COMT genetic variation confers risk for psychotic and affective disorders: a case control study. *Behavioral and Brain Functions*, **1**, 19.

9. Winje, E., Willoughby, K. and Lask, B. (2008) Season of birth bias in eating disorders: fact or fiction? *International Journal of Eating disorders*, **41** (6), 479–490.

10. Davis, G.E. and Lowell, W.E. (2006) Solar cycles and their relationship to human disease and adaptability. *Medical Hypotheses*, **67**, 447–461.

11. Yang, C., Kim, H., Seo, H. *et al.* (1998) Paired like homeodomain proteins, Phox 2a and Phox 2b, are responsible for noradrenergic cell-specific transcription of the dopamine 41-hydroxylase gene. *Journal of Neurochemistry*, **103**, 1813–1826.

12. Hultman, C.M., Ohman, A., Cnattingius, S. *et al.* (1997) Prenatal and neonatal risk factors for schizophrenia. *British Journal of Psychiatry*, **170**, 128–133.

13. Favaro, A., Tenconi, E. and Santonastaso, P. (2006) Perinatal factors and the risk of developing anorexia nervosa and bulimia nervosa. *Archives of General Psychiatry*, **63**, 82–88.

14. Bremner, J., Krystal, J., Southwick, S. and Charney, D. (1996) Noradrenergic mechanisms in stress and anxiety: II. *Clinical studies Synapse*, **23**, 39–51.

15. Mitchell, D.A., Lambert, G., Secher, N.H. *et al.* (2009) Jugular venous overflow of noradrenaline from the brain: a neurochemical indicator of cerebrovascular sympathetic nerve activity in humans. *Journal of Physiology*, **587** (11), 2589–2597.

16. Marzo, A., Bai, J. and Otani, S. (2009) Neuroplasticity regulation by noradrenaline in mammalian brain. *Current Neuropharmacology*, **7**, 286–295.

17. Frampton, I., Watkins, E., Gordon, I. and Lask, B. (2010) Do abnormalities in regional cerebral blood flow in anorexia nervosa resolve after weight restoration? *European Eating Disorders Review* (Article first published online: 7 Oct 2010).

18. Ture, U., Yasargil, M.G., Al Mefty, O. and Yasargil, D.C.H. (2000) Arteries of the insula. *Journal of Neurosurgery*, **92**, 676–687.

19. Edvinsson, L. and Hamel, E. (2002) Perivascular nerves in brain vessels, in *Cerebral Blood Flow and Metabolism*, 2nd edn (eds L. Edvinsson and D.N. Krause), Lippincott Williams & Wilkins, Philadelphia, PA, pp. 43–67.

20. Hamel, E. (2006) Perivascular nerves and the regulation of cerebrovascular tone. *Journal of Applied Physiology*, **100**, 1059–1064.

21. Gordon, I., Lask, B., Bryant-Waugh, R. *et al.* (1997) Anorexia nervosa in children: evidence of a primary limbic abnormality. *International Journal of Eating Disorders*, **22**, 159–165.

22. Chowdhury, U., Gordon, I., Lask, B. *et al.* (2003) Early onset anorexia nervosa: evidence of limbic system imbalance. *International Journal of Eating Disorders*, **33**, 388–396.

23. Frampton, I., Nunn, K., Fuglset, T. and Lask, B. (2010) The neurobiology of anorexia nervosa. Material presented at Plenary Session of Eating Disorders Research Society 2010, Cambridge, MA, paper in preparation.

24. Nunn, K., Gordon, I., Frampton, I. *et al.* (2008) Anorexia nervosa: the fault is not in her parents but in the insula. *European Eating Disorders Review*, **16**, 355–360.

25. Nunn, K., Frampton, I., Fugslet, T. *et al.* (2010) Anorexia nervosa and the insula. *Medical Hypotheses*, in press.

26. Naidich, T.P., Kang, E., Fatterpekar, G.M. *et al.* (2004) The insula: anatomic study and MR imaging display at 1.5 T. *American Journal of Neuroradiology*, **25**, 222–232.

27. Dronkers, N.F. (1996) A new brain region for coordinating speech articulation. *Nature*, **384**, 159–161.

28. Dronkers, N.F., Wilkins, D.P., Van Valin, R.D. *et al.* (2004) Lesion analysis of the brain areas involved in language comprehension. *Cognition*, **92**, 145–177.

29. Damasio, A. (1999) *The Feeling of What Happens: Body, Emotion and the Making of Consciousness*, Heinemann, London.

30. Sisk, C. and Foster, D. (2004) The neural basis of puberty and adolescence. *Nature Neuroscience*, **7**, 1040–1047.

31. Tchanturia, K., Davies, H., Lopez, C. *et al.* (2008) Neuropsychological task performance before and after cognitive remediation in anorexia nervosa: a pilot case series. *Psychological Medicine*, **38** (9), 1371–1373.

32. Damasio, A. (2010) *Self Comes to Mind: Constructing the Conscious Brain*, Pantheon Books, New York, NB.

33. Fawcett, J. (1995) *Analysis and Evaluation of Conceptual Models of Nursing*, F. A. Davis Company, Philadelphia, PA.

34. Kaye, W., Frank, G. and McConaha, C. (1999) Altered dopamine activity after recovery from restricting-type anorexia nervosa. *Neuropsychopharmacology*, **21**, 503–506.

35. Treasure, J., Macare, C., Mentxaka, I. and Harrison, A. (2010) The use of a vodcast to support eating and reduce anxiety in people with eating disorder: a case series. *European Eating Disorders Review*, **18**, 515–521.

36. Gu, Q. (2002) Neuromodulatory transmitter systems in the cortex and their role in cortical plasticity. *Neuroscience*, **111**, 815–835.

37. Brewerton, T., Frampton, I. and Lask, B. (2009) The neurobiology of anorexia nervosa. *US Psychiatry*, **2**, 57–60.

38. Shelley, B. and Trimble, M. (2004) The insular lobe of Reil: its anatamico-functional, behavioural and neuropsychiatric attributes in humans: a review. *World Journal of Biological Psychiatry*, **5**, 176–200.

39. Tanner, J. and Preece, M (eds) (1989) *The Physiology of Human Growth*, Society for the Study of Human Biology Symposium, Vol. **29**, ambridge University Press, Cambridge (England), New York.

40. Tanner, J.M., Whitehouse, R.H. and Takaishi, M. (1966) Standards from birth to maturity for height, weight, height velocity, and weight velocity: British children, 1965. I. *Archives of Disease in Childhood*, **41** (219), 454–471.

41. Shaw, P., Kabani, N., Lerch, J. *et al.* (2008) Neurodevelopmental trajectories of the human cerebral cortex. *The Journal of Neuroscience*, **28**, 3586–3594.

42. Hart, M., Wilkins, B., Sibbritt, D. *et al.* (2010) Tyrosine repletion in young people with anorexia nervosa. Current PhD study at the University of Newcastle, New South Wales, Australia.

43. Caria, A., Veit, R., Sitaram, R. *et al.* (2007) Regulation of anterior insular cortex activity using real-time fMRI. *NeuroImage*, **35** (3), 1238–1246.

9 Neurobiological models: implications for patients and families

Ilina Singh[1] and Alina Wengaard[2]

[1]*London School of Economics and Political Science, London, UK*
[2]*Regional Eating Disorders Service, Oslo University Hospital, Oslo, Norway*

9.1 Introduction

This chapter addresses the consequences of the development of neurobiological models for patients' and families' understandings of eating disorders and their receptivity to treatments. In this chapter we focus on anorexia nervosa (AN) because this condition has been the main focus of recent neuroscientific research, the current status of which is addressed substantively elsewhere in this book. We begin by presenting a brief introduction to the emergence of neurobiological models of AN. We then outline the current state of knowledge about the impact of illness representations on patients with AN and their families. We refer also to the general biases to which neurobiological knowledge is susceptible when presented in public arenas, as well as in the professional environment. Finally, we integrate research and concepts from the field of 'neuroethics' to evaluate the potential influence of neurobiological models of AN and the technologies used to develop them (such as brain imaging and genetic testing) on patients' and families' understanding of the disorder.

9.2 The emergence of neurobiological models

Originally, aetiological theories of eating disorders were heavily informed by psychoanalytic ideas, including an emphasis on psychogenic factors in the 1930s. During the 1960s and 1970s, a focus on the so-called 'anorexogenic family' emerged [1]. During the 1980s there was a greater focus on the sociocultural perspective, including a feminist discourse in sociology and psychology that emphasised cultural factors in AN. *Fat Is a Feminist Issue* by Susie Orbach was published in 1980 [2], and in 1994

Eating Disorders and the Brain. Edited by Bryan Lask and Ian Frampton.
© 2011 John Wiley & Sons, Ltd. Published 2011 by John Wiley & Sons, Ltd.

Fallon *et al.* published *Feminist Perspectives on Eating Disorders* [3]. These robust sociological and feminist critiques of AN focused on the Western cultural obsession with thinness and fitness for women, which is seen to encourage and perhaps to cause abnormal cognitions and behaviours around food. Yet social and cultural factors are insufficient to explain why only a very limited number of females develop AN.

With the advent of more sophisticated biotechnologies, recent research on the aetiology of AN has focused on its neurobiology. Studies on neurotransmitter function, genetics, neuroimaging and neuropsychology aim therefore to identify underlying neuroanatomical and pathophysiological bases for AN. Growing importance is placed on identifying genetic pathways to illness behaviours and cognitions, in line with growing interest in and research on the genetic understanding of health and illness. Studies have identified genetic markers associated with enhanced susceptibility to AN. Comorbid individual and familial psychological traits, such as anxiety and obsessionality, have also been identified, and these may provide further clues to the genetic and epigenetic processes that are associated with AN [4].

Although many of the identified brain abnormalities are due to the effects of starvation, neuroscience research has shown that there appear to be some trait-related characteristics that predispose an individual to develop AN [5]. Better understanding of neurobiological contributions to AN is expected to inform treatments. Once biological risks are identified, more precise treatments based on biomarkers and cognitive profiles may become possible. Though it is unlikely that it will be possible anytime soon to determine from a brain scan alone whether a person has a condition like AN, future diagnostic schema may include clinically reliable biomarker information and other factors that will allow us to generate an individual risk profile and thereby improve the accuracy of diagnosis [6] (current Diagnostic and Statistical Manual (DSM) working groups have been charged with identifying promising biomarkers that could have clinical utility in the decades to come; this is in keeping with the development of the US National Institute of Mental Health-based Research Domain Criteria (RDoC) Project (http://www.nimh.gov)).

9.3   Anorexia nervosa and illness representations

Illness representations are the theories that people have about their illnesses, and include a sufferer's beliefs and knowledge about the nature of their illness and its causes, and their emotional response to the illness. The impact of a neurobiological understanding of AN is likely to affect these representations. In this section we review the literature on AN illness representations in order to illustrate the importance of illness concepts to patients' sense of self, to caregivers' beliefs and attitudes towards patients, and to patients' receptivity to treatments. An illness representation is guided by three sources of information [7]: (i) the general pool of 'lay' information formed through social communications and cultural perceptions of illness; (ii) significant others or authoritative sources such as a doctor or parent; and (iii) current experience of illness. Leventhal *et al.* [8] claim that making sense of the illness is a process in which links are made between abstract and concrete sources of information. The sufferer tries to label the experienced symptoms using concepts or labels that are available to him or her, and at the same time existing schemas/concepts influence the interpretation of the symptoms. Leventhal *et al.* imply that this symmetry rule linking symptoms with diagnosis is automatic and intuitive [8]. Across a wide range of physical illnesses, illness representations are important in influencing levels of illness distress, engagement in treatment, utilisation of services and outcome of treatment [9]. Although developed to assess perceptions of physical illness, the construct has been shown to be relevant to depression and schizophrenia. It has been suggested that modifying illness representations may effect change in mental illness [9].

Attributions

The lack of a clear, coherent conceptualisation of AN produces a lack of understanding among patients, who tend to ascribe idiosyncratic meanings to the illness [10]. A patient's response to AN is embedded in the meanings the patient and his or her family give to the illness and its symptoms. For example, the belief that the illness is caused by the patient's personality is associated with reduced warmth among caregivers. If it is seen as a 'hunger strike', parents may feel guilty, anxious and overprotective; if the illness is seen as a suicide attempt, self-destruction, life-threatening or revenge, this may result in criticism and hostility from the parents towards the patient [10]. Other studies have suggested that when patients and their families see the cause of AN as a personality factor, fewer positive appraisals of the patient are made [11]. In general, individuals with conditions that are thought to be more under their control (for example drug misuse) are more likely to elicit anger and less likely to elicit helping behaviours in others, when compared to individuals whose conditions are thought to be outside their control, such as childhood cancers [12].

Motivation and illness representations

Knowledge about emotional and cognitive representations – the way patients understand and feel about their illness, its functions, causes, consequences and likely course – is important for understanding what motivates patients to change [9]. Lack of motivation presents a major challenge to the management of AN, yet little research has been done on factors that may influence motivation to change in eating disorders [9]. A few studies have explored the relationship between illness representations and stages of change [13], showing that consequences, treatment control and personal control, as well as cyclical timeline perceptions (developing a realistic perspective that eating disorders are characterised by relapse) [9], account for a significant amount of variance in readiness to change scores. This finding pinpoints some of the factors that can motivate change in the patient and that can be included in the therapeutic work.

Stockford *et al.* [9] found a significant relationship between illness representations and stage of change, suggesting that illness representations may be worth considering in therapeutic work. For example, the stage of precontemplation is associated with fewer perceived consequences, less personal control, less control over treatment/cure and lower levels of emotional representations. Readiness to change is predicted by more perceived personal and treatment control as well as less illness coherence. Predictors of change included understanding consequences of the illness, a sense of personal control, self-confidence and being understood by friends, family and professionals, as well as having control over the treatment. However, this study [9] could not infer whether introducing change in illness perceptions would result in movement to a particular stage of change. Therefore, longitudinal studies are required to assess change and the factors that influence change over time.

Holliday *et al.* [14] have reported that illness representations are important to outcome. They found that participants with AN view their disorder as chronic, uncontrollable and not amenable to cure, as compared to the more optimistic perception of lay study participants. The perspective of AN as chronic was correlated with negative perceptions of illness controllability and curability. Attributing cause of illness to psychological stress, together with strong illness identity and low perception of control, was associated with poor mental health and poor functional ability.

Acceptance that AN is not due to chance or bad luck is also a predictive factor for readiness to change. When patients receive feedback after neuropsychological testing about some of the underlying traits associated with illness, for example neuropsychological styles such as cognitive rigidity and weak central coherence, they want to share this information with their family members, thus forging a shared understanding of the problem [10]. Giving patients information about the nature of the illness may help sufferers develop a different perspective on the illness and on their role in it [10].

Stigma

As discussed earlier, patients' illness representations are formed through different sources of information. Among these, cultural perceptions of illness are highly influential in how patients understand their illness. The general public still tends to oscillate between thinking that individuals with AN can pull themselves together and have only themselves to blame [14], and envying AN sufferers' 'self-discipline' around food [12]. Alarmingly, however, medical and nursing stuff are inclined to perceive patients with AN as responsible for their condition [12]. Such negative perceptions constitute stigma, which presents a major obstacle to identification and treatment of AN.

While there are numerous studies on the problem of stigma in other psychiatric illnesses, such as schizophrenia, depression and bipolar disorder, there are considerably fewer studies on stigma in eating disorders [12]. The few studies that have been conducted on the stereotypes, prejudice and stigma in the public perception of AN conclude with the need for more information campaigns about the biological aspects of the illness [12]. Media representation of AN is one of the targets of the proposed information programmes. In North American media coverage, AN is frequently presented as part of entertainment news about celebrities. In this context, AN makes for 'soft news' about an illness that is framed as a personality-driven condition [4]. Improving media communication by acknowledging the complexity of the interplay between the biological and social factors in AN may eventually help to reduce stigma and ease the patient experience [4].

9.4   Impact of a neurobiological model on families' understandings of anorexia nervosa

The family is central to the management of AN and, understandably, parents experience intense levels of anxiety, guilt and helplessness [15]. Yet family members report having insufficient information and skills to support patients, especially in relation to tackling challenging behaviours [10]. Indeed, there is considerable misunderstanding of the illness amongst lay persons, including family members. As families play a major role in determining whether or not patients may recover, clearly a family approach to the treatment of AN is essential. This should include containment of anxiety, education about the illness and the discussion, and implementation of relevant strategies for tackling the illness [15].

A biological explanation of AN may make an additional supportive contribution to these therapeutic endeavours. For example, the guilt, shame and blame experienced by some parents may be alleviated by a biological explanation. As Treasure *et al.* [10] have stated, this explanation may help to dismantle myths and misattributions around AN, thereby rendering the meaning of this illness less idiosyncratic [10]. Further, this process may in time help reduce the stigma surrounding eating disorders.

Impact of a neurobiological model on the self–illness relationship

Research involving neurotechnology such as functional magnetic resonance imaging (fMRI) and genetic tools such as gene sequencing, candidate gene searches and animal models are used increasingly to understand the biological bases of complex disorders such as AN. The knowledge produced by such methods is valuable, but the impact of the neurobiological models of AN generated by these tools on how patients conceptualise their illness in relation to personal identity is still largely unknown.

Studies of various psychiatric disorders suggest that exposure to neuro and genetic accounts and technologies affects how aspects of personal identity are viewed by patients and by the public. These dimensions of identity include the capacity to take personal responsibility for antisocial or pathological behaviours, personal authenticity (Who do I take myself to be? What kind of person am I?) and personal agency (Can I act to influence myself and my world?). How patients perceive the relationship between self and illness along these dimensions can in turn influence the way they cope with their illness and their receptiveness to treatment.

It is also important to note that these aspects of personal identity have neurobiological dimensions, which can be affected by the presence of disease. An inability to perceive oneself as an agent (i.e. to have influence) is a specific feature in many illnesses, but it has a distinctive element in illnesses that directly affect cognitive functioning. For example, schizophrenic patients experience a loss of ability to attribute their own actions and thoughts to themselves. Nonattributed or misattributed thoughts and actions become material for delusional interpretations and delirium [16]. In AN, agency is relevant to several features of the illness. For example, patients with obsessionality often experience a loss of self-control and sense of agency. Investigation of the mechanisms underlying agency is important therefore in explaining some features of illnesses such as schizophrenia and AN.

Exposure to biological treatments can affect patients' and families' experiences and understandings of the illness. However, evidence suggests that such exposure does not necessarily translate into reductionist accounts of identity, agency or personal responsibility. Empirical research in this area has investigated the role of psychotropic drug treatments in patients' self-understandings [17, 18]. For example, Singh's research on stimulant drug treatment of young people with attendtion deficit hyperactivity disorder (ADHD) has found that stimulants are recruited into their explanatory narratives of brain function, mental disorder and personhood. In this case, however, these narratives do not confirm ethical concerns that drug treatment threatens young people's sense of an authentic self, notions of personal responsibility over behaviour or perceptions of personal agency [18, 19]. In other words, young people taking stimulants for ADHD do not appear to favour deterministic, biological explanations of behaviour, even though psychotropic drugs do moderate children's perceptions of personal responsibility, self-control and beliefs about an 'authentic' self.

Research into how people respond to genetic risk information also suggests that biological explanations have less deterministic influence than is often feared by critics. For example, the ApoE4 gene is associated with an increased risk of contracting Alzheimer's disease (AD), and with a higher risk of early onset of AD: seven to nine years earlier than average. There is a genetic test for ApoE4. Despite the replicated discovery of a strong genetic component to the timing and development of AD, neither family members of AD patients nor clinicians working with these families report substantive changes in their behaviours as a result of knowing about this genetic component. In one study, few clinicians told family members about the ApoE4 gene and few family members reported knowing about the gene. Those who did know tended not to want to be tested, as they mistrusted the power of a genetic explanation for AD, or felt that knowing their risk of developing AD was fruitless given the absence of a cure and all the other genetic and environmental variables that affect susceptibility [20].

Not only does the availability of genetic information appear not to have a deterministic, negative impact on patients, it has several positive consequences for them [21]. Genetic risk information galvanises patient groups to organise around common health concerns, providing support to sufferers and research funds to improve understanding of the biological roots of particular illnesses. This organising, networking and fundraising process is seen to represent a 'political economy of hope' [22] in which genetic risk information is translated into positive social and psychological processes, rather than operating deterministically to burden the sufferer.

Neuroessentialism

'Neuroessentialism' refers to the reduction of complex behaviours to neurobiology. Despite the findings discussed above, sociologists and ethicists have worried about the authority that biological explanations of mental disorder can have over other explanations. Neuroimaging tools such as fMRI are thought to contribute to this process of reduction. Neuroimaging enables significant advances in understanding the neurobiology of psychiatric illnesses and offers new insights into brain structure and function. The ability to visualise brain structure and function also enables researchers to ask questions that were previously impossible to answer.

But interpreting such neuroscientific data is a complex process both for scientists and for the lay public [23]. While many researchers using neuroimaging data are sensitive to the possibility of misinterpretation, media accounts – from which the general public receives much of its information about brain scans – tend to flatten complexity into attractive two-dimensional pictures. The scan data may be interpreted as though they represent something real or fundamental, located statically inside the brain [24, 25]. Such interpretations of neuroimaging data are thought to raise the risk of neuroessentialism. Neuroessentialist critiques are not antipsychiatry critiques;

that is, they do not question the reality of mental illnesses. Rather, this literature is concerned with the lack of neuroscientific elaboration of the mutually shaping interactions between biological and environmental factors.

Indeed, some of the concerns about neuroimaging are shared by neuroscientists, social scientists and ethicists, who have raised questions about the interpretation of neuroimaging data, particularly in relation to the translation of raw statistical data into significant findings. Analysis of neuroimaging is no more immune to statistical manipulation than any other science. Vul *et al.* [26] have carefully outlined the ways in which the use of particular statistical methods to interpret brain scan data resulted in significant findings according to some methods and insignificant findings according to others. However, the great majority of the lay public are unaware that fMRI technology is based on computational physics, that the colourful pictures generated are a result of complex statistical data processing, and that therefore fMRI images are highly susceptible to misrepresentation. For example, coloured images of localised functions in the brain have the potential for being interpreted by the public to mean that complex psychological processes occur in one specific region of the brain [23]. The media often encourage this interpretation. This sort of 'phrenological' thinking could also be used to support the idea that brain structure can reveal different categories of persons [23]. Of course, the brain is not a static structure and the phenomenon of localised functions should not be taken out of the context of the complex dynamism that is involved in brain structures and processes. For example, Brocha's area is specific to expressive speech (a localised function), but expressive speech is also part of a complex and dynamic process involving many other brain structures.

The media, and therefore the general public, have a tendency to attribute more credibility to explanations for behaviour or psychological processes when a brain image is attached [27]. This response is thought to be due to various factors, such as a tendency to favour reductionistic models of complex psychological processes and the simple visual power of brain images. Neuroscientific information is hypothesised to function as a seductive detail in the processing of information [27]. One study showed that participants rated bad explanations which included some neuroscientific information as good or satisfactory compared to better explanations that were unaccompanied by such information. In spite of the strength of the seductive-detail effect, it is unclear why lay participants find bad information 'with neuroscience' to be more convincing [27].

As a mode of critique, neuroessentialism is valuable because it raises questions about techniques and methods that have power within science, and about the re-creation of knowledge produced from a limited set of methodological and theoretical orientations. However, it is unclear whether neuroessentialism is a relevant concern for patients. For example, if neuroessentialism is in fact a perspective found in patients exposed to fMRI, is this perspective harmful or simply incorrect? Does sustained exposure to fMRI in a research project confirm this reductionist perspective, or do patients begin to question the persuasive power of the technology as their participation in the research demystifies fMRI?

Moreover, the specific psychiatric condition a patient has is also likely to play an important role in shaping the individual's experience of fMRI. To date, the debate about neuroscience technologies and identity has infrequently taken into account the distinctive features of psychiatric disorders – and of individuals with those disorders – that might moderate the ways in which brain-based accounts and interactions with scanning technology are integrated. In the case of AN, distinctive features such as anosognosia (denial that there is anything wrong) may moderate outcomes of participation in fMRI research in relation to perceptions of the relationship of self to illness. The persuasive power of fMRI is therefore likely to be moderated by the particularities of the condition, and it is only through empirical research that such nuances of interaction can be identified and analysed.

There may even be a benefit to exposure to fMRI and/or a brain-based explanation of AN. The fusion of personal identity and the illness is a therapeutic challenge. Therapy is frequently organised around effecting some distance between the self and the illness. A biological model of AN, as presented by fMRI, and reinforced by participation in fMRI, may over time assist that process, with positive implications for treatment acceptability and treatment outcomes. There is some evidence that feedback from neuropsychological testing has this effect in those with AN [28] (earlier, we pointed out that a neurobiological model of AN might relieve the guilt and blame within families of patients with AN. There is also evidence that identifying AN as a 'real' illness may relieve the guilt and shame patients feel over their own behaviours [10]).

Chapter 10 further elaborates the clinical implications of neuroscientific knowledge of eating disorders. These potential clinical benefits make up an important, and largely unexplored, dimension in social science and bioethical research on the individual and social impact of neuroimaging technology and genetic research in psychiatry. More must be done by those scholars who are positioned as critical observers of the potentially reductionist processes in child and adolescent psychiatry. Social scientists and ethicists should partner with neuroscientists and psychiatric geneticists conducting research in this area, so that empirical evidence can contribute to normative judgements about the impact of these technologies on the patient with AN and his or her family. An important component of such partnerships should be the development of formal strategies for educating patients and families about how to interpret biomarker information, with emphasis on the multicausal pathways of complex behavioural disorders, gene–environment interactions in determining phenotypes and the probabilistic nature of biomarker information.

Commercialisation of biomarkers: implications for patients and families

Improved public understanding of biomarker information is especially important in an age in which commercial companies enable individuals and families to undergo fMRI scans and genetic tests that provide them with risk information for a wide range of disorders. In the United States, companies such as Cephos (www.cephoscorp.com), the 'world leader in fMRI commercialisation', and 23andMe (www.23andme.com), 'a retail DNA testing service', have a thriving business providing biomarker information to the public. Once the neurobiology of AN is clearer, it is likely that these companies will include AN biomarkers in their information. 23andMe currently provides disease risk status for childhood conditions such as ADHD (for which biomarker evidence is too weak to be included in DSM-5) and includes 'food preference' and 'response to diet and exercise' in its list of genetically identified traits. If AN comes to be known as a hereditary biological condition, it is possible that concerned mothers with a personal history of eating disorders, or families in which one sibling is diagnosed with AN, will seek to test undiagnosed children's susceptibility for AN or associated traits. Without a firm awareness that genetic results from such tests, or results of a brain scan, will not be deterministic, families may come to enact controlling behaviours around food and eating in an effort to protect an 'at-risk' child – with possible paradoxical effects on that child's ability to establish a positive relationship with food and eating.

Participation in neuroscience and genetic research into eating disorders

Social science and bioethics investigations of the impact of neurobiological narratives for patients with eating disorders and their families should focus more on patients' participation in neuroscience and genetic research studies. Participation in research involving these technologies has ethical dimensions about which too little is currently known. For example, given the public misperceptions about the interpretive power of neuroimaging, what steps should researchers take to ensure that patients understand the potential harms and benefits of participation in research that involves these technologies? Consent processes should ensure that patients and their families are sufficiently well informed to enable autonomous decision-making about research participation.

A further consequence of participation in fMRI research is the possibility of incidental findings that are individually significant, such as a brain tumour. Patients and families must be informed of this possibility and be told how the research group will handle such a situation, or state their preferences about the communication of such information. Of course, it is possible that an incidental finding in a neuroimaging study could save a patient's life (e.g. [29]). We do not have good data currently on how best to inform patients about the possibility of incidental findings, or how to support their decision-making about their preferences regarding disclosure of such information.

9.5 Conclusion

There is still a tendency among the general public, aggravated by the media, to view AN as caused by personal problems, difficult life situations or the need to be thin [14], despite all the emerging research that points to a neurobiological basis. These public perceptions of AN fuel the social stigma of the disease, and inevitably create more suffering for patients and their families. In this chapter we have tried to demonstrate the need for, and the importance of, research that investigates the impact of a neurobiological account of AN on patients and their families. We have focused on how novel neuro and genetic technologies are currently positioned to support this account, and we have argued that exposure to such technologies even through research participation may affect patients' and families' understanding of illness, as well as self-understandings and the relationship between illness and identity. This is currently an under-researched area in AN (and in eating disorders in general) but there is considerable potential to build an evidence base from interdisciplinary research collaborations involving eating-disorder specialists, neuroscientists, psychiatric geneticists, social scientists and ethicists.

References

1. Minuchin, S., Baker, L. and Rosman, B.L. (1978) *Psychosomatic Families: Anorexia Nervosa in Context*, Harvard University Press, Cambridge, MA.
2. Orbach, S. (1978) *Fat Is a Feminist Issue*, Paddington Press, New York.
3. Bordo, S. (2004) *Unbearable Weight: Feminism, Western Culture, and the Body*, University of California Press, Berkeley.
4. O'Hara, S.K. and Smith, K.C. (2007) Presentation of eating disorders in the news media: what are the implications for patient diagnosis and treatment? *Patient Education and Counseling*, **68** (1), 43–51.
5. Brewerton, T., Frampton, I. and Lask, B. (2008) The neurobiology of anorexia nervosa. *European Review of Psychiatry*, **1**, 59–64.
6. Singh, I. and Rose, N. (2009) Biomarkers in psychiatry. *Nature*, **460** (7252), 202–207.
7. Hagger, M.S. and Orbell, S. (2003) A meta-analytical review of the common-sense model of illness representations. *Psychology and Health*, **18** (2), 141–184.
8. Leventhal, H., Brissette, I. and Leventhal, E.A. (2003) *The Common-Sense Model of Self-Regulation of Health and Illness: The Self-Regulation of Health and Illness Behaviour*, Routledge, New York.
9. Stockford, K., Turner, H. and Cooper, M. (2007) Illness perception and its relationship to readiness to change in the eating disorders: a preliminary investigation. *The British Journal of Clinical Psychology*, **46** (Pt 2), 139–154.
10. Treasure, J., Sepulveda, A.R., MacDonald, P. *et al.* (2008) The assessment of the family of people with eating disorders. *European Eating Disorders Review*, **16** (4), 247–255.
11. Whitney, J., Haigh, R., Weinman, J. and Treasure, J. (2007) Caring for people with eating disorders: factors associated with psychological distress and negative caregiving appraisals in carers of people with eating disorders. *The British Journal of Clinical Psychology*, **46** (Pt 4), 413–428.
12. Crisafulli, M.A., Von, H.A. and Bulik, C.M. (2008) Attitudes towards anorexia nervosa: the impact of framing on blame and stigma. *The International Journal of Eating Disorders*, **41** (4), 333–339.
13. Cooper, M., Stockford, K. and Turner, H. (2007) Stages of change in anorexic and bulimic disorders: the importance of illness representations. *Eating Behaviors*, **8** (4), 474–484.
14. Holliday, J., Wall, E., Treasure, J. and Weinman, J. (2005) Perceptions of illness in individuals with anorexia nervosa: a comparison with lay men and women. *The International Journal of Eating Disorders*, **37** (1), 50–56.
15. Lask, B. and Bryant-Waugh, R. (2007) *Eating Disorders in Childhood and Adolescence*, Routledge, London and New York.
16. Farrer, C., Franck, N., Frith, C.D. *et al.* (2004) Neural correlates of action attribution in schizophrenia. *Psychiatry Research*, **131** (1), 31–44.
17. Singh, I. (2005) Will the 'real boy' please behave: dosing dilemmas for parents of boys with ADHD. *The American Journal of Bioethics*, **5** (3), 34–47.
18. Singh, I. (2007) Clinical implications of ethical concepts: moral self-understandings in children taking methylphenidate for ADHD. *Clinical Child Psychology and Psychiatry*, **12** (2), 167–182.
19. Singh, I., Kendall, T.,Taylor, C. *et al.* (2010) Young people's experience of ADHD and stimulant medication: a qualitative study for the NICE guideline. *Child and Adolescent Mental Health* (Article first published online: May 2010), doi: 10.1111/j.1475-3588.2010.00565.
20. Lock, M., Lloyd, S. and Prest J. (2006) *Genetic Susceptibility and Alzheimer's Disease: The Penetrance and Uptake of Genetic Knowledge. Thinking about Dementia*, Rutgers University Press, Rutgers, NJ, pp. 123–152.

21. Hedgecoe, A.M. (2001) Ethical boundary work: geneticization, philosophy and the social sciences. *Medicine, Health Care, and Philosophy*, **4** (3), 305–309.
22. Novas, C. (2006) The political economy of hope: patients' organisations, science and bio-value. *BioSocieties*, **1** (3), 289–305.
23. McCabe, D.P. and Castel, A.D. (2008) Seeing is believing: the effect of brain images on judgments of scientific reasoning. *Cognition*, **107** (1), 343–352.
24. Bell, E. and Racine, E. (2009) Enthusiasm for functional magnetic resonance imaging (fMRI) often overlooks its dependence on task selection and performance. *The American Journal of Bioethics*, **9** (1), 23–25.
25. Dumit, J. (2004) *Picturing Personhood: Brain Scans and Biomedical Identity*, Princeton University Press, Princeton, NJ.
26. Vul, E., Harris, C., Winkielman, P. and Pashler, H. (2009) Puzzling high correlations in fMRI studies of emotions, personality and social cognition. *Perspectives on Psychological Sciences*, **5** (4), 274–290.
27. Weisberg, D.S., Keil, F.C., Goodstein, J. *et al.* (2008) The seductive allure of neuroscience explanations. *Journal of Cognitive Neuroscience*, **20** (3), 470–477.
28. Lopez, C., Roberts, M.E., Tchanturia, K. *et al.* (2008) Using neuropsychological feedback therapeutically in treatment for anorexia nervosa: two illustrative case reports. *European Eating Disorders Review*, **16** (6), 411–420.
29. O'Brien, A., Hugo, P., Stapleton, S. *et al.* (2001) 'Anorexia saved my life': coincidental anorexia nervosa and cerebral meningioma. *The International Journal of Eating Disorders*, **30** (3), 346–349.

10 Implications for treatment

Camilla Lindvall[1] and Bryan Lask[1, 2, 3]

[1]*Regional Eating Disorders Service, Oslo University Hospital, Oslo, Norway*
[2]*Ellern Mede Service for Eating Disorders London, UK*
[3]*Great Ormond Street Hospital for Children, London, UK*

10.1 Introduction

The neuroscience of eating disorders has traditionally been perceived as mysterious, complex and even irrelevant to treatment. In this chapter we demonstrate how such knowledge can be applied in the clinical setting. Specifically, we focus on the implications of neuroscience for our understanding of academic ability and school performance, and how this perspective can inform treatment, particularly the use of medication and the development of a novel approach aimed at remediating neurocognitive deficits: cognitive remediation therapy (CRT). A clinician's perspective and the implications of neuroscience knowledge on understanding, attitudes and stigma are discussed in Chapters 1 and 9, respectively.

Eating disorders are possibly amongst the most misunderstood of all illnesses, in part because of the long-held belief that the main reason for their development relates to Western society's emphasis on thinness as an ideal. Public attitudes tend to the view that thinness is to be admired. There is considerable attention paid to the physical appearance of female celebrities, with negative comments for weight gain and positive comments for thinness. However, once thinness tends to emaciation, reactions become more critical, with little understanding that anorexia nervosa (AN) has developed. This lack of recognition is reinforced by the subject's anosagnosia for her condition, and the general tendency to consider those who become overly preoccupied with their weight and shape, and seemingly 'choose' to be very thin, as self-centred and indulgent. An equally negative response occurs in relation to bingeing and overeating, while purging is reacted to with incomprehension and disgust. Consequently, in contrast to most illnesses, there is considerable stigma attached to having an eating disorder.

Knowledge that there is a neurobiological basis to the eating disorders should, in time, go some way to altering the erroneous perceptions of those who believe that the attitudes and behaviours of those with eating disorders are primarily volitional.

Eating Disorders and the Brain. Edited by Bryan Lask and Ian Frampton.
© 2011 John Wiley & Sons, Ltd. Published 2011 by John Wiley & Sons, Ltd.

Even so, some have a concern that knowledge of a biological underpinning might reduce the patient's sense of personal responsibility and thus detract from personal effort to overcome the illness. This argument lacks any logical or empirical support. The same concern might be applied to such conditions as lung cancer, heart disease or kidney stones. Each of these has a clear and proven biological basis that we do not (indeed cannot) conceal from our patients. Whether or not they choose to take as much responsibility as possible for their health care is influenced by a number of factors. There is no evidence that these include the simple knowledge that their illness has a biological basis.

Our clinical experience indicates quite the opposite. In contrast to the general negativity of patients with eating disorders towards any attempts to help them, when presented with the neuroscientific basis of their disorder, for example the results of neuropsychological testing and of neuroimaging, patients show considerable interest and indeed enthusiasm to learn more, and even to participate in our neuroscience research. We all have a responsibility to update ourselves with current neuroscientific understandings and to provide patients and their carers with as much knowledge as possible. These issues are discussed in more depth in Chapter 9.

We turn now to the application of neuroscience knowledge in the management of those with eating disorders. There are three main areas of application: psychopharmacology, the educational context and psychological treatment.

10.2   Psychopharmacology

There are three aspects of the use of medication in the management of eating disorders: (i) treatment of the eating disorder itself; (ii) treatment of comorbidity; and (iii) relief of distress.

Treatment of the eating disorder

A number of psychopharmacological agents have been used in the treatment of eating disorders, but with variable effectiveness, determined to some extent by the particular disorder. In AN, antidepressants, antipsychotics, lithium and appetite stimulants have all been tried. A meta-analysis of antidepressant studies in AN concluded that antidepressants are no more effective than placebo for improving or maintaining weight gain, reducing eating-disorder psychopathology or enhancing associated functioning.

First-generation antipsychotics such as chlorpromazine, haloperidol, pimozide and sulpiride have all failed to be shown to be superior to placebo. Second-generation antipsychotics, such as olanzapine, respiridone and quetiapine, have the potential for being of more value than the first generation, given their effects on cognition and affect, mediated to some extent through the dopamine system, and their side effect of weight gain. Trials have indeed shown increased weight gain when compared with placebo, but not maintained over time. Open trials have shown some improvement in cognition, affect and eating-disorder psychopathology. However, support from the few randomised controlled trials conducted is not yet forthcoming [1]. Neither lithium nor appetite stimulants have shown any value.

In brief, the use of psychopharmacological agents for AN has very limited value and care needs to be taken with regard to potential side effects, especially in relation to the metabolic upheaval associated with starvation and purging. It is to be hoped that an improved understanding of the neurobiological basis for AN may lead ultimately to the development of more effective agents.

The value of psychopharmacology in the treatment of bulimia nervosa (BN) and binge-eating disorder (BED) is better established. The pharmacological treatment of choice for BN is fluoxetine, with alternative specific serotonin reuptake inhibitors (SSRIs) being considered in the case of poor tolerance or poor response [2]. Although BED responds better to cognitive behavioural therapy (CBT) [3], practical and cost implications may lead to the use of medications instead. There is some evidence that SSRIs are superior to placebo and may have some value [4].

Of the conditions specific to childhood and adolescence, such as food-avoidance emotional disorder (FAED), selective eating (SE) and functional dysphagia (FD), there have been no substantial studies upon which guidance can be based. It is possible that anxiolytics are of value in FD and there are reports of a good response to olanzapine (O'Toole 2010, personal communication). Both anxiolytics and antidepressants may have some value in FAED. The treatment of SE may also be enhanced by the use of anxiolytics in those children motivated to try new foods but too anxious to do so. Formal studies are needed to evaluate psychopharmacological agents for children and adolescents with eating disorders.

For now, there may be an indication for the use of antidepressants and antipsychotics for comorbid conditions, but not for the AN itself. Finally, there is some emerging evidence for the value of hydroxyzine, an antihistamine with established anxiolytic effects and a very low side-effect profile [5].

Treatment of comorbidity

Some of the above agents are of value in the treatment of comorbid conditions such as depression (specifically the SSRIs), anxiety (anxiolytics and both first- and second-generation antipsychotics) and obsessive–compulsive disorder (SSRIs).

Relief of distress

The most common scenario is that of intense anxiety at mealtimes. In such circumstances the short-term use of anxiolytics is indicated.

With the considerably enhanced understanding of the neuroscience and particularly the neurochemistry of eating disorders (see Chapter 5), it is to be hoped that novel and more effective treatments will be developed.

10.3   The educational context

Our increasing understanding of consistent neuropsychological profiles associated with eating disorders (see Chapter 4) has important implications for our patients' experiences in school. Problems with visuospatial memory, central coherence and executive functioning are likely either to impair performance or to impose additional strain on young people who typically have perfectionist tendencies. However, such subtle difficulties are unlikely to be recognised without formal cognitive assessment, especially given the hard-working and conscientious approach many young people with eating disorders typically adopt towards schoolwork. Consequently, such patients often experience covert stress, additional to the overall burden, which in turn is likely to contribute to the maintenance of their illness.

Awareness of these cognitive styles and their effects can be shared with patients, relatives and teachers and be used to assist with academic work. In the first instance, it may be helpful for parents and teachers to help the young person reduce their self-imposed high academic standards and to devote their energy to fighting back against their eating disorder. In some cases, the adults may need to take academic decisions on behalf of the young person, who is too unwell to make their own choices: perhaps to delay examination entry or to repeat a school year once physical and psychological recovery are underway.

As well as reducing the overall demands of the academic environment, awareness of each patient's unique profile of cognitive strengths and weaknesses can be used to design individualised learning-support programmes to help remediate specific difficulties in visual memory, planning and organisation. Such school-based approaches to individual learning support share a common heritage with the clinical application of such remedial strategies in eating disorders: that is, CRT.

10.4 Psychological treatment

From brain lesions to eating disorders: the remediating power of cognitive training

The literal meaning of the term 'remediation' is the act or process of correcting a fault or deficiency. Cognitive remediation is a relatively new form of therapy within eating disorders, focused on correcting, or *remediating*, cognitive deficits or impairments. The technique was originally conceptualised and developed as an intervention for patients with brain lesions during the Second World War. Led by the Russian neuropsychologist Luria [6], a team of researchers made significant advances in the field of brain surgery and in the restoration of brain functions after trauma. In the search for ways to compensate psychological dysfunction in patients suffering from brain lesions, it was noted that the implementation of simple cognitive and behavioural exercises could rehabilitate neuropsychological deficits in specific brain regions. It was also noted that surrounding brain regions were affected, resulting in improvements in compensatory functions.

The pioneering work of Luria laid the groundwork for the development of CRT during the second half of the twentieth century. During the course of the last 50 years, the use of cognitive enhancement exercises has been gradually adapted, and today the term CRT is being used as an umbrella expression covering a wide variety of tasks and exercises related to cognitive training. Within it we find a number of different interventions based on the original concept of the reorganisation of neural networks, also referred to as *neuroplasticity*.

Neuroplasticity is the brain's ability to change, and although most apparent during the early developmental stages of the brain, it occurs throughout an individual's lifespan. Plasticity, that is neural changes, allows the brain to be continually responsive to environmental changes and to adapt accordingly. Such changes and adaptations are the core features of CRT, hypothesised to work by strengthening and refining already existing neural circuits, but also by creating new neural connections in the brain [7, 8]. CRT is believed to work both by boosting and altering active cognitive processes, and by 'jump-starting' dormant cognitive skills and capacities, thus allowing new thinking styles and strategies to emerge. Why these processes may be essential to the sustained recovery from eating disorders, and especially from AN, will be discussed below.

CRT for AN has developed out of a tradition of neuropsychological assessment and has been adapted to remedy the maladaptive thinking styles often associated with the illness. On the basis of neuropsychological evidence and clinical observations, functional deficits in a wide range of cognitive domains have been revealed in patients suffering from AN [9, 10]. While some of these deficits revert to normal with weight restoration, others seem to persist. Amongst these, executive-function deficits such as *set-shifting difficulties* [11, 12], *weak central coherence* [13] and *visuospatial impairments* [14, 15] are the most commonly reported, and appear to be the least likely to resolve after refeeding.

Set-shifting, central coherence and visuospatial processes have all been dealt with in Chapter 4. However, their relevance to CRT is of the utmost importance, and hence they will be briefly revisited below.

Impaired set-shifting (sometime referred to as poor cognitive flexibility) refers to difficulties with shifting or changing mental strategies and rules according to changing demands of the environment. This inflexibility can manifest as an inability to adapt to changing circumstances and in difficulty in overriding well-learned cognitive and behavioural patterns. In patients with AN, deficits in this particular domain lead to concrete and rigid approaches to problem solving, and to the perseverance of maladaptive thinking and behavioural patterns.

Central coherence refers to the processing of information in terms of the whole gestalt – the big picture – as well as the fine detail. Many patients with AN have a tendency to focus only on the fine detail at the cost of the big picture [16, 17]. This tendency can be seen both as a weakness in global information processing, but also as a strength in detail-focused processing. However, in AN, the balance between global and local information processing is disrupted, resulting in an excessive preoccupation with detail, order and symmetry. This detail-focused approach is reflected in the excessive attention paid to the finest details of weight, shape, calorie and fat content.

The *visuospatial domain* refers to object recognition (What is it?), spatial location (Where is it?) and visual memory (What did it look like?). Several studies have yielded evidence of persistently impaired visual memory as well as deficits in spatial processing in patients with AN [10]. Difficulties in this domain can help explain yet another characteristic feature of AN, the distortion of body image. This inaccurate internal representation of body may be explained in part by the weakness in spatial processing and visual memory.

These cognitive deficits, if not addressed, may contribute to the difficulty in treating AN and its poor prognosis. CRT is a promising intervention aimed at improving these characteristic neuropsychological deficits and associated cognitive styles.

The principles of CRT

CRT is an interactive treatment which addresses the *process* of thinking rather than the *content*, thus helping patients develop a metacognitive awareness of their own thinking style. The aim is to identify and target the cognitive impairments specific to each patient, and to motivate the patient to engage in metacognitive processes; that is, to consider their cognitive/thinking styles and to explore alternative strategies, which in turn might lead to behavioural changes. By becoming aware of problematic cognitive styles, the patient can reflect on how these affect everyday life and learn to develop new strategies. These are then practised in treatment and related to everyday life.

During CRT sessions, no effort is made to discuss or explore emotionally charged themes such as food, weight and calories. Should patients raise such issues, they are explored within the context of the cognitive styles. In this way, CRT differs from most other forms of therapy for AN. However, it is in no way thought to replace any of the existing treatments, but rather to complement them.

How is CRT delivered?

CRT has mainly been delivered to patients with AN, rather than other eating disorders, and usually through individually based therapy sessions. The therapy structure has largely been developed for adults with AN [18] and full details can be found in the manual by Tchanturia and Davies [19]. This consists of a wide variety of exercises, mainly focusing on set-shifting and central coherence, and provides the therapist with the theoretical rationale for delivering CRT (i.e. the empirical neuroscientific background) and guidelines regarding task administration. The manual proposes 10 once- or twice-weekly sessions, each lasting approximately 30–40 minutes. During these sessions, the goal is to (i) identify the patient's cognitive style(s) and acknowledge the strengths and weaknesses of these during information processing, (ii) challenge ineffective thinking patterns and explore new ways of thinking, (iii) promote thinking about thinking (i.e. metacognition) and (iv) implement small behavioural changes as a result of all of the above.

Given the relative novelty of CRT for AN, its content and method of delivery is still evolving. Lately, a number of eating-disorder services in the UK have experimented with group-based [19, 20] and family-based CRT [21]. Three modes of delivery (individual, group and family) seem applicable and each appears to have its own advantages. Individually delivered CRT allows for in-depth exploration of each participant's cognitive styles and difficulties. Group-based delivery encourages peer-group support, enhances the morale of the whole group and appears to be both time- and resource-efficient. Family-based delivery helps parents to understand better their child's difficulties and also draws attention to the fact that parents commonly share the same characteristic thinking styles.

Given CRT was originally developed for adults and tends to use adult-oriented materials, it has become necessary to develop more age-appropriate materials for children and adolescents. Toys, games and puzzles all seem to be well received by this younger population.

Clinicians can adopt various approaches when deciding which domain(s) to focus upon. The first approach, which for many might appear the most logical, is to select tasks and puzzles on the basis of neuropsychological test results (e.g. from the Ravello Profile). By doing so, the CRT exercise programme will be individually tailored, evidence-based and address the core features of the patient's cognitive style. However, clinicians might also experience patients to be, for example, extremely rigid despite scoring in the normal range on tests assessing flexibility and set-shifting. Thus, another approach assesses neurocognitive abilities *clinically* during the course of CRT. For now, these two approaches can work as guiding principles, leaving the therapist flexible in choice of methods.

Increasing cognitive flexibility

Set-shifting, or cognitive flexibility, is one of the most important executive functions, and allows people to shift back and forth between different information units, or 'mental sets'. Generally, those who are good at flexible thinking are also good at multitasking, and are able continuously to alter their thoughts and behaviours according to shifting environmental demands. For many patients with AN, being flexible is often considered somewhat challenging, and it also represents quite the opposite of the usual thinking style associated with the illness. Thus, during the initial stage of CRT, it is important to establish whether the patient is able successfully to shift between different mental categories, rules and behaviours, and if not, how this affects their everyday lives.

In essence, the patient is presented with a set of tasks or games, and is asked to follow the therapist's instructions in solving them. If the patient experiences difficulties in solving these, the therapist and patient together try to figure out *why* the task is difficult to solve, *how* it might be solved in a different or more efficient way, and what the pros and cons of the different strategies may be for the task and for everyday functioning. Two tasks focusing on cognitive flexibility – Token Tower and Up & Down – are presented below. These two tasks were originally presented in the CRT manual by Tchanturia and Davies [19]. Here, these and other tasks have been modified to suit a younger patient population.

Token tower

The aim of this task is to construct a tower consisting of building 'blocks' represented by tokens of various shapes, sizes and colours (Figure 10.1). The purpose of the exercise is to practise shifts (set-shifting) while building the tower.

Commonly, the therapist lays the first token, using a 'hidden' rule (based on either the colour of the token, its size or its shape, or a combination of these). The patient then has to figure out what rule is being used, and follow it until it changes (i.e. the therapist changes the routine of building the tower). As with all CRT exercises, the aim is not to obtain immaculate task performance, but to identify the process for tackling the task. The Token Tower is a simple and playful game where turn-taking, set-shifting and multitasking abilities are established, practised and reflected upon. This game is designed to prevent elicitation of anxiety commonly associated with the desire of performing flawlessly, and is delivered in a fashion making it more play-like and amusing than serious. As with all other games and puzzles focusing on increasing cognitive flexibility, the aim is to identify *how* the patient goes about solving these tasks, and whether the process is efficient. If it is not, discussions and metareflection are used to figure out *why* the task was difficult to solve, *how* it might be solved in a different or more efficient way, and how different ways of thinking can have different effects on everyday life.

Figure 10.1   Token tower (in real life, the various figures are coloured).

Up & down

The aim of this task is for the patient to practise set-shifting following two different arrow directions (up or down). The patient is presented with the picture in Figure 10.2 and is asked to follow these instructions:

> *The picture shows a monkey climbing up and down a palm tree. I want you to tell me how he climbs (up or down) by starting counting in the upper-left corner. Start with 1, and keep on counting upwards until you encounter an arrow. When you encounter an arrow, instead of keeping counting, state the direction in which the arrow points (up or down). When you have done this, the direction of the arrow will inform you whether you should continue counting upwards (arrow pointing up), or if you should shift, starting to count downwards (arrow pointing down). The arrows at the right and left of the ladders indicate where to continue at the end of a row.*

In the picture presented above, the correct sequence would be: 1, 2, 3, *down*, 2, 1, *up*, 2, 3, 4, 5, *down*, 4, 3, 2, 1, *up*, 2, 3, *down*, 2, 1, 0, *up*, 1, 2, 3, 4, *down*, 3, *up*, 4. As in the Token Tower task, completion of this task is followed by discussion and reflection regarding the process by which the patient tackled the task.

Boosting global information processing

The ability to process information globally enables people to perceive themselves and their surroundings as whole, rather than separate or detached units. Further, this ability also allows for interpretation of details contextually, and gives a fuller understanding of the integration of and relationship between them. Neurocognitive studies exploring central coherence in patients with AN have yielded evidence of a decreased ability to

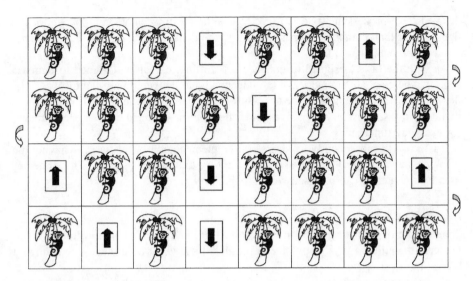

Figure 10.2 Up & down.

'see the wood for the trees'. This expression indicates the inability to interpret stimuli in a gestalt manner, and describes excessive focus on details in perceptual processes, when interpreting internal and external stimuli and when guiding thoughts, feelings and behaviours. Three exercises designed to practise 'seeing the bigger picture' – Geometric Figures, Optical Illusions and Summarising – are presented below. As with the two set-shifting tasks, the original versions of these central coherence tasks are to be found in the CRT manual by Tchanturia and Davies [19]. Here, new versions of the original tasks are presented.

Geometric figures

The patient is presented with a collection of different geometric figures (Figure 10.3) and is asked to choose one of them, unseen by the therapist. The patient is then asked to describe the figure to the therapist, whose job is to draw a picture guided by the patient's words. The patient cannot see what the therapist is drawing and the therapist is not allowed to ask any questions. Patient and therapist then compare their images, and explore the strategies used to describe the figure. Commonly in AN, a

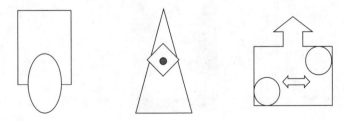

Figure 10.3 The geometric figures task.

detailed local-processing style is used, concentrating on separate components of the figure rather than combining separate entities and depicting full figures (e.g. a square, an oval, a rectangle, etc.).

As with the tasks designed to enhance set-shifting, exercises designed to increase central coherence are simple, easy to understand and delivered in a playful way. The therapist and patient together try to identify the cognitive style used to tackle these particular tasks, consider alternatives and reflect on the pros and cons of each strategy for everyday functioning.

It is possible subsequently to reverse the implementation of this task by having the therapist deliver the description and the patient try to draw the diagram. The strategies used by the patient can be discussed in a similar way.

Optical illusions

An example of an optical illusion is presented in Figure 10.4. This illustration could be depicting either a vase or two facial profiles 'looking' at each other, depending on where one focuses.

Illusions are powerful tools for identifying detailed versus holistic information processing, and are usually used by the therapist to gain information regarding a specific thinking style related to the eating disorder. Commonly, the therapist starts by asking the patient to describe what they see at a first glance. If the patient sees only one aspect of the picture, this particular way of processing visual information is discussed and reflected upon. The patient is then encouraged to study the picture again, and to explore whether there are additional objects, figures or details 'hiding' in the picture. In doing so, the patient explores alternative strategies when solving the task, and these alternative strategies are then explored and related to everyday life coping strategies.

Summarising

In this task, the patient is asked to read a document or story and to summarise it. Usually, the therapist starts off by asking the patient to use their own words when summarising the text. As the patient becomes more comfortable with the process of summarising, the difficulty of the tasks increases, and the therapist might ask the patient to summarise in, for example, five sentences, five bullet points or a text message using no more than a few words. An example of such a story is the tale of the 'Twelve Dancing Princesses'.

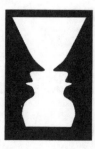

Figure 10.4   Optical illusion.

The Twelve Dancing Princesses

Once there lived a King, who had twelve beautiful daughters. They all lived together in a big palace. The kingdom was at peace, and everyone in the palace lived happily together. There was just one strange thing. Every morning when the twelve princesses came downstairs to breakfast they looked exhausted, as if they had hardly slept at all, and their new silk shoes were completely worn out, as if they had danced all night.

The King could not understand how this could be. Their bedroom had no windows, and he personally locked the only door every night. The King simply had to find out what was happening. So he sent out a message to every corner of his kingdom. Anyone in the whole kingdom could come to the palace for three days and three nights. Whoever could solve the mystery could marry whichever princess he chose, and would reign as the next King. But if they failed, they would be put to death.

The first person to try was the tall and handsome Count of Brel. For three days and three nights he kept watch on the princesses, following them every day and watching over them every night. But on each morning, the princesses' shoes were completely worn out and he had no idea why. People came from far and wide to try to solve the puzzle. But all failed, and all were put to death.

As with other tasks, strategies are explored and discussed and are related to everyday life.

Enhancing visuospatial abilities

CRT tasks focusing on visuospatial abilities aim at improving the patient's ability to recognise different objects (object recognition) and to remember what objects look like (visual memory) and where they were situated (spatial location). Impairments in this domain in AN are common and may affect body image. Hence, practicing or enhancing visuospatial abilities during CRT sessions might alter or change an erroneous body image. Two tasks focusing on visuospatial processes and memory – The Grid and Finding Your Way – are presented below.

The grid

In this task, the patient is asked to look at, and memorise, various objects or figures presented in a grid (Figure 10.5). The patient is given a preset amount of time (depending on the task's level of difficulty) to memorise what is seen, and is then presented with an empty grid in which to fill in the recalled figures. As with all CRT tasks, the golden rule is to start with an easy task, and gradually to increase the level of difficulty. When patients struggle, the strategy being used is discussed and alternatives are explored. The pros and cons of each strategy are then considered in relation to everyday life.

Finding your way

In this visuospatial task, the patient is asked to find the way from one end of a 'maze' to the other, and while doing so, to keep count of the left and right turns (Figure 10.6). The task would be presented as follows:

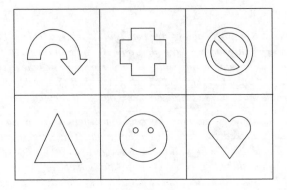

Figure 10.5 The grid.

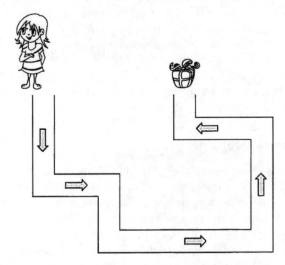

Figure 10.6 Finding your way.

> *The girl in the picture is waiting to receive her birthday present. Can you see the girl and the gift? All right, imagine you're the girl, and to receive the present, you have to find your way through this maze. On your way to the gift, please try to remember how many left and right turns you make. Do you understand the task? Ok, let's begin!*

After having completed the task, discussion and reflection follows regarding the process by which the patient tackled the task. The choice of strategy, its pros and cons, and how one might relate this way of handling a task to everyday life are also elaborated upon.

The metacognitive process: how did I tackle the task?

The construct of neuroplasticity provides a theoretical rationale for encouraging a 'metacognitive' perspective in CRT. It is believed that by reflecting on one's cognitive styles, noting ineffective strategies and learning new ones, existing neural circuits are strengthened and new ones are created. Thus the essence of CRT involves exploring the strategies used to tackle a task, considering possible alternatives and reflecting on the pros and cons of everyday life. It is not whether the task was successfully completed that matters most but *how* it was attempted. The metacognitive component in CRT is encouraged throughout the entire treatment process, and is designed to help patients explore their cognitive styles and where necessary to enhance them. Having understood *how* one's own thinking styles operate and how these might influence various aspect of daily life, it then becomes possible to explore the potential for change.

To help the patient engage in the metacognitive process during CRT, all tasks are accompanied and followed by questions encouraging thinking about one's own thinking. Small variations of a predetermined set of questions can be used throughout the CRT programme, allowing for fruitful reflections and discussion. A few of the most commonly used questions are given in Table 10.1.

Homework

An important part of CRT is to explore how the knowledge acquired in therapy can be transferred to real-life settings. To enable this, small homework tasks can be introduced once the patient seems ready. The aim is for the patient to use the knowledge acquired during CRT sessions and to experiment with this knowledge outside the therapy context. The tasks are fairly simple and relate to everyday routines, which are easy to alter and reflect upon. The exercises are not supposed to elicit strong emotional reactions, and are usually not related to the explicit features of the illness (e.g. food, calories, weight, body). These small experiments are designed to help the

Table 10.1 Questions designed to encourage metacognitive reflections.

---

1. What did you think of this task/puzzle/game?
    Was it easy or difficult?
    In what way was it easy/difficult?
    Did you like it/dislike it?
2. How did you go about trying to solve it?
    Did you use any particular strategy/technique/trick?
    How did that particular strategy/technique/trick work for you?
    Could you have completed it in a different way?
    What would have been different if you had chosen a different strategy/technique/trick?
    If you had been given the same task again, how would you have tackled it?
3. Did you learn anything about your own thinking style while tackling the task/puzzle/game?
    If yes, what did you learn?
4. Would you say that this particular thinking style is one that you use in other areas of your
    life as well (outside therapy sessions)?
    Can you give me an example of an event or a situation where you might use the same
        'thinking style' or the same strategy/technique/trick in your day-to-day life?
    What usually happens when you use that strategy/technique/trick in your daily life?
    Could you approach challenges/tasks/chores differently in your daily life?
    What do you think would happen if you did?
    What do you think are the pros and cons of each strategy/technique/trick?

Table 10.2   Examples of homework.

When you get dressed, put on your clothes in a different order than usual.
Try describing the route from home to school/work/the store/your favourite café to someone else.
Create a new playlist on your iPod (or other music device), and listen to this instead of your old one.
Choose another route when visiting a friend or going to school or work.
Brush your teeth with your nondominant hand.
Try writing a birthday invitation to a friend in no more than a few words.
Change the background picture on your mobile phone or computer.
Go to/rent a movie that you usually would not have chosen to see.
Take a different route to school/work/a friend, and show someone else how you got there on a map.
Read a newspaper or magazine starting from the back instead of the front.
Change the colour of your nail polish/lipstick/rouge.
Wear your watch on the other wrist for a day.
Try remembering what you wore one/two/three days ago, and describe your outfit to someone else.
Watch a movie and describe the plot to a friend or a family member using no more than five sentences.
Collect leaves/flowers/shells/pictures and make a collage.
Describe yourself by first writing a short text about yourself, then shorten it down to a few sentences, and finally, summarise the text in a few words.

patient to explore alternative strategies and implement those that seem helpful. A few examples of behavioural tasks are listed in Table 10.2. The tasks are focused on either set-shifting, central coherence or visuospatial abilities. The selection of tasks is best based on the therapist's clinical judgement, and should address issues related to the particular patient's cognitive style or difficulties.

The effect of CRT and future directions

Although CRT for AN is a fairly new intervention, preliminary evidence regarding the efficacy of the treatment is encouraging. Results have shown improved cognitive performance and reduction of eating-disorder psychopathology [12, 22] and support the use of CRT as an additional treatment component for patients suffering from AN. Qualitative feedback through 'goodbye letters' has also shown that patients value the intervention, improve their metacognitive skills and are successful in making behavioural changes in their everyday life as a result of their newly acquired skills [23]. These findings refer to studies focusing on the effect of CRT for adults, and there are no reported studies using CRT with children and adolescents with eating disorders. Also, the administration of CRT has largely been based on the manual developed for adults by Tchanturia and Davies [19]. When treating a younger population, age-appropriate materials are required. Consequently, we have recently developed a CRT resource pack for children and adolescents [24].

Early clinical impressions are encouraging, but randomised controlled studies will be needed to allow conclusions to be drawn regarding the efficacy of the treatment, whether for adults or the younger population. It will also be of interest to compare efficacy between modes of delivery: individual, group and family. Outcome measures should include neuropsychological test performance (using a standardised test battery such as the Ravello Profile [25]), eating-disorder psychopathology, physical parameters and evidence of comorbidity.

10.5 Conclusion

The poor prognosis for so many patients with eating disorders may to some extent be explained by the failure to address the underlying neurobiological contribution to their pathogenesis and maintenance. Recent advances in our understanding of the neuroscience basis of eating disorders could have significant clinical implications. In this chapter we have focused on three areas: psychopharmacology, the educational context and psychological treatment. Psychopharmacological agents have limited value but as we learn more about the neurotransmitter disturbances it is likely that more effective medications will be developed. The neurocognitive deficits that are commonly identified have implications in the educational setting. Awareness of and attention to such weaknesses could have beneficial effects on anxiety, educational performance and self-esteem, each of which could in turn improve psychological well-being. CRT shows considerable promise as a novel, theoretically sound, easily applicable and user-friendly approach.

References

1. Claudino, A.M., Silva de Lima, M., Hay, P.J. *et al.* (2006) Antidepressants for anorexia nervosa. *Cochrane Database of Systematic Reviews*, (1), (Article No.CD004365), doi: 10.1002/14651858.CD004365pub2
2. Broft, A., Berner, L.A. and Walsh, T.B. (2010) Pharmacotherapy for Bulimia Nervosa, in *The Treatment of Eating Disorders: A Clinical Handbook* (eds C.M. Grilo and J.E. Mitchell), The Guilford Press, New York, pp. 388–413.
3. Grilo, C.M., Masheb, R.M. and Wilson, G.T. (2005) Efficacy of cognitive behavioural therapy and fluoxetine for the treatment of binge eating disorders: a randomized double-blind, placebo-controlled trial. *Biological Psychiatry*, **57**, 301–309.
4. Reas, D.L. and Grilo, C.M. (2008) Review and meta-analysis of pharmacotherapy for binge eating disorders. *Obesity*, **16**, 2024.
5. Lesser, J., Mangham, D., Gorius, J. and Jahraus, J. (2010) Hydroxyzine in eating disorders: a new use for an old medication. Paper presented at the Academy for Eating Disorders Annual Meeting 2010.
6. Luria, A.R. (1972) *The Man with a Shattered World: The History of a Brain Wound*, Harvard University Press, Cambridge, MA.
7. Demily, C. and Franck, N. (2008) Cognitive remediation: a promising tool for the treatment of schizophrenia. *Expert Review of Neurotherapeutics*, **8** (7), 1029–1036.
8. McGurk, S.R., Twamley, E.W., Sitzer, D.I. *et al.* (2007) A meta-analysis of cognitive remediation in schizophrenia. *American Journal of Psychiatry*, **164** (12), 1791–1802.
9. Frampton, I. and Hutchinson, A. (2007) Eating disorders and the brain, in *Eating Disorders in Childhood and Adolescence*, 3rd edn (eds B. Lask and R. Bryant-Waugh), Routledge Press, pp. 125–147.
10. Brewerton, T.D., Frampton, I. and Lask B. (2009) The neurobiology of anorexia nervosa. *US Psychiatry, Touch Briefings*, **2** (1), 57–60.

11. Roberts, M.E., Tchanturia, K., Stahl, D. *et al.* (2007) A systematic review and meta-analysis of set-shifting ability in eating disorders. *Psychological Medicine*, **37** (8), 1075–1084.

12. Tchanturia, K., Davies, H. and Campbell, I.C. (2007) Cognitive remediation therapy for patients with anorexia nervosa: preliminary findings. *Annals of General Psychiatry*, **6**, 14.

13. Lopez, C., Tchanturia, K., Stahl, D. and Treasure, J. (2008) Central coherence in eating disorders: a systematic review. *Psychological Medicine*, **38** (10), 1393–1404.

14. Lask, B., Gordon, I., Christie, D. *et al.* (2005) Functional neuroimaging in early-onset anorexia nervosa. *The International Journal of Eating Disorders*, **37**, S49–S51.

15. Lena, S.M., Fiocco, A.J. and Leyenaar, J.K. (2004) The role of cognitive deficits in the development of eating disorders. *Neuropsychology Review*, **14** (2), 99–113.

16. Gillberg, I.C., Gillberg, C., Rastam, M. and Johansson, M. (1996) The cognitive profile of anorexia nervosa: a comparative study including a community-based sample. *Comprehensive Psychiatry*, **37** (1), 23–30.

17. Lopez, C., Tchanturia, K., Stahl, D. *et al.* (2008) An examination of the concept of central coherence in women with anorexia nervosa. *The International Journal of Eating Disorders*, **41** (2), 143–152.

18. Tchanturia, K. and Hambrook, D. (2010) Cognitive remediation therapy for anorexia nervosa, in *The Treatment of Eating Disorders: A Clinical Handbook*, 1st edn (eds C.M. Grilo and J.E. Mitchell), New York, The Guilford Press, pp. 130–149.

19. Tchanturia, K., Davies, H., Reeder, C., and Wykes, T. (2010) *Cognitive Remediation Therapy for Anorexia Nervosa*. Unpublished work.

20. Wood, L., Al-Khairulla, H. and Lask B. (2010) Group-based cognitive remediation therapy for children and adolescents with anorexia nervosa. *Clinical Child Psychology and Psychiatry*. **16** (2), in press.

21. Lask, B. and Owen I. (2010) Family-based cognitive remediation therapy with children and adolescents with anorexia nervosa, in preparation.

22. Pretorius, N. and Tchanturia, K. (2007) Anorexia nervosa: how people think and how we address it in cognitive remediation therapy. *Therapy*, **4** (4), 423–433.

23. Whitney, J., Easter, A. and Tchanturia, K. (2008) Service users' feedback on cognitive training in the treatment of Anorexia Nervosa. *The International Journal of Eating Disorders*, **6** (41), 542–550.

24. Owen, I., Lindvall, C. and Lask, B. (2011) Cognitive Remediation (CRT) for Children and Adolescents: The CRT Resource Pack. www.ellernmede.org, www.rasp.no.

25. Rose, M., Davis, J., Frampton, I. and Lask, B. (2011) The Ravello Profile: development of a global standard neuropsychological assessment for young people with anorexia nervosa. *Clinical Child Psychology and Psychiatry*, **16** (2), in press.

11 Future directions

Ian Frampton[1] and Bryan Lask[2, 3, 4]

[1]*College of Life and Environmental Sciences, University of Exeter, UK*
[2]*Regional Eating Disorder Service, Oslo University Hospital, Oslo Norway*
[3]*Ellern Mede Service for Eating Disorders, London, UK*
[4]*Great Ormond Street Hospital for Children, London, UK*

11.1 Introduction

As we noted in the Introduction, the very fact that an entire book can now be devoted to the neuroscience of eating disorders is by itself an indication of how far the field has progressed. To some extent, an increasing focus on the potential neurobiological basis for eating disorders reflects a more general trend in psychiatry and psychology research and practice. The 'decade of the brain' has helped to make neuroscience more accessible to the wider public and fuelled increased media interest in this area.

On the other hand, an increased focus on the role of the brain in psychiatric disorders also points back to the historical origins of neuropsychiatry and neurophysiology. With the advent of neuroimaging technologies that Helmholtz, James and other pioneers of neuropsychology could only have dreamed of, we are now in a position to understand the neurobiological basis of mental life as never before.

These new technologies and increased understanding about the neurobiological bases of psychological processes give us a unique opportunity to construct a more complete neuroscientific account of eating disorders. This description should be able to tell us something about the underlying cause, assessment and diagnosis, treatment, prevention and future research priorities for eating disorders.

11.2 Cause

Watkins notes in Chapter 2 that searching for a single cause for eating disorders is a fruitless task. As she suggests, eating disorders are a complex, multifactorial 'final common pathway' of interacting biological, psychological and sociocultural risk factors. While a neuroscience-based account may not be able to add much to the last of these (although as Singh and Wengaard point out in Chapter 9, even here a neuroscience perspective can add something), it can clearly add to our understanding of the biological and psychological risk factors.

For the biological factors, Nunn (Chapter 5) begins with typical erudition from the premise that 'we and the universe are a single fabric', by which he hopes to remind us that we are made entirely of molecules taken in from the world around us as food. In his noradrenergic hypothesis, he suggests that an underlying genetically determined error in noradrenalin production in the brain could be the fundamental cause of anorexia nervosa (AN). Alternative causal hypotheses have been developed through the use of positron emission tomography (PET) neuroimaging techniques that have implicated the neurotransmitters serotonin and dopamine, both in the acute illness and as underlying trait risk factors. As neuroimaging techniques continue to develop and our understanding of the interplay between genes and neurotransmitters improves, neuroscience will have an increasing prominence in causal theories of all psychiatric disorders, including restricting, binge–purging and overweight disorders of eating.

In any case, as Rose and Frampton point out (Chapter 7), any competent theoretical model of eating disorders (neuroscientific or otherwise) will need to account for their developmental nature. They propose that the more comprehensive models have incorporated an account of how genetic and environmental factors in early brain development confer predisposing risk factors that interact with later psychological and social precipitating factors. In all these models, neurobiological changes associated with puberty seem to play a central role, helping to account for the natural history and epidemiology of eating disorders that emerge predominantly in the second decade of life.

A neuroscience perspective may also lead us to reframe psychological causal factors at a neurobiological level. There is a risk here that *everything psychological becomes biological*, something that Wood (Chapter 1) cautions in his thoughtful and thought-provoking contribution. Nevertheless, many of the precipitating psychological risk factors that Watkins (Chapter 2) identifies – attachment and interpersonal relationships, body dissatisfaction, dieting reward – can themselves be restated as neurobiological factors. For example, as Øverås suggests (Chapter 6), the beguiling pathognomic feature of body-image disturbance that contributes to body dissatisfaction may itself be the result of underlying impairments in neuropsychological processes of perception and memory for the body.

Causal neuroscience accounts should also be able to say something about the specific comorbidities we see in patients. Why is it that some comorbidities are common (obsessive–compulsive disorder (OCD), depression), whereas others are extremely rare (schizophrenia, dementias)? Hopefully neuroscience will help us to understand more about what these disorders have in common to account for why they tend to occur together.

11.3   Assessment and diagnosis

There is a broad consensus that the current diagnostic systems for eating disorders are in a mess: Fairburn [1] points out that any diagnostic system resulting in most patients fitting the residual category (eating disorders not otherwise specified, EDNOS) is in trouble; Nicholls *et al.* [2] remind us that childhood-onset eating disorders and the developmental factors that underlie them are poorly served by current, adult-oriented thinking. In recent years a great deal of effort has been devoted to reforming eating-disorder diagnoses for the upcoming Diagnostic and Statistical Manual 5 (DSM-5) for both adult and child patients [3–5].

However, we suggest that these proposed reforms, while having the virtue of retaining continuity with the current diagnostic systems (and hence supporting continuity in basic science and treatment-related research), do not go far enough in taking account of the current level of neuroscientific understanding reviewed by the contributors to this book. Building future diagnostic systems on existing descriptors constrains us forever to base the clinical identification of eating disorders on an archaic taxonomic system that groups psychiatric illnesses according to their observable *surface characteristics* (such as weight, number of purging events per week, and self-report of thoughts, feelings and behaviours). However, the neuroscience of eating disorders now enables us to define underlying biomarkers that are potentially identifiable before the illness becomes manifest. Potential candidates include the trait neuropsychological endophe-notypes, described by Steinglass and Glasofer (Chapter 4), and the neurotransmitter abnormalities and specific patterns of neurocognitive functioning identified through neuroimaging studies reviewed by Fuglset and Frampton (Chapter 3).

In collaboration with the eating-disorders research community, we have recently developed a common global neuropsychological assessment battery, the Ravello Pro-file [6] (www.ravelloprofile.org). We hope that this easy-to-obtain and -administer package of neuropsychological tests will promote collaborative research and support neuroscientifically informed clinical practice in eating disorders. In this endeavour, we very obviously 'stand on the shoulder of giants' who have gone before us and have contributed to our current understanding of neuropsychological factors in AN and bulimia nervosa (BN).

Basing future diagnostic systems on the assessment of neuropsychological and neu-robiological functioning would, as Singh and Wengaard point out (Chapter 9), have a profound effect on the way we understand and treat eating disorders. Such a paradigm shift would in their view also radically alter the way that patients and their fami-lies themselves understand, attribute and respond to eating disorders. The risk here is that such seductive *neuroessentialist* accounts reduce the unique complexity of each individual's experience of an eating disorder to the simplistic 'blobology' of a brain image taken by a scanner. On the other hand, as the authors point out, there may well be significant benefits from 'brain-based' explanations of eating disorders, such as relieving guilt and blame. Interdisciplinary research involving eating-disorder special-ists, neuroscientists, psychiatric geneticists, social scientists and ethicists is urgently needed to explore the complex issues raised by the neuroscience.

In any event, neuroscience-based assessment and diagnosis has been promoted by the US National Institute of Mental Health in its Research Domain Criteria (RDoC) Project [7], launched in 2010. This project begins from the premise that: '. . . in ante-dating contemporary neuroscience research, the current [DSM] diagnostic system is not informed by recent breakthroughs in genetics and molecular, cellular and systems neuroscience'. The project has defined a matrix of five major *domains of function-ing* (negative affect, positive affect, cognition, social behaviour and arousal/regulatory systems) that can be studied in six *classes* (genes, molecules, cells, neural circuits, behaviours and self-reports).

The RDoC Project acknowledges that to date the science is not yet well enough developed to permit neuroscience-based classification. However, the authors suggest that it is necessary to start to develop such approaches if the field is ever to reach the point where advances in genomics, pathophysiology and neuroscience can inform diagnosis in a meaningful way. They hope that the RDoC Project represents the beginning of such a long-term ambition.

For eating disorders, collaborative initiatives such as the Ravello Profile could make a valuable contribution to future systems of assessment and diagnosis from this perspective. Such reform could lead to a totally new way of classifying eating disorders on the basis of common patterns of underlying biomarkers rather than the current conventional distinction between AN and BN. It may also result in the *fractionation* of current diagnostic entities. For example, preliminary analysis of Ravello Profile data of more than 300 patients with a clinical diagnosis of AN suggests that from a neuropsychological perspective, three distinct clusters of patients of approximately equal size can be determined with common profiles of neuropsychological strengths and weaknesses [8].

11.4 Treatment

The treatment implications of such diagnostic reform are obvious. For example, the cognitive remediation therapy (CRT) approaches reviewed by Lindwall and Lask (Chapter 10) could be targeted for patients with specific neuropsychological profiles. Based on the pioneering work of Tchanturia and her colleagues at the Institute of Psychiatry, University of London [9], this approach initially developed for patients with schizophrenia has recently been successfully adapted for use in eating-disorder treatment.

Beyond this specific treatment example, Rose and Frampton (Chapter 7) point out that any adequate neuroscientific model of eating disorders must define potential treatment implications. In the series of models they review, suggestions are made for novel pharmacological and psychological treatments. To date, pharmacological treatments for AN have proved to be strikingly ineffective, which could serve to undermine the argument for a neuroscience approach in the first place: if eating disorders truly have a neurobiological basis, presumably they should be amenable to pharmacotherapy? In response, it is worth pointing out that to date, the medications that have been used clinically 'off licence' and tested in clinical trials are drugs that were developed for other conditions such as depression or anxiety, rather than specifically for eating disorders.

As Fuglset and Frampton note (Chapter 3), PET imaging evidence of reduced serotonin activity in the synapse in patients with acute AN accounts for the ineffectiveness of specific serotonin reuptake inhibitor (SSRI) medication. Since there is already a reduced activity and depleted supply in the synapse as a result of malnutrition, preventing the presynaptic reuptake of serotonin will not help. On the other hand, there is some evidence that olanzapine (and potentially other atypical antipsychotic medication) could be beneficial in low doses. In the longer term, new drugs will need to be designed on the basis of pharmacokinetic models that have yet to be specified.

Of the current models, the insula hypothesis of Nunn and colleagues [10, 11] predicts that vasodilatory agents that improve regional blood flow in the brain could be effective, although this assertion has not yet been tested. The same authors also suggest that novel drugs that act on specific neurotransmitter systems could be helpful, but their model does not specify which. There has been interest recently in the possibility that low doses of hydroxyzine (an antihistamine drug) could be useful because of its anxiety-reducing effect, and also because it has few negative side effects.

Taken together, it is probably fair to say that in the case of AN, there is still considerable scope for advances in neuroscience to contribute to the design of effective drug treatments. For BN, the picture is somewhat more positive, although the drugs that have been shown to be effective in clinical trials (primarily SSRIs) were of course not developed on the basis of a neuroscience model of the eating disorder, but rather on the venerable method in psychiatry of 'let's try it and see if it works'. Again, there is future scope here for a more sophisticated approach to designing and testing drugs on the basis of theoretical pharmacology.

Turning to psychological treatments, neuroscience may be valuable in helping to account for why to date no effective first-line approach for AN has been identified. If, as many of the neuroscience models predict, the underlying basis for the disorder is neurobiological (for example, the rate-limiting disconnection of neural networks proposed in the insula hypothesis), then intervening at a cognitive-behavioural level is unlikely to be effective. Recently developed models such as that of Hatch and colleagues [12] also predict that therapies targeted at conscious thought processes (cognitive therapy and psychotherapy) are less likely to be effective if the fundamental underlying problem lies in 'lower-level' prelinguistic emotion-processing networks.

On the other hand, the neuroscience models of eating disorders do predict alternative psychological treatments that should be effective. For example, Hatch and colleagues suggest that novel 'emotion-processing' psychological treatments will need to be developed; other modellers have recommended treatments that increase emotional intelligence. Rather more specifically, mindfulness-based treatments that specifically address awareness of the emotional state of the body are predicted to be effective by the insula hypothesis [11]. This is a promising suggestion, since it has been shown that Buddhist meditators have more grey matter than expected in their right insula, an area involved in interoceptive awareness [13].

If advances in neuroscience identify specific neural circuits that are impaired in eating disorders, it should be possible to develop targeted treatments designed to improve their functioning. For example, Caria and colleagues [14] recently demonstrated that it is possible to learn to control local brain activity with operant training by using real-time functional magnetic resonance imaging (rtfMRI)-based neurofeedback. In their study, a group of healthy participants were provided with continuously updated information about the level of activation of their right anterior insula cortex by visual feedback while in the scanner. All participants were able to successfully regulate blood oxygen level detection (BOLD)-magnitude activation in this region within three sessions of 4 minutes each. Training resulted in a significantly increased activation cluster that was specific to the region. This extraordinary study is the first to investigate the volitional control of emotionally relevant brain region by using rtfMRI training and confirms that self-regulation of local brain activity with rtfMRI is possible, with potentially profound treatment implications.

11.5   Prevention

The eating-disorders research community has been justifiably challenged for its failure to attend to prevention by focusing almost exclusively on patients who are manifestly unwell. On the other hand, it is fair to argue that techniques to identify high-risk individuals and to develop secondary-prevention approaches are difficult to develop when many of the risk factors are common (body dissatisfaction) or virtually universal (growing up in a social context that values thinness and attractiveness).

Neuroscience may add to prevention efforts by identifying reliable biomarkers conferring increased risk that can be detected prior to the development of the manifest disorder. For example, online short-form versions of the Ravello Profile could be developed as a universal screener to identify young people with the 'high-risk' cognitive style of set-shifting difficulties, extreme detail focus and poor visual memory. Genetic screening could be developed once we know more about the genetic basis of neurotransmitter abnormalities, although the help of the neuroethicists will be urgently required at that point, as recommended by Singh and Wengaard (Chapter 9).

11.6   Future directions

What does the future hold for the neuroscience of eating disorders? Clearly, as the work described in this book continues to develop, the whole field will diversify and hopefully new connections will form, leading to fresh insights and innovation, ultimately for patient benefit. At this current state of the neuroscience, it might be useful to consider future directions in each of the classes defined by the NIMH RDoC Project: genes, molecules, cells, neural circuits, behaviours and self-reports.

Genes

Since about one third of the genome is devoted to the central nervous system, we can hope that many future advances in gene science will be applicable to eating disorders. Twin studies have helped to identify to what extent genes versus environment are relevant; in the next phase of research we will need to find out more about the genetic control of early brain development in determining its structural integrity (the wiring) as well as the role of genes in neurotransmitter production and processing (the chemistry). As Nunn and colleagues note (Chapter 8), it will be helpful to pay attention to those genes responsible for programming foetal brain development (the homeobox genes, including PAX and PHOX) and how epigenetic factors such as sunlight/UV or temperature at time of conception could modify their expression, and so help us to understand the strange season-of-birth effect in eating disorders [15].

Consistent results from several studies indicate strong genetic factors in AN that may be linked to the commonly associated personality traits of obsessionality, perfectionism, anxiety and behavioural inhibition [16]. This suggests that as well as contributing to possible deficits in the wiring, genes may be involved in the higher-level expression of psychological attributes, which is worthy of further study.

Genomewide association studies (GWASs) are a powerful method for discovering genetic risk factors by investigating the whole genome rather than focusing on a restricted number of candidate genes. An international collaborative GWAS in AN is currently underway, and the findings of this study will help neuroscientists by identifying future directions for genetic research. Finally, neuroscience approaches to defining potential endophenotypes of eating disorders developed by Treasure's group at the University of London's Institute of Psychiatry, in particular the consistent neuropsychological profiles seen in patients and their first-degree relatives, will continue to be a helpful way to link underlying genetic risk factors to eating-disorder psychopathology.

Molecules

Nunn makes a compelling case in Chapter 5 that *we are what we eat*. If a disorder alters what we eat, it will also change us at a molecular level. Understanding more about the biochemistry of starvation could be a promising route towards the development of new drug treatments. He counsels against following fads in the latest 'chemical of the day or neurotransmitter in fashion' and presents an alternative model for exploring candidate neurochemicals that could be adopted by future studies.

The current PET neuroimaging technique used to track neurotransmitter activity has significant negative side effects (as described by Fuglset and Frampton in Chapter 3), including poor temporal and spatial resolution as well as the complexities involved in creating, transporting and injecting radioactive ligands; we will need to develop new approaches for researching brain chemistry. Magnetic resonance spectroscopy (MRS) has been used for more than 10 years in research in AN and BN and may have further potential to help us explore metabolic processes in the brain. Dual-energy X-ray absorptiometry (DXA) scanning may also be a more helpful way to accurately quantify body fat composition and its role in triggering other metabolic and endocrine processes, such as reproductive maturity, together with pelvic ultrasound [17], rather than the tyranny of simply weighing patients as a metric of recovery [18].

Cells

Studies of neuron function have helped us to understand how genetically determined cellular impairments at the terminal junction contribute to reduced serotonin availability. Cell-biology studies have also recently identified anatomical and functional impairment of the retina and optic nerve in patients with AN without vision loss [19], suggesting that we will need to continue to explore a wide range of central nervous system cell types to understand more fully the impact of eating disorders at the cellular level.

Circuits

Among the neuro models reviewed by Rose and Frampton (Chapter 7), three make clear predictions about candidate neural networks that are implicated in eating disorders. Kaye's model defines a ventral and dorsal neural circuit dysfunction (incorporating insula and striatum) that he relates to altered serotonin and dopamine metabolism. March and colleagues, in linking AN and BN to a broad spectrum of neurodevelopmental disorders including OCD and Tourette's syndrome, invoke the so-called cortico–striatal–palladal–thalamic (CSPT) network, which has previously been implicated in these other disorders [20]. Finally, Nunn *et al.* [10, 11] 'go out on a limb' by invoking a more widely distributed network incorporating neocortex, basal ganglia, insula and thalamus.

It is important that different models predict different neurocircuitry involvement, since this will make it possible to directly test them against each other using common functional imaging paradigms. The use of functional connectivity (FC) paradigms in fMRI will help to detect brain structures operating together by using multiple 'seeds' to identify functionally interconnected networks. Such advanced image-processing and statistical techniques are developing rapidly and will become a powerful methodology to test theoretically predicted neural networks.

As well as using such imaging technologies to identify structures that are 'firing together' in a network, we also need to demonstrate that the structures are physically connected to each other and so are 'wiring together'. The use of diffusion-tensor imaging techniques in MRI will help to test whether predicted neural networks are in reality 'cabled' together.

It is also worth pointing out that the definition of 'circuits' adopted by the RDoC Project is not confined to the neural networks described above. The guidance notes that 'circuits' can refer to measurements of particular circuits as studied by neuroimaging techniques (as above), as well as to other measures validated by animal models or functional neuroimaging (e.g. emotion-modulated startle, event-related potentials). Future research efforts in eating-disorder neuroscience could gain a lot by investigating these basic processes alongside more 'elaborate' functional imaging paradigms.

Behaviours

In the NIMH RDoC, 'behaviour' can refer to behavioural tasks (such as a working memory task) or to behavioural observations. For the former category, we really do need to agree a common core corpus of standard neuropsychological assessment tasks (as envisioned by the Ravello Profile collaboration) to facilitate collaborative research. Particularly in the case of AN, fortunately a relatively rare disorder, clinically oriented research teams working very intensively with small numbers of patients simply do not have the throughput required to generate large datasets. The AN GWAS collaboration is a shining example of how researchers can work together with well-resourced support (in their case from the Wellcome Trust). Eating-disorder neuroscience researchers will need to collaborate in submitting bids to governmental and independent funding organisations as a first step toward working together on the subsequent data collection and analyses.

Regarding the second definition of behaviour offered by the RDoC, recent promising innovations reviewed by Steinglass and Glasofer, such as *delay discounting* paradigms, offer a new direction for experimental studies of psychological processes in eating disorders. In an era of high-technology neuroimaging techniques, there is still room for elegant experimental studies bringing together methods from a broad base of science – in this case, behavioural economics.

Self-reports

In the case of AN, the most striking self-report from patients is their willingness to describe their body-image disturbance. Øverås presents a very clear model for how neuroscience approaches can be used to deconstruct and explore these phenomenological accounts (Chapter 6). In her analysis, neuropsychological constructs (visuospatial perception and memory) from the *behaviour* class can be used to investigate phenomena at the *self-report* level.

In the future it should be possible to explore such 'cross-coding' between RDoC classes even further. For example, the cognitive architecture supporting representation of the body has been extensively studied, both in normally developing and special populations, such as people who have suffered a stroke. These studies have contributed to our understanding about how the representation of the body contributes to our subjective awareness of how we feel [21], and even to the experience of consciousness itself [22]. Crucially, it has been argued that the insula cortex is at the centre of these networks, creating a valuable link to existing theories of eating disorders that implicate the insula [10, 11, 23] and creating a focus for future research activity.

A word about obesity

Before concluding this section on future directions for eating-disorder neuroscience, it is important to focus briefly on obesity. Obesity is not reviewed elsewhere in this book and this probably reflects a continued and well-intentioned commitment by clinicians and researchers not to view obesity as a psychiatric disorder (at the 2009 Eating Disorder Research Society Annual Meeting, a proposal to consider including obesity in the draft guidance for DSM-5 was overwhelmingly opposed).

However, by maintaining such a clear diagnostic distinction between psychiatric eating disorders (AN and BN) and obesity, there is a risk that our understanding of the neuroscience will suffer. There may be common elements such as delay discounting, food reward, hunger and satiety monitoring and body representation that could benefit from shared exploration. At the very least, it will be important for researchers in eating-disorder neuroscience to keep up to date with developments in obesity research, and vice versa, if we are not to miss potentially vital connections.

11.7   Conclusion

Eating-disorder neuroscience is at a very interesting stage of development. Recent advances in technology have been accompanied by a surge of research activity. Most importantly, perhaps, we have now reached a critical point whereby studies are no longer confined to empirical, essentially descriptive endeavours, albeit using very sophisticated measuring instruments such as MRI scanners. Research groups are now beginning to propose and test specific hypotheses about the cause and maintenance of eating disorders. In the case of AN, work by Connan and colleagues [24], reviewed in Chapter 7, has led to a series of sophisticated models being developed by this group that have significantly enhanced our understanding of potential endophenotypes. These 'biomarkers' could prove to be essential in helping to link together the classes of the RDoC and may become a more accurate way of defining clinical status than the current, purely descriptive approaches.

Kaye and colleagues [23] have devised a series of elegant studies to develop a comprehensive model for AN, encompassing components as diverse as genes and appetitive function. Importantly, their model is focused on the role of the serotinergic (5-HT) and dopaminergic (DA) systems and as such can be contrasted with the recent model proposed by Nunn and colleagues in Chapter 8, which implicates noradrenaline. Other theorists have concentrated their attention on other components of the hypothalamic–pituitary–adrenal (HPA) axis. Such clear differences between theoretical models will facilitate direct head-to-head comparisons in experimental trials that only one of the models can survive. By collaborating in the design and implementation of such studies, we will be able to develop and refine eating-disorder neuroscience.

As well as helping us to understand more about the factors that cause and maintain eating disorders, ultimately these endeavours will help to develop novel treatment approaches for the benefit of patients.

Much further ahead we can anticipate the development of '*connectomics*': an emerging field that is to neuroscience as genomics is to genes [25]. Where genetics considers individual genes or groups of genes, genomics looks at the entire genetic complement of an organism. Connectomics makes a similar leap, from studying individual cells to mapping regions of the brain containing millions of cells. Such maps could ultimately shed more light on early brain development and on the pathogenesis of eating disorders. In the meantime we hope that this volume has shed sufficient light on contemporary knowledge to enlighten and enthuse the reader.

References

1. Fairburn, C. (2005) Evidence-based treatment of anorexia nervosa. *International Journal of Eating Disorders*, **37**, S26–S30.
2. Nicholls, D., Chater, R. and Lask, B. (2000) Children into DSM don't go: a comparison of classification systems of eating disorders for children. *International Journal of Eating Disorders*, **28** (3), 317–324.
3. Becker, A.E., Eddy, K.T. and Perloe, A. (2009) Clarifying criteria for cognitive signs and symptoms for eating disorders in DSM-V. *International Journal of Eating Disorders*, **42**, 611–619.
4. Bravender, T., Bryant-Waught, R., Herzog, D. *et al.*, Workgroup for Classification of Eating Disorders in Children and Adolescents (WCEDCA) (2007) Classification of child and adolescent eating disturbances. *International Journal for Eating Disorders*, **40**, S117–S122.
5. Bravender, T., Bryant-Waugh, R., Herzog, D. *et al.* (2010) Classification of eating disturbance in children and adolescents: proposed changes for the DSM-V. *European Eating Disorders Review*, **18**, 79–89.
6. Davis, J., Rose, M., Frampton, I. and Lask, B. (2011) The Ravello profile: development of a global standardized neuropsychological assessment for young people with anorexia nervosa. *Clinical Child Psychology and Psychiatry*, in press.
7. National Institute of Mental Health (2010) Research Domain Criteria, http://www.nimh.nih.gov/research-funding/rdoc.shtml.
8. Rose, M. (2010) Preliminary cluster analysis of the Ravello profile. Presentation to the Eating Disorders Research Society Annual Meeting, Boston, MA.
9. Tchanturia, K., Davies, H. and Campbell, I.C. (2007) Cognitive remediation for patients with anorexia nervosa: preliminary findings. *Annals of General Psychiatry*, **14**, 1–6.
10. Nunn, K.P., Frampton, I., Gordon, I. and Lask, B. (2008) The fault is not in her parents but in her insula: a neurobiological hypothesis of anorexia nervosa. *European Eating Disorders Review*, **16**, 355–360.
11. Nunn, K., Frampton, I., Fuglset, T. *et al.* (2011) The insula hypothesis of anorexia nervosa: conceptual and empirical support. *Medical Hypotheses* (Article first published online: 17 Nov 2010).
12. Hatch, A., Madden, S., Kohn, M. *et al.* (2010) Anorexia nervosa: towards an integrative neuroscience model. *European Eating Disorders Review*, **18**, 156–179.
13. Hölzel, B.K., Ott, U., Gard, T. *et al.* (2008) Investigation of mindfulness meditation practitioners with voxel-based morphometry. *Social Cognitive and Affective Neuroscience*, **3**, 55–61.
14. Caria, A., Veit, R., Sitaram, R. *et al.* (2007) Regulation of anterior insular cortex activity using real-time fMRI. *NeuroImage*, **35** (3), 1238–1246.

15. Winje, E., Willoughby, K. and Lask, B. (2008) Season of birth in eating disorders: fact or fiction. *International Journal of Eating Disorders*, **41**, 479–490.
16. Brewerton, T.D., Frampton, I. and Lask B. (2009) The neurobiology of anorexia nervosa. *US Psychiatry, Touch Briefings*, **2** (1), 57–60.
17. Allan, R., Sharma, R., Sangani, B. *et al.* (2010) Predicting the weight gain required for recovery from anorexia nervosa with pelvic ultrasonography: an evidence-based approach. *European Eating Disorders Review*, **18**, 43–48.
18. Lask, B. and Frampton, I. (2009) Anorexia nervosa: irony, misnomer and paradox. *European Eating Disorders Review*, **17**, 165–168.
19. Moschos, M.M., Gonidakis, F., Varsou, E. *et al.* (2010) Anatomical and functional impairment of the retina and optic nerve in patients with anorexia nervosa without vision loss. *British Journal of Ophthalmology* (Article first published online: 19 Oct 2010), doi: 10.1136/bjo.2009.177899.
20. Woolley, J., Heyman, I., Brammer, M. *et al.* (2008) Brain activation in paediatric obsessive–compulsive disorder during inhibitory control. *British Journal of Psychiatry*, **192**, 25–31.
21. Craig, A.D. (2002) How do you feel? Interoception: the sense of the physiological condition of the body. *Nature Reviews Neuroscience*, **3**, 655–666.
22. Craig, A. (2008) How do you feel – now? The anterior insula and human awareness. *Nature Reviews Neuroscience*, **10**, 59–70.
23. Kaye, W.H., Fudge, J.L. and Paulus, M. (2009) New insights into symptoms and neurocircuit function of anorexia nervosa. *Nature Reviews: Neuroscience*, **10**, 573–584.
24. Connan, F., Campbell, I.C., Katzman, D. *et al.* (2003) A neurodevelopmental model for anorexia nervosa. *Physiology and Behaviour*, **79**, 13–24.
25. www.wired.com/science/discoveries/news/.../connectomics.

Index

Eating Disorders and the Brain. Edited by Bryan Lask and Ian Frampton.
© 2011 John Wiley & Sons, Ltd. Published 2011 by John Wiley & Sons, Ltd.